Handbook of
Interventional
Radiologic
Procedures

Handbook of Interventional Radiologic Procedures

Second Edition

Krishna Kandarpa, M.D., Ph.D.

Associate Professor of Radiology, Harvard Medical School; Co-Director of Cardiovascular and Interventional Radiology, Brigham and Women's Hospital, Boston

John E. Aruny, M.D.

Assistant Professor of Radiology, Eastern Virginia Medical School of the Medical College of Hampton Roads; Attending Radiologist and Director of Vascular and Interventional Radiology, DePaul Medical Center, Norfolk, Virginia

Forewords by
Herbert L. Abrams, M.D.
Professor of Radiology, Stanford University School of Medicine, Stanford, California; Philip H. Cook Professor of Radiology, Emeritus, Harvard Medical School, Boston

Barry T. Katzen, M.D.
Clinical Professor of Radiology, University of Miami School of Medicine; Medical Director, Miami Vascular Institute at Baptist Hospital, Miami

Little, Brown and Company
Boston   New York   Toronto   London

Library of Congress Cataloging-in-Publication Data
Handbook of interventional radiologic procedures / [edited by] Krishna
   Kandarpa, John E. Aruny. — 2nd ed.
        p.   cm.
    Rev. ed. of: Handbook of cardiovascular and interventional radiologic
procedures. 1st ed. © 1989.
    Includes bibliographical references and index.
    ISBN 0-316-48256-0
    1. Radiology, Interventional—Handbooks, manuals, etc.
I. Kandarpa, Krishna.   II. Aruny, John E.
    [DNLM: 1. Cardiovascular System—radiography—handbooks.   WG 39
H2359 1995]
RD33.55.H36   1995
617′.05—dc20
DNLM/DLC
for Library of Congress   95-332
                                                                                                          CIP

Printed in the United States of America
RRD-VA

Second Printing

Editorial: Tammerly J. Booth, Kristin L. Odmark
Production Editor: Marie A. Salter
Copyeditor: Cathleen Cote
Indexer: Alexandra Nickerson
Production Supervisor/Cover Designer: Mike Burggren

To our families

Contents

Foreword

There are a few superb single- and multivolume reference texts in the area of cardiovascular and interventional radiology. These contain a wealth of information about the technical aspects of the diseases to be studied and the usefulness of diagnostic and therapeutic approaches. Nevertheless, for both the novice and the more experienced radiologist, a systematic approach to many technical details that is immediately available in the laboratory setting represents an important addition to our work environment.

In recognizing this gap, Dr. Kandarpa performed a major service by providing us with the first edition of this handbook in 1989. This new edition retains many of the features that made the first edition successful. A telegraphic style is used throughout, rendering the sequence of steps to be taken crystal clear and doing it with a thoughtfulness and thoroughness that have been widely appreciated by all who have used the book. Great pains are taken to simplify matters, and helpful elements such as the form used to record some of the basic data on each patient—a necessary part of each procedure—are included. In each chapter, the indications, contraindications, preprocedure preparation, procedural aspects, catheterization, postprocedure management, results and complications to be anticipated, and methods of preventing complications are succinctly summarized. Alert to the trends of modern medicine, the editors again include a section on outpatient angiography, one that many radiologists in community hospitals and in larger institutions have found immensely useful for a quick review of what is required.

In the broadening field of interventional procedures, the book lucidly depicts the precise sequence of steps in addition to the precautions and technical maneuvers required. Under angioplasty, the success rates in the various arterial beds encountered are summarized and the complications that may occur described. Moving from the vascular bed to such important techniques as nephrostomy, biliary decompression, and abscess drainage, this impressive handbook develops a solid body of technical knowledge and advice.

The subsequent sections on materials, imaging methods, nursing management, and drugs and dosages constitute an invaluable storehouse of information that has been helpful for all patients who come to the vascular and interventional laboratory, as well as for every radiologist involved in the procedures.

Handbook of Interventional Radiologic Procedures, Second Edition, is an impressive and brilliant expansion that responds to the ever-increasing scope of vascular and interventional radiology. There are now forty chapters—an increase of thirteen—with new material on upper limb and renal venography, atherectomy, stents and stenting, transjugular intrahepatic portosystemic shunts, fallopian tube recanalization, and many other essential subjects. Each treatment lives up to the superb quality of the sections of the first edition. Furthermore, the valuable lists of references at the end of each chapter have been fully updated, and provide the reader with an excellent resource for further exploration.

I noted in my foreword to the first edition that "this is a volume that belongs in every cardiovascular and interventional laboratory, no matter what the level of experience of those involved." Questions may arise in the minds of those conducting procedures, but it is clear that such questions will be readily answered by this text; its handy size only increases its usefulness. The fact that all of the sections are strong and carefully structured stands out in a multiauthored book, one in which Dr. Kandarpa has obviously had the major role both in organization and in writing the material.

Herbert L. Abrams, M.D.

Foreword

The discipline of vascular and interventional radiology has matured significantly in the past decade and is now recognized as a subspecialty of radiology by the American Board of Radiology and the American Board of Medical Specialists. Certificates of Added Qualification (CAQ) were recently developed and the first examinations conducted. While interventional radiology continues to evolve, the large body of information on standards in techniques and standards of care continues to grow. The scope of interventional radiology is quite broad, and many have suggested that the interventional radiologist might be the "general surgeon" of the next millennium.

With this in mind, the authors have developed a text that will be of great value to the interventional radiologist, both as a practical reference and a teaching manual. Its straightforward, concise, "how-to" approach to problem-solving will be appreciated by the experienced interventionalist seeking a quick reference and will serve as a useful instructional guide —indeed, a genuine "handbook"—to the fellowship trainee. Techniques are described simply and are well illustrated. Though techniques may differ from institution to institution, the descriptions in this text bring together those principles common to their application regardless of local variations.

Handbook of Interventional Radiology, Second Edition, begins with a discussion of fundamentals of diagnostic angiography and venography; a chapter on cardiac catheterization is also included. The chapters that follow are organized by area of common practical application within the vascular and nonvascular areas. The section on vascular intervention is up to date and organized both from a technical and practical, clinical point of view, as demonstrated by the chapters on the treatment of acute mesenteric ischemia and transcatheter arterial embolization. The entire gamut of nonvascular interventional procedures is addressed, and important sections on noninvasive assessment and issues related to contrast media are included. An extensive guide to both disposable equipment (needles, guidewires, catheters, and stents) and angiographic hardware is also included.

Perhaps most important in this text is the inclusion of pharmacologic and patient care information, which is extremely useful when providing conscious sedation and antibiotic therapy. The information in this section represents the maturation of interventional radiology as a clinical specialty and emphasizes the integrated care that should be provided by interventionalists in everyday practice.

It is a pleasure for me to write the foreword for this handbook, which will undoubtedly become an indispensable tool for all interventionalists.

Barry T. Katzen, M.D.

From inability to let well alone, from too much zeal for the new and contempt for what is old; from putting knowledge before wisdom, science before art, and cleverness before common sense, from treating patients as cases and from making the cure of the disease more grievous than the endurance of the same, Good Lord, deliver us.

Sir Robert Hutchinson
Correspondence regarding
modern treatment in the *British
Medical Journal,* March 21, 1953,
p. 671

Preface

The preface to the first edition began with the statement, "Cardiovascular and interventional radiology is a rapidly evolving field"—this edition is proof of that fact as well as the swift pace of these advancements. We have extensively revised the book but have endeavored to stay true to the original purpose by emphasizing material on practical procedural details and patient management. *Handbook of Interventional Radiologic Procedures,* Second Edition, complements the spectrum of educational materials needed for the complete training of the interventional radiologist. There are other textbooks available for those interested in learning more about the pathophysiologic mechanisms and diagnostic details of the diseases discussed here, and still others provide more detailed technical information on surmounting procedural difficulties. In the final analysis, however, no book can substitute for practical clinical experience.

Handbook of Interventional Radiologic Procedures is directed primarily at residents and fellows in training, but it will also be useful for community radiologists who are several years out of formal training and have the skills required for performing interventional procedures. This book will help cardiovascular and interventional nurses and special procedure technologists perform their tasks more efficiently by complementing their own skills and knowledge. Finally, as minimally invasive therapies enter the mainstream of modern medicine, the referring physician and house officer, who increasingly consult with the interventional radiologist, will find this book useful in comprehending the ramifications of these procedures for their patients.

The contents of the *Handbook* are extensively reorganized and expanded and only the rarest of procedures are excluded. The focus is on adult cardiovascular and nonvascular interventional procedures. As in the first edition, chapters addressing materials required for performing procedures, imaging methods, nursing management, and drugs and dosages are included. Newer procedures, such as arterial stenting, atherectomy, and transjugular intrahepatic portosystemic shunting, have also been included, and there is a new chapter on the use of contrast agents in the patient with renal dysfunction. We have, to the best of our ability, corrected mistakes and oversights in the first edition.

We realize that there is no single way to perform a procedure and do not mean to imply that the descriptions here are the only correct ones. The intent is to provide a framework that the interventionalist can use and build on as more experience is gained. Each chapter has been organized in a consistent outline format in order to facilitate easy access to specific sections on indications and contraindications, preprocedure preparation, procedural protocol, postprocedure care, and the results and complications to be expected. This latter information is especially useful while the procedure is being discussed with the patient before obtaining informed consent.

In addition to all of the contributors to the first edition, we are most grateful to the present contributors for their efforts in creating what we hope will be a successful handbook. We are also grateful to Kristin Odmark of Little, Brown and Company, for her helpful suggestions.

K.K.
J.E.A.

Contributing Authors

John E. Aruny, M.D.
Assistant Professor of Radiology, Eastern Virginia Medical School of the Medical College of Hampton Roads; Attending Radiologist and Director of Vascular and Interventional Radiology, DePaul Medical Center, Norfolk, Virginia

Michael A. Bettmann, M.D.
Professor of Radiology, Dartmouth Medical School, Hanover, New Hampshire; Chief of Cardiovascular and Interventional Radiology, Dartmouth-Hitchcock Medical Center, Lebanon, New Hampshire

John A. Bittl, M.D.
Associate Professor of Medicine, Harvard Medical School; Director of Interventional Cardiology, Brigham and Women's Hospital, Boston

Eileen M. Bozadjian, B.S., R.N.
Nurse Manager, Department of Radiology and Cardiac Catheterization Laboratory, Brigham and Women's Hospital, Boston

Albert L. Bundy, M.D., J.D.
Boston Ultrasound Consultants, P.C., Brookline, Massachusetts

Paul M. Chetham, M.D.
Assistant Professor of Anesthesiology, University of Colorado Health Sciences Center; Staff Anesthesiologist, University Hospital, Denver

Maria M. Damiano, R.T. (R) (CV)
Director of Education and Training, Department of Radiology, Brigham and Women's Hospital, Boston

Michael G. Flater, R.N.
Instructor in Medicine, University of Connecticut School of Medicine; Clinical Coordinator for Cardiac Electrophysiology, University of Connecticut Health Center, Farmington, Connecticut

Geoffrey A. Gardiner, Jr., M.D.
Associate Professor of Radiology, Jefferson Medical College of Thomas Jefferson University; Director of Cardiovascular and Interventional Radiology, Thomas Jefferson University Hospital, Philadelphia

Clement J. Grassi, M.D.
Assistant Professor of Radiology, Harvard Medical School; Attending Interventional and Cardiovascular Radiologist, Brigham and Women's Hospital, Boston

Susan Grossman, M.D.
Associate Professor of Clinical Medicine, New York Medical College, Valhalla, New York; Attending Nephrologist and Associate Director of Internal Medicine, St. Vincent's Medical Center of Richmond, Staten Island, New York

Maria G. M. Hunink, M.D., Ph.D.
Associate Professor of Decision Sciences, University of
Gronigen, Gronigen, The Netherlands; Adjunct Associate
Professor, Harvard University School of Public Health,
Boston

Krishna Kandarpa, M.D., Ph.D.
Associate Professor of Radiology, Harvard Medical School;
Co-Director of Cardiovascular and Interventional Radiology,
Brigham and Women's Hospital, Boston

DuckSoo Kim, M.D.
Associate Professor of Radiology, Harvard Medical School;
Director of Cardiovascular and Interventional Radiology,
Beth Israel Hospital, Boston

Oun J. Kwon, M.D.
Assistant Professor of Radiology, State University of New
York, Health Science Center at Syracuse, School of Medicine;
Interventional Radiologist, SUNY Health Science Center at
Syracuse, Syracuse, New York

Leonard J. Lind, M.D.
Associate Professor of Clinical Anesthesia, University of
Cincinnati College of Medicine; Attending Anesthesiologist,
University Hospital, Cincinatti

Albert A. Maniscalco, M.D.
Associate Clinical Professor of Medicine, New York Medical
College, Valhalla, New York; Chief of Nephrology,
St. Vincent's Medical Center of Richmond, Staten Island,
New York

Michael F. Meyerovitz, M.D.
Associate Professor of Radiology, Harvard Medical School;
Co-Director of Cardiovascular and Interventional Radiology,
Brigham and Women's Hospital, Boston

Joseph F. Polak, M.D., M.P.H.
Associate Professor of Medicine, Harvard Medical School;
Director of Noninvasive Vascular Imaging, Brigham
and Women's Hospital, Boston

Kathleen Reagan, M.D.
Associate Professor of Clinical Radiology, Columbia
University College of Physicians and Surgeons; Co-Director
of Cardiac Radiology, Columbia-Presbyterian Medical Center,
New York

Mohsin Saeed, M.D.
Assistant Clinical Professor of Radiology, University of
California, San Diego, School of Medicine, San Diego; Vice-
Chairman, Department of Radiology, Scripps Clinic and
Research Center, La Jolla, California

Sanjay Saini, M.D.
Associate Professor of Radiology, Harvard Medical School;
Director of Computed Body Tomography, and Associate
Radiologist, Massachusetts General Hospital, Boston

Stuart G. Silverman, M.D.
Assistant Professor of Radiology, Harvard Medical School;
Director of Cross-Sectional Interventional Service, Brigham
and Women's Hospital, Boston

Stuart J. Singer, M.D.
Clinical Assistant Professor of Radiology, State University of
New York, Health Sciences Center at Syracuse, School of
Medicine; Attending Radiologist, Crouse-Irving Memorial
Hospital, Syracuse, New York

Julie M. Sniffen, M.S.
Infection Control Practitioner, Brigham and Women's
Hospital, Boston

Abbreviations

ABI	Ankle-brachial index
ACE	Angiotensin-converting enzyme
ACT	Activated clotting time
ADH	Antidiuretic hormone
AMI	Acute mesenteric ischemia; acute myocardial infarction
AP	Anteroposterior
ASA	Acetylsalicylic acid
AST	Access site thrombosis
AV	Arteriovenous
BNF	Bird's nest filter
BP	Blood pressure
bpm	Beats per minute
Bq	Becquerel
BUN	Blood urea nitrogen
CAD	Coronary artery disease
CBC	Complete blood count
cc	Cubic centimeter
CCU	Cardiac care unit
CFA	Common femoral artery
CFX	Circumflex
CHF	Congestive heart failure
CIA	Common iliac artery
CNS	Central nervous system
COPD	Chronic obstructive pulmonary disease
CPR	Cardiopulmonary resuscitation
Cr	Creatinine (serum)
CT	Computed tomography
CXR	Chest x-ray
D5W	5% dextrose solution
D5½NS	5% dextrose, half-normal saline solution
DP	Dorsalis pedalis
DSA	Digital subtraction angiography
DVT	Deep vein thrombosis
ECG	Electrocardiogram
EIA	External iliac artery
ESWL	Exracorporeal shock wave lithotripsy
FDA	Food and Drug Administration
FFP	Fresh-frozen plasma
FNTC	Fine needle transhepatic cholangiography
Fr.	French size
FSH	Follicle stimulating hormone
GFR	Glomerular filtration rate

GW	Guidewire
Hct	Hematocrit
Hgb	Hemoglobin
HIV	Human immuno-deficiency virus
IA	Intraarterial
ID	Internal diameter
IDDM	Insulin-dependent diabetes mellitus
II	Image intensifier
IIA	Internal iliac artery
IM	Intramuscular
IMA	Inferior mesenteric artery; internal mammary artery
IPA	Internal pudendal artery
IPG	Impedence plethysmography
IU	International units (enzyme activity)
IV	Intravenous
IVC	Inferior vena cava
IVP	Intravenous pyelogram
keV	Kiloelectron volt
K-G	Kimray-Greenfield
Kr.	Krypton
KUB	Kidney, ureter, bladder film
KVO	Keep vein open
kV(p)	Kilovolt (peak)
LA	Left atrium
LAD	Left anterior descending
LAO	Left anterior oblique
lat	Lateral
LDH	Lactic dehydrogenase
LH	Luteinizing hormone
LPO	Left posterior oblique
LV	Left ventricle
MAO	Monoamine oxidase
mCi	Millicurie
MI	Myocardial infarction
MRA	Magnetic resonance angiography
MRI	Magnetic resonance imaging
NG	Nasogastric
NOMI	Nonocclusive mesenteric ischemia
NPO	Nothing by mouth
NS	Normal saline
NSAID	Nonsteroidal antiinflammatory drug
NTG	Nitroglycerin

OP	Outpatient
PA	Pulmonary artery
PBI	Penile-brachial index
PCN	Percutaneous nephrostomy
PCWP	Pulmonary capillary wedge pressure
PE	Pulmonary embolism
PFA	Profunda femoral artery
PG	Percutaneous gastrostomy
PGJ	Percutaneous gastro-jejunostomy
PIOPED	Prospective investigation of pulmonary embolism diagnosis
PO	By mouth
PRBC	Packed red blood cells
prn	As needed
PSE	Partial splenic embolization
psi	Pounds per square inch
PT	Prothrombin time
PTA	Percutaneous transluminal angioplasty
PTCA	Percutaneous transluminal coronary angioplasty
PTHBD	Percutaneous transhepatic biliary drainage
PTRA	Percutaneous transluminal angioplasty of renal artery
PTT	Partial thromboplastin time
PV	Portal venous
PVC	Premature ventricular contraction
PVR	Pulse volume recording
q	Every
qid	Four times per day
qod	Every other day
RA	Right atrium
RAO	Right anterior oblique
RAS	Renal artery stenosis
RBBB	Right bundle branch block
RCA	Residual cortical activity; right coronary artery
RPO	Right posterior oblique
RV	Right ventricle
RVEDP	Right ventricular end diastolic pressure
RVH	Renovascular hypertension
RVR	Renal vein renin
SC	Subcutaneous
SCM	Sternocleidomastoid
SFA	Superficial femoral artery
SGOT	Serum glutamic oxaloacetic transaminase
SK	Streptokinase
SMA	Superior mesenteric artery
SMV	Superior mesenteric vein
SNF	Simon nitinol filter
SVC	Superior vena cava
TIA	Transient ischemic attack
tid	Three times per day
tPA	Tissue plasminogen activator
UK	Urokinase
US	Ultrasound
VMA	Vanillylmandelic acid
VT	Ventricular tachycardia
V̇/Q̇ scan	Ventilation-perfusion scan
WBC	White blood cell count

Diagnostic Angiographic Procedures

Notice

The indications and dosages of all drugs in this book have been recommended in the medical literature and conform to the practices of the general medical community. The medications described do not necessarily have specific approval by the Food and Drug Administration for use in the diseases and dosages for which they are recommended. The package insert for each drug should be consulted for use and dosage as approved by the FDA. Because standards for usage change, it is advisable to keep abreast of revised recommendations, particularly those concerning new drugs.

Angiography

General Principles

Krishna Kandarpa
Geoffrey A. Gardiner, Jr.

Indications

1. Diagnosis of primary vascular disease (e.g., vascular occlusive disease, vasospastic disorders, aneurysms, arteriovenous malformation, arteriovenous fistulas).
2. Diagnosis and localization of small vascular tumors (e.g., parathyroid adenomas, pancreatic insulinomas).
3. Preoperative definition of vascular anatomy (e.g., for revascularization procedures, local tumor resection, organ transplantation).
4. Diagnosis and treatment of vascular complications of disease or surgery.
5. Performance of percutaneous endovascular procedures (e.g., thrombolysis, balloon angioplasty, atherectomy, stenting, embolization, infusion of pharmaceuticals).

Contraindications (peripheral angiography)

ABSOLUTE

Medically unstable patient with multisystem dysfunction. (If angiography is absolutely necessary, underlying abnormalities should be corrected, and preventive measures against anticipated complications should be taken.)

RELATIVE

1. Recent myocardial infarction, serious arrhythmia, substantial serum electrolyte imbalance.
2. Serious documented past contrast reaction (see Chap. 28).
3. Impaired renal status.
4. Coagulopathies or seriously altered coagulation profile.
5. Inability to lie flat on angiography table due to congestive heart failure or compromised respiratory status.
6. Residual barium in abdomen from recent examination (will obscure details of visceral angiography).
7. Pregnancy, because of risk of exposure of fetus to ionizing radiation.

Preprocedure Preparation

1. Evaluate history and physical examination and document the appropriateness of performing the procedure. Complete a patient data sheet (Fig. 1-1). All prior imaging studies and physiologic tests (e.g., noninvasive vascular tests and radionuclide scans) should be available to the angiographer at the time of the study.
2. Obtain informed consent [1–3] (see Chap. 35).

Name _____   Age _____ Sex _____
Number _____   Location _____
Radiologist _____   Referring MD _____
                          Date _____

Clinical data

Procedure and indication _____
_____

Complaints/symptoms _____
_____

Medical Hx:
  — Heart disease (CAD, MI, CHF, arrhythmia,
    valvulopathy) _____

  — Peripheral vascular disease _____
  — Hypertension _____
  — Diabetes _____
  — Renal disease _____
  — Coagulopathy _____
  — TIA/stroke/seizures _____
  — Cancer _____
  — Other (hepatic dysfunction, multiple myeloma,
    pheochromocytoma, sickle cell disease, homocystinuria)
    _____

Surgery Hx:
_____
_____

Current medications _____
Allergies (drug sensitivity) _____
Prior contrast reaction _____

Physical findings

Blood pressure __ Pulse _____ Temp _____ Respiration rate _____
Cardiac examination _____
_____

	Pulses:	Rad	Ax	Fem	Pop	DP	PT
	L	___	___	___	___	___	___
	R	___	___	___	___	___	___

	Bruits:	Carotid	Abdomen	Femoral
	L	___	___	___
	R	___	___	___

Other: _____

Laboratory Results

ECG _____
Creat _____ BUN _____ Hct _____ Hb _____
PT _____ PTT _____ Plat _____ WBC _____
Previous imaging studies _____
_____

Fig. 1-1. Patient data sheet.

Noninvasive studies _____

_____

Procedure plan (see Appendix C)

Puncture site: (check for inguinal hernia, recent surgery or surgical scar, local infection, femoral artery aneurysm, iatrogenic arteriovenous fistula) _____

1. Needle: _____
2. Wires: _____
   _____
   _____
3. Catheters: _____
   _____
   _____
4. Special instructions/precautions to nurses and technologists _____
   _____
   _____

Fig. 1-1 (continued)

3. Check laboratory results: blood urea nitrogen (BUN), creatinine (Cr), hematocrit/hemoglobin (Hct/Hgb), prothrombin time (PT), partial thromboplastin time (PTT), platelets, etc. (See Appendix C for the appropriate choice of parameters for individual patients.) The need for routine evaluation of coagulation parameters prior to transfemoral angiography has been questioned [4]. Hypertension and improper technique were confirmed to be the most important risk factors for hemorrhage after arterial puncture. This study suggested limiting the determination of the coagulation profile to patients who have clinical evidence of a bleeding disorder or liver disease, and to those who are anticoagulated.

4. Limit oral intake to *clear liquids only* after midnight preceding the day of the examination or 8 hours prior to angiography. Oral medications may be continued.

5. Start IV fluids the night before the angiogram in order to hydrate the patient (e.g., D5½NS at 150 ml/hour) [5]. Avoid unnecessary dextrose in diabetic patients. Monitor fluid status. (See Chap. 30 for a more detailed approach to the hydration of a patient with underlying renal disease.)

6. **On-call orders** for the floor:
   a. Premedicate with diazepam (Valium) 10 mg PO given on-call to angiography (optional). Reduce dose for elderly and pediatric patients. (See Chaps. 38 and 39.)
   b. Patient must void urine before leaving for the angiography suite.
   c. Transfer patient to angiography with identification plate, chart, and latest laboratory reports on chart. *The front cover of the chart should list all precautionary measures needed to protect the patient and personnel.*

7. Considerations for **patients with specific diseases or conditions.** Consult with referring or managing clinician, or both, on all items listed below. For more specific details see the appropriate cited chapters.

   a. Heparinized patient. Stop heparin infusion 4 hours prior to the arterial puncture in order to normalize the coagulation status. A PTT of 1.2 × control is acceptable, barring other bleeding abnormalities. Alternatively, activated clotting time (ACT) may be followed. Since this test can be performed at the bedside, the timing of catheter removal and reinstitution of heparin can be more accurately determined. Heparin may be restarted 6–12 hours after removal of the catheter and puncture-site compression [6], or sooner in selected cases.

   b. Warfarinized patient. Stop warfarin sodium (Coumadin) several days prior to arterial puncture if possible. For patients with persistently elevated PT, treat with FFP (fresh-frozen plasma is fast-acting and its effect is short-lived) or vitamin K (25–50 mg IM 4 hours prior to puncture) [6]; onset and duration of effect are both prolonged (PT ≤ 15 seconds is acceptable).

   c. Thrombocytopenic patient. For transfemoral or transaxillary punctures, the functional platelet count should be greater than 75,000/ml [6].

   d. Insulin-dependent diabetic patient. (See also Chaps. 30, 38, and 39.) In consultation with the referring physician, cut the morning insulin dose by half. Schedule the patient for the first case (around 8:00 A.M.). A slow infusion of 5% dextrose (D5W) may be started prior to the procedure. Return the patient to the floor by midday for resumption of oral food intake and reestablishment of insulin requirements. Blood glucose levels should be monitored during prolonged procedures; insulin dose may need to be titered before resumption of usual regimen. If a diabetic patient on NPH (neutral protamine hagedorn) insulin receives heparin during the procedure, do not reverse the heparin with protamine sulfate, since this may cause a fatal anaphylactic reaction [7]. Patients with diabetes (with or without nephropathy) should be well hydrated in order to lower the increased risk of acute tubular necrosis [8]:

   e. Renal dysfunction (see Chap. 30).

   f. Precautionary measures. The front cover of a patient's chart should list the precautions necessary to protect both the patient (especially if immunocompromised) and the personnel who may come in contact with a patient with infectious disease (e.g., HIV, infectious hepatitis, methicillin-resistant staphylococcal infection).

   g. Lidocaine hypersensitivity (local infiltration) (see Chap. 39). Consider

      (1) Local skin test and, if negative, proceed with local infiltration, *or*

(2) Procaine hydrochloride (an ester-linkage local anesthetic), *or*

(3) Infiltrate sterile normal saline alone.

8. Medication precautions (see Chaps. 38, 39, and 40).

   a. Most angiography and interventional procedures can be completed safely and expeditiously with a judicious combination of midazolam and fentanyl, which provide adequate conscious sedation and analgesia [9].

   b. Age. Reduce medication doses by 30–50% for elderly patients.

   c. Severe coronary artery or cerebrovascular disease. Avoid drugs that cause excessive drop in blood pressure or cardiac output [6,10].

   d. Seizures. Avoid drugs that lower seizure threshold (e.g., meperidine [Demerol], phenothiazines) [6].

   e. Hepatic dysfunction. Avoid drugs such as barbiturates, which are metabolized by the liver [6]. Reduce initial doses of sedatives and analgesics.

   f. Renal dysfunction. Extreme caution should be used in administering meperidine. Accumulation of its metabolite in these patients may lead to CNS excitation and seizures.

   g. Pheochromocytoma. Patients with labile blood pressure need alpha-blockade: Dibenzyline 10 mg PO qid given for 1 week prior to the angiogram [6]. Phentolamine (Regitine) should be available for treating potential hypertensive crisis, which occurs in 8% of these patients during the procedure [11]. *Anesthesia consultation is recommended.*

   h. Multiple myeloma. As with patients with diabetic nephropathy, these patients should be well hydrated in order to prevent acute tubular necrosis [6,8].

   i. Sickle cell anemia and polycythemia vera. Patients may suffer thromboembolic complications following angiography [10,12].

Procedure

RETROGRADE FEMORAL ARTERY CATHETERIZATION,
SELDINGER TECHNIQUE

1. Preparation

   a. Sterile puncture-site preparation (iodinated scrub following groin shave) and draping of patient. The patient must be in a comfortable position that can be tolerated for the duration of the procedure prior to preparation.

   b. All patients subjected to any angiographic or interventional procedure under conscious sedation should have continuous physiologic monitoring (see Chaps. 38 and 39).

   c. Infuse local anesthesia with 2% lidocaine (Xylocaine) (without epinephrine) at the skin entry site.

   (1) Skin wheal at the entry site (using 25-gauge, 5/8-in. needle) and deep on each side of the artery in an inverted cone distribution (using 22-gauge, 1½-in. needle).

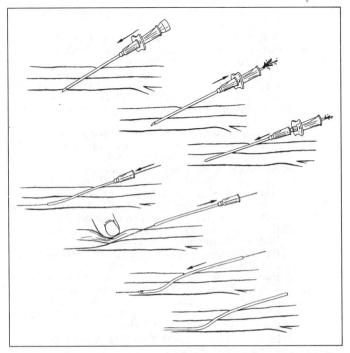

Fig. 1-2. Schematic of the Seldinger puncture technique using a needle covered by a plastic sheath. (1) Needle and stylet are introduced as a unit into the artery; (2) stylet is removed and needle is withdrawn until brisk pulsatile backflow of blood is noted; (3) inner metallic cannula is removed; (4) a wire is introduced through the plastic sheath; (5) wire is fixed and sheath is removed with compression over the puncture site; (6) the track is dilated; and (7) a catheter is placed over the wire. (From IS Johnsrude, DC Jackson, and NR Dunnick. *A Practical Approach to Angiography* [2nd ed.]. Boston, 1987. P. 36. Published by Little, Brown and Company.)

(2) Avoid entering the artery or vein and injecting lidocaine into wall of artery. Slow, gentle injection will save the patient considerable discomfort. Wait 1–2 minutes after injection before making a superficial skin incision (3 mm long × 3 mm deep) with a No. 11 scalpel blade.

(3) Use a curved 5-in. Mosquito forceps to spread the subcutaneous tissues; avoid spreading down to the artery.

d. Check that fluoroscopy is working before the artery is punctured.

2. **Femoral artery puncture** (Fig. 1-2)

a. Locate the femoral artery and inguinal ligament (which runs from the anterior superior iliac spine to the pubic tubercle) by palpation (Fig. 1-3). The true position of the inguinal ligament is about 1–2 cm below the location estimated by palpation or fluoroscopy [13,14].

b. The artery should be punctured over the middle of the medial third of the femoral head; the skin entry site should be over the lower femoral neck. A window of only 3–5 cm is available for safe common femoral artery puncture (Fig. 1-4).

c. For difficult cases, localize the puncture site by fluoroscopy over the femoral head [13,14] or with specific palpation techniques for anatomic localization [15], in order to

　　(1) Prevent high arterial punctures that may lead to uncontrollable bleeding [16].

　　(2) Prevent low arterial punctures that may result in pseudoaneurysm of the superficial femoral artery (SFA) [17].

d. The Seldinger needle (thin-wall 18-gauge, 2³/₄-in. long) should be angled to parallel the course of the femoral artery, approximately at 40 degrees with respect to the skin. Note:

　　(1) In obese patients and in those with prior local surgery, the anatomic landmarks may be markedly different from those expected.

　　(2) If difficulty is encountered in puncturing the artery, fluoroscopy may be used to direct the needle.

　　(3) Calcium in the wall of the artery will occasionally provide a target.

e. Double- or single-wall punctures are acceptable techniques. Single-wall punctures are useful when directly puncturing grafts [18], when the patient has abnormal clotting parameters, or when prevention of any puncture-site bleeding is mandatory. Double-wall punctures frequently are used with impunity. Improper technique can result in vessel wall trauma regardless of the type of needle used [19].

f. For a right-handed physician puncturing a right femoral artery: Place the left middle and index fingers above and below the skin incision. Support the Seldinger needle with the right middle and index fingers on each flange and the thumb over the stylet. Advance the needle until the arterial pulsations are felt or are transmitted through the needle. Enter the artery with a steady forward thrust.

g. Remove the stylet from the Seldinger needle. Once there is good pulsatile blood return through the needle, a guidewire should be *gently* advanced up the femoral artery, through the iliac arteries, and into the aorta under fluoroscopic guidance.

　　(1) If the blood return is nonpulsatile, rule out: a venous puncture (then puncture more laterally if necessary); needle partially intramural (reposition); severe occlusive disease (check with small hand injection of contrast before proceeding).

　　(2) If difficulty is experienced in passing the wire out the end of the needle, **do not force the wire.** Gentle manipulation is permissible, but it is better to pull out, hold pressure for 3–5 minutes, and start again.

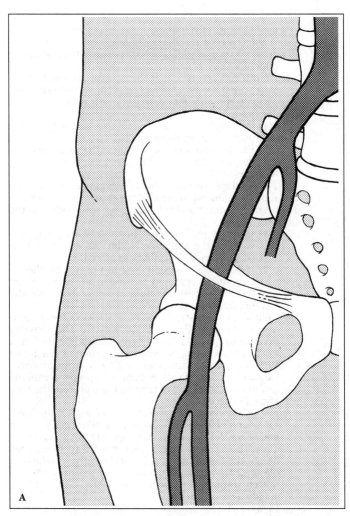

Fig. 1-3. Anatomic relationships of the femoral artery. A. Shows the common femoral artery crossing over the medial third of the femoral head. The vein (not shown) is approximately 0.5–1.5 cm medial to the femoral artery. Arterial and venous puncture sites should be over the femoral head and well below the inguinal ligament, which is shown crossing diagonally from the anterior-superior iliac spine to the superior pubic tubercle. B. A lateral view of the same region illustrates how the external iliac artery and vein (not shown) dive deep into the pelvis above the inguinal ligament. A puncture site above the ligament cannot be compressed and could result in a large pelvic hemorrhage.

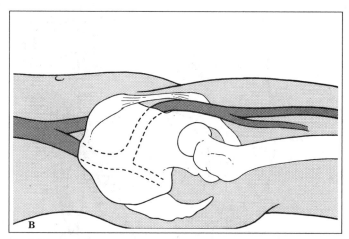

Fig. 1-3 (continued)

      (3) If the guidewire cannot be advanced through the iliac arteries, a 5 Fr. dilator can be introduced into the femoral artery over the wire, and, if brisk back-bleeding is noted, contrast may be gently injected by hand to evaluate the problem.

      (4) Knowledge of the wires available and their uses will be helpful in negotiating tortuous or difficult iliac arteries (see Chap. 31).

3. Catheterization

  a. Once the wire is advanced into the aorta, an appropriate dilator is introduced over the wire, and the dilator is subsequently exchanged for the desired catheter.

      (1) Advancing the catheter may be difficult if the entry route is too vertical or if subcutaneous tissues have not been adequately spread.

      (2) In obese patients, use a large (0.038 in.) wire (heavy duty, if necessary) to avoid subcutaneous buckling. Taping back the lower abdominal pannus away from the groin is often useful.

  b. Always confirm the position of the tip of the catheter fluoroscopically prior to power injection.

      (1) Check for free backflow.

      (2) Inject a test amount of 2–3 ml of contrast, if necessary.

      (3) Avoid injection into the intercostal and lumbar arteries.

4. Injection.
Inform nurse and technologist of desired contrast, volume, and flow rate (see Chap. 32).

5. Imaging.
Inform technologist of desired filming sequence, positions, etc. Useful techniques for optimizing lower extremity arteriography are summarized by Daray [20] (see Chap. 32).

6. Other arterial and venous accesses

  a. Antegrade femoral artery puncture (Fig. 1-5). The

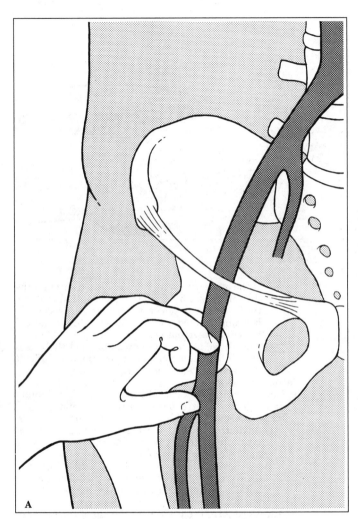

Fig. 1-4. Localization of femoral artery puncture site. A. Frontal view showing palpation by hand below inguinal ligament. B. A hemostat is placed, and proper position is checked fluoroscopically (optional, but can also serve to test fluoroscopy before puncture). C. Lateral view showing relationship of skin incision site to vessel-wall puncture site. D. Seldinger needle in the vessel. E. Lateral view showing needle tip within lumen and stylet removed. F. Guidewire is passed through needle into vessel and up into the aorta. Wire is used to dilate the tract and place the catheter (not shown).

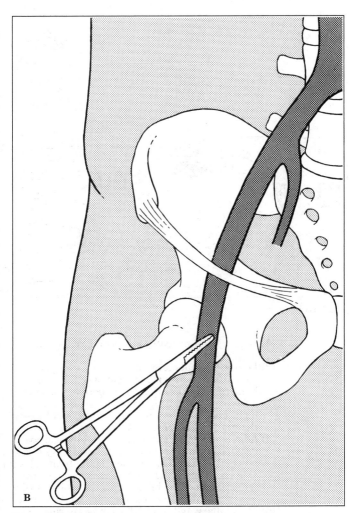

Fig. 1-4 (continued)

skin incision (*not* the arterial puncture site) may have to be above the inguinal ligament in some patients. In obese patients, the pannus should be upwardly retracted and secured. Arterial puncture site, angle of entry, and technique are similar to retrograde approach.

b. **Left axillary artery or high brachial artery puncture.** Used when there is no femoral artery access, and if there is no substantial atherosclerotic narrowing in the subclavian or axillary arteries [21,22].

  (1) Abduct the left arm to its extreme and place the hand under the patient's head.

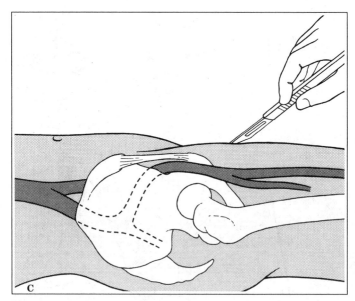

Fig. 1-4 (continued)

(2) Obtain baseline axillary, brachial, radial, and ulnar pulses.

(3) Locate the puncture site of the axillary artery along the lateral axillary fold over the proximal humerus (neck) so that the underlying bone provides support during compression (Fig. 1-6). A high brachial artery puncture site would be over the proximal humeral shaft.

(4) Administer local anesthesia carefully and avoid deep penetration because of the proximity of the brachial plexus. One of the complications of an axillary artery puncture is a hematoma causing compression of the brachial plexus, which is why a high brachial artery puncture is often preferred.

(5) The axillary and brachial arteries are easily displaced sideways. Therefore, fix the artery firmly at the intended puncture site with your (left) index and middle fingers on either side. Use of an intraarterial sheath while using a brachial artery access may decrease the incidence of complications [21].

(6) The Potts-Cournand needle, having a sharp stylet with a perforated hub, will allow easy single-wall entry.

(7) Angle the needle at 45 degrees with respect to the skin and gently advance it as a unit. When arterial blood is seen exiting from the stylet hub, remove the hub and place the catheter with the usual Seldinger exchange technique.

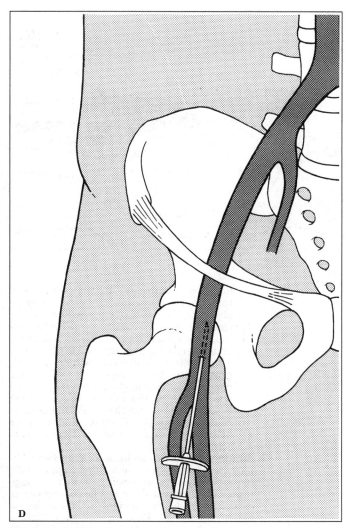

Fig. 1-4 (continued)

    c. Femoral vein puncture
       (1) The femoral vein is located about 0.5–1.5 cm me-
          dial to the femoral artery (see Fig. 1-3). Prepara-
          tion is similar to arterial puncture described
          above.
       (2) Seldinger needle technique:
          (a) Seldinger needle (18-gauge) is used to obtain
             access to the vein. It is often useful to have
             the patient perform the Valsalva maneuver
             in order to distend the vein while trying to

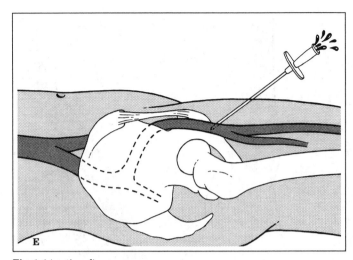

Fig. 1-4 (continued)

puncture it. Skin entry site and venous puncture site should be medial to the artery by about 1 cm and below by about 1 cm.

(b) Once the needle is down to the periosteum of the femoral head, the inner stylus is removed and a 20-ml syringe is attached to the needle. The needle is then slowly withdrawn with gentle intermittent aspiration. When free nonpulsatile flow of dark blood is seen, the needle tip is in the vein. A wire may then be advanced through the needle and into the vein. Subsequent dilatation and catheter placement is similar to arterial technique described above.

(3) Single-wall needle technique: With this technique an 18-gauge single-wall bevel-tipped needle (no inner stylet) is attached to a 20-ml syringe filled with heparinized saline. The femoral vein is located as previously described, and the patient is asked to perform a Valsalva maneuver ("take a deep breath, and bear down as if you are going to have a bowel movement"), during which time the needle-syringe assembly is advanced toward the femoral vein with gentle intermittent suction. When the anterior wall of the vein has been crossed, a gush of dark venous blood will be noted in the syringe. Gently detach the syringe while keeping the position of the needle firmly fixed. If small droplets of venous blood are noted emanating from the needle hub, the wire is advanced into the femoral vein. From this point, the procedure is continued as described previously.

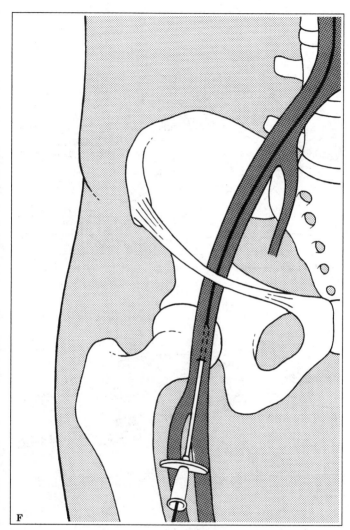

Fig. 1-4 (continued)

(4) At the end of a venous procedure, groin pressure for 5–10 minutes is usually sufficient.

Postprocedure Management [1]

1. Compression of arterial puncture (20 minutes). If the patient has been heparinized during the procedure, make sure the coagulation parameters have normalized (PTT close to control value or ACT of approximately 150 seconds)

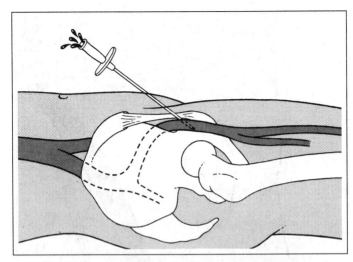

Fig. 1-5. Proper needle position for an antegrade femoral puncture in lateral view.

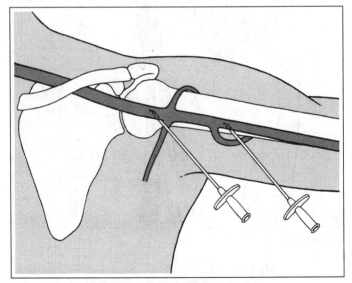

Fig. 1-6. Anatomic relationship of the axillary artery to the humeral head and location of axillary and high brachial artery puncture sites.

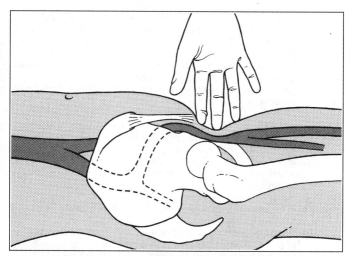

Fig. 1-7. Lateral view of a right hand compressing a right femoral artery against the femoral head. The middle finger rests over the arterial puncture site, the index finger is above, and the ring finger is below. Compression should not obliterate the vessel lumen.

before the catheter is removed and the puncture site is compressed. (New devices for unattended groin compression and for immediate "sealing" of the puncture site with collagen plugs are undergoing preliminary clinical trials. Their clinical success should shorten the time spent by the physician compressing the puncture site.)

   a. Make sure the patient is comfortable, because cooperation is essential during compression.

   b. Remove the catheter and allow about 2 ml of blood to back-bleed. A wire should be placed to straighten the curl of a pigtail catheter before it is removed.

   c. Use impermeable gloves during compression. No sponges or towels should be used. Any bleeding should be visible.

   d. Compress the actual puncture site with the middle finger. Compress above the site with the index finger and below it with the ring finger (Fig. 1-7).

   e. Do not obliterate the pulse. Distal pulses should be faintly palpable.

   f. Apply steady moderate pressure for 15 minutes. Then gently reduce pressure over the next 5 minutes. Never remove compression abruptly.

   g. If rebleeding occurs, repeat compression for 20 minutes.

   h. At termination of compression, palpate all distal pulses and compare to baseline examination.

2. Compression of venous puncture (10 minutes). Apply steady pressure as above, easing off gently toward the end.

3. Bed rest, with legs extended, should be ordered for 8 hours (the head of the bed may be elevated slightly using power controls); patient may be allowed to "log roll" with assistance.
4. Check groin for bleeding or hematoma, q15min × 4 hours, q30min × 4 hours, qh × 4 hours.
5. Check blood pressure and pulse q30min × 4 hours, qh × 4 hours.
6. IV fluids 1000 ml D5½NS at 250 ml/hour, then 1000 ml D5½NS at 150 ml/hour. Adjust fluid administration according to patient's cardiopulmonary and renal status (see Chaps. 30, 38, 39, and 40).
7. If the patient is unable to void and is in urinary distress, a urinary catheter may be placed until the patient is able to ambulate.
8. Resume diet and previous orders.
9. If heparinization is needed, restart IV infusion after 6–12 hours [6].
10. The angiographer should visit all inpatients on the evening of and the day after the procedure in order to assess and manage any untoward effects of the procedure.

Prevention and Management of Complications

1. The incidence of complications (Table 1-1) increases with the patient's age and the duration of the procedure [6,23–31]; therefore, expeditious procedures are the goal.
2. Thrombosis
   a. Is usually due to the catheter; factors include size (relative to arterial lumen) and type of material [6], length of catheter exposed to blood (50% of patients demonstrate significant thrombus on catheter on pull-out angiograms [25,28–30]).
   b. The occurrence is also related to extent of intimal damage, vasospasm, and the patient's coagulation status [6].
   c. Heparinization reduces risk of thrombosis [31].
3. Hemorrhage (puncture-site hematoma)
   a. Locate puncture site accurately over the femoral head, because compression of the artery is best at that site; arterial punctures above and below the femoral head are difficult to compress adequately [13,14,16,17].
   b. Always compress above skin entry site (gentle, nonocclusive compression with one finger above, one finger at, and one finger below skin entry site is best).
   c. If the angle of the needle is too flat, puncture of the posterior wall may be above the inguinal ligament; this will predispose to retroperitoneal hematoma [16].
   d. Using smaller sized catheters (5 Fr. and below) may reduce the degree of hemorrhage [32].
   e. Reversal of anticoagulation to baseline status by monitoring ACT can minimize this risk.
   f. Management of **puncture-site hematoma or uncontrollable bleeding**
      (1) If a groin hematoma is present, trace its margins

Table 1-1. Complications of angiography—types and incidence [11,16,24–27]

Complication	Site (%) Femoral	Axillary
Overall incidence	1.73	3.29
Death[a]	0.03	0.09
Systemic		
Cardiac	0.29	0.26
Cardiovascular collapse	0.03	0.04
Neurologic (overall)	0.17	0.46
Seizures	0.06	0.15
Renal failure	0.01	
Fever/chills	0.004	
Puncture-site		
Hemorrhage[b]	0.26	0.68
Thrombosis/obstruction[c]	0.14	0.76
Pseudoaneurysm	0.05	0.22
Arteriovenous fistula	0.01	0.02
Limb amputation	0.01	0.02
Total	0.47	1.7
Catheter- and guidewire-related		
Perforation/contrast extravasation	0.44	0.37
Distal embolism	0.10	0.07
Breakage	0.10	0.02
Idiosyncratic contrast reaction [26]		
Overall incidence	4.0	
Requiring hospitalization	0.1	
Fatal outcome (1/20,000)	0.006	

[a]About 25% of deaths are due to aortic dissection or rupture; 18% are due to cardiac complications.
[b]Comprise about 25% of complications requiring surgery. However, hemorrhage is the most common complication *not* requiring surgery.
[c]Comprise about 50% of complications requiring surgery. The incidence of asymptomatic thromboembolism is higher [25].

with unwashable ink, and follow any increase in size.
(2) Notify the vascular surgeon in cases of uncontrollable puncture-site bleeding, diminution or loss of pulses, neurologic symptoms in the extremity, or suspicion of a retroperitoneal hematoma (in this case, obtain an abdominal CT scan to confirm or rule out the diagnosis quickly).
4. Pseudoaneurysm
   a. Avoid superficial femoral artery puncture (low puncture) [17]; adequate groin compression becomes difficult without support of the femur underneath.

b. If suspected, a color Doppler US examination should be performed and, if necessary, obliteration by compression should be attempted [33]. Failing this, surgical repair may be needed.

5. Embolization. To prevent sequelae of distal embolization [34,35], consider
  a. Immediate thrombectomy.
  b. Selective thrombolysis, depending on the severity and progression of symptoms [36].

6. Contrast-induced nephropathy. Use of low-osmolality contrast agents may decrease the incidence of this complication [37,38]. Adequate hydration and minimization of the amount of contrast used also are recommended. (See Chaps. 28 and 29 for a detailed approach to minimizing and managing this risk.)

References

1. Standards of Practice Committee, Society of Cardiovascular and Interventional Radiology. Standard for diagnostic arteriography in adults. *J Vasc Interv Radiol* 4:385–395, 1993.
2. Bundy AL. *Radiology and the Law.* Rockville, MD: Aspen Systems, 1988. Pp. 109–135.
3. Webber MM. Informed consent in research and practice. *Radiology* 144:939–941, 1982.
4. Wilson NV, Corne JM, Given-Wilson RM. Critical appraisal of coagulation studies prior to transfemoral angiography. *Br J Radiol* 63:147–148, 1990.
5. Eisenberg, RL, Bank WO, Hedgkock MW. Renal failure after major angiography can be avoided with hydration. *AJR* 136:855–861, 1981.
6. Rose JS. *Invasive Radiology: Risks and Patient Care.* Chicago: Yearbook, 1983. Pp. 19–29.
7. Cobb CA, Fung DL. Shock due to protamine hypersensitivity. *Surg Neurol* 17:245–246, 1982.
8. Lang EK, et al. The incidence of contrast medium induced ATN following angiography: A preliminary report. *Radiology* 138:203–206, 1981.
9. Cragg AH, et al. Randomized double-blind trial of midazolam/placebo and midazolam/fentanyl for sedation and analgesia in lower-extremity angiography. *AJR* 157:173–176, 1991.
10. Johnsrude IS, Jackson DS, Dunnick NR. *A Practical Approach to Angiography* (2nd ed). Boston: Little, Brown, 1987.
11. Hessel SJ, Adams DF, Abrams HL. Complications of angiography. *Radiology* 138:273–281, 1981.
12. Rao VM, et al. The effect of ionic and nonionic media on the sickling phenomenon. *Radiology* 144:291–293, 1982.
13. Rupp SB, et al. Relationship of the inguinal ligament to pelvic radiographic landmarks: Anatomic correlation and its role in femoral angiography. *J Vasc Interv Radiol* 4:409–413, 1993.
14. Grier D, Hartnell G. Percutaneous femoral artery puncture: Practice and anatomy. *Br J Radiol* 63:602–604, 1990.
15. Millward SF, Burbridge BE, Luna G. Puncturing the pulseless femoral artery: A simple technique that uses palpation of anatomic landmarks. *J Vasc Interv Radiol* 4:415–417, 1993.

16. Kaufman JL. Pelvic hemorrhage after percutaneous femoral angiography. *AJR* 143:335–336, 1984.
17. Rapaport S, et al. Pseudoaneurysm: A complication of faulty technique in femoral arterial puncture. *Radiology* 154:529–530, 1985.
18. Smith DC, Grable GS, Shipp DJ: Safe and effective catheter angiography through prosthetic vascular grafts. *Radiology* 138:487, 1981.
19. Frood LR, et al. Use of angiographic needles with or without stylets: pathologic assesment of vessel walls after puncture. *J Vasc Interv Radiol* 2:269, 1991.
20. Darcy MD. Lower-extremity arteriography: Current approach and techniques. *Radiology* 178:615–621, 1991.
21. Watkinson AF, Hartnell GG. Complications of direct brachial artery puncture for arteriography: A comparison of techniques. *Clin Radiol* 44:189–191, 1991.
22. McIvor J, Rhymer JC. 245 Transaxillary arteriograms in arteriopathic patients: Success rates and complications. *Clin Radiol* 45:390–391, 1992.
23. Waugh JR, Sacharias N. Arteriographic complications in the DSA era. *Radiology* 182:243, 1992.
24. Barnes RW, et al. Complications of percutaneous femoral arterial catheterization: Prospective evaluation with the Doppler ultrasonic velocity detector. *Am J Cardiol* 33:259–263, 1974.
25. Barnes RW, Slaymaker EE, Hahn FJY. Thromboembolic complications of angiography for peripheral arterial disease: Prospective assessment by Doppler ultrasound. *Radiology* 122:459–461, 1977.
26. Shehadi WH. Contrast media adverse reactions: Occurrence, recurrence and distribution patterns. *Radiology* 143:11, 1982.
27. Shawker TH, Kluge RM, Ayella RJ. Bacteremia associated with angiography. *JAMA* 229:1090–1092, 1974.
28. Formanek G, Frech RS, Amplatz K. Arterial thrombus formation during clinical percutaneous catheterization. *Circulation* 41:833–839, 1970.
29. Dawson P, Strickland NH. Thromboembolic phenomena in clinical angiography: Role of materials and techniques. *J Vasc Interv Radiol* 2:125, 1991.
30. Strickland NH, et al. Contrast media-induced effects on blood rheology and their importance in angiography. *Clin Radiol* 45:240–242, 1992.
31. Antonovic R, Rosch J, Dotter CT. The value of systemic arterial heparinization in transfemoral angiography: A prospective study. *AJR* 127:223–225, 1976.
32. Cragg AH, et al. Hematoma formation after diagnostic arteriography: Effect of catheter size. *J Vasc Interv Radiol* 2:231–233, 1991.
33. Fellmeth BD, et al. Postangiographic femoral artery injuries: Nonsurgical repair with US-guided compression. *Radiology* 178:671, 1991.
34. van Andel GJ. Arterial occlusion following angiography. *Br J Radiol* 53:747–753, 1980.
35. Bolasny BL, Killen DA. Surgical management of arterial injuries secondary to angiography. *Ann Surg* 174:962–964, 1971.
36. Mills JL, et al. Minimizing mortality and morbidity from iatrogenic arterial injuries: The need for early recognition and prompt repair. *J Vasc Surg* 4:22–27, 1986.
37. Lautin EM, et al. Radiocontrast-associated renal dysfunction: Incidence and risk factors. *AJR* 157:49–58, 1991.

38. Lautin EM, et al. Radiocontrast-associated renal dysfunction: Comparison of lower-osmolality and conventional high-osmolality contrast media. *AJR* 157:59–65, 1991.

Outpatient Angiography

Kathleen Reagan
Stuart J. Singer

The literature suggests that outpatient arteriography is safe and cost-efficient [1–7].

Selection Criteria

1. The patient should have the mental capacity to detect symptoms of complications and to follow given instructions.
2. A responsible adult companion who can take the patient home and watch him or her on the night of discharge should be available.
3. The patient should be within one hour of a medical facility that can attend to possible complications on the night of discharge.

Exclusion Criteria

Screen patient with referring physician at the time of scheduling. Exclude patients with:
1. Insulin-dependent diabetes mellitus (IDDM), especially when poorly controlled. Some authors [6] do not find stable IDDM to be a contraindication to outpatient arteriography when iopamidol 300 (Isovue 300) is used as a contrast medium.
2. Patients on anticoagulant medication, and those with coagulopathies or electrolyte imbalances.
3. Uncontrolled hypertension (possible increased risk of hematoma formation).
4. Renal insufficiency (increased risk of contrast-induced nephropathy).
5. Symptomatic cardiopulmonary failure.
6. History of severe allergy or previous reaction to contrast media.

Preprocedure Evaluation and Planning

1. Bloods are drawn on the day the patient is evaluated prior to the procedure.
   a. Complete blood count (CBC) with platelets.
   b. BUN, Cr.
   c. PT, PTT.
2. Patient is evaluated in the cardiovascular and interventional radiology outpatient clinic on the day he or she is visiting the referring physician. An outpatient arteriography form including chief complaint, brief medical history,

significant past medical history, allergies, previous surgical procedures, and current medications is completed. At this time, the procedure is explained, informed consent is obtained, and a brief physical examination is performed. The patient is given the instructions highlighted below.
3. Arrangements for admission, should it become necessary, are discussed with the referring physician.

Instructions to Patient

1. The patient is instructed to arrive at 8 A.M. at the angiography reception area with another adult who will later drive the patient home.
2. Planned same-day admissions: Occasionally a patient will be admitted to the hospital from the angiography suite for surgery on the next day. Such patients are also scheduled for angiography early in the day. The referring physician arranges for such admissions. These are patients who technically have "outpatient" angiography but are inpatients from there on.
3. Clear liquids are permitted after midnight on the night prior to the examination. The patient is instructed to continue taking regularly scheduled medication. If the patient takes aspirin or dipyridamole (Persantine), or both, these medications are held on the day of the procedure.

Preprocedure Evaluation on Arrival

The patient is quickly reevaluated in the angiography department on the day the study is scheduled. Routine preprocedural vital signs are obtained, and IV fluids are started. Standard preparation for angiography is done as discussed above.

Arteriography

1. Puncture site: Femoral approach is common; high brachial approach also may be used. Single-wall needle technique is recommended because it theoretically causes less damage to the artery. Small caliber arterial access kits are commercially available (Cook, Inc., Bloomington, IN).
2. Use 4 Fr. or 5 Fr. catheter; new pediatric 3 Fr. systems are available for single leg runoff or intraarterial digital subtraction angiography (IA DSA) studies.
3. At the end of the procedure, following successful puncture-site compression, the patient is transferred to the recovery room, accompanied by a nurse or physician.

Postprocedure Recovery and Follow-up

1. Recovery room: Observe vital signs, distal pulses, puncture site, and intake and output for 4 hours. IV fluids are continued, and oral fluid intake is encouraged. Prior to discharge, the patient should have stable vital signs and be alert, oriented, ambulatory, and able to tolerate oral fluids and to urinate. If the patient and puncture site remain stable

for 4 hours, the angiographer discharges the patient to the care of an adult companion with the following instructions:

a. Limit activity, especially of the limb with the puncture site, for the rest of the day (e.g., if the patient has stairs at home, they should be climbed only once, one at a time, favoring the affected limb).

b. Encourage oral fluid intake.

c. If bleeding or other complications occur, call the angiographer. The phone number and beeper number of the angiographer on call, and the address of nearest emergency room are given to the patient prior to discharge.

2. Follow up by phone at 24–48 hours to check on the status of the patient, the puncture site, or pertinent complaints. Next follow-up phone call at 1 month.

Complications

If after 4 hours in the recovery room, puncture-site bleeding continues, the patient is unstable, or complications related to procedure are suspected, immediate appropriate action is taken, and the patient is admitted to the hospital if necessary.

References

1. Adams PS, Roub LW. Outpatient arteriography and interventional radiology: Safety and cost benefits. *Radiology* 151:81–82, 1984.
2. Saint-Georges G, Aube M. Safety of outpatient angiography: A prospective study. *AJR* 144:235–236, 1985.
3. Rogers WF, Moothart RW. Outpatient angiography and cardiac catheterization: Effective alternatives to inpatient procedures. *AJR* 144:233–234, 1985.
4. Wolfel DA, et al. Outpatient arteriography: Its safety and cost effectiveness. *Radiology* 153:363–364, 1984.
5. Fierens E. Outpatient coronary arteriography. *Cathet Cardiovasc Diagn* 10:27–32, 1984.
6. Dyet JF, et al. Outpatient Arteriography—A safe and practical proposition? *Clin Radiol* 42:114–115, 1990.
7. Standards of Practice Committee, Society of Cardiovascular and Interventional Radiology: Standard for diagnostic arteriography in adults. *J Vasc Interv Radiol* 4:385–395, 1993.

Venography

Krishna Kandarpa
John E. Aruny

Leg Ascending Venography

Indications [1,2]

Suspected acute deep vein thrombosis (DVT). Clinical signs of DVT have a greater than 50% false-positive rate, and anticoagulant therapy is associated with a morbidity rate of 3–8% [1].

Relative Contraindications

1. Previous severe contrast reaction (premedicate if necessary).
2. Pregnancy (consider noninvasive test first; if clearly normal, venography is unnecessary).
3. Elderly patients with severely compromised cardiopulmonary status (consider noninvasive tests first).

Preprocedure Preparation

1. Restrict oral intake to clear liquids.
2. Check renal status (BUN, Cr) and hydration, especially in diabetic patients.
3. Give a coherent explanation of the procedure and risks, and obtain informed consent [3].
4. Reduce patient anxiety by reassurance and, if necessary, sedation with diazepam (Valium) 10 mg PO (or other appropriate sedative).
5. Obtain results of prior noninvasive tests or venograms.

COMMENTS

1. Documented previous serious contrast reaction. Premedicate as described in Chap. 28.
2. Swollen foot
   a. Elevate extremity for several hours prior to the procedure, *and/or*
   b. Wrap foot in elastic bandage for 30–60 minutes or longer, as necessary.
3. Collapsed, poorly visible veins
   a. Keep the extremity in a dependent position, *and/or*
   b. Apply warm compresses to the dorsum of the foot.
   c. On rare occasions, surgical cutdown is necessary to expose the vein.
4. Prevention of calf pain during venography. Add 2 ml of lidocaine (Xylocaine 2%) to 50 ml of contrast [4]. The use of nonionic low-osmolar contrast agents appears to produce less discomfort during the procedure than conventional contrast agents [5].

Procedure

1. **Fluoroscopic tilt.** Table with 6–12-in.-high footrest for contralateral leg support. Ipsilateral foot is unsupported, dependent, and relaxed. Table at approximately 45 degrees.
2. **Needle.** 19–23-gauge stainless steel Butterfly.
3. Infusion setup with three-way stopcock, with inputs from contrast syringe and heparinized saline bag, and output port to patient.
4. **Puncture site.** Peripheral vein on dorsum of foot, needle directed toward the foot. Puncture carefully and ensure free reflux of blood and easy injection of contrast. If subcutaneous extravasation occurs (pain and local swelling), stop injection and assess severity of extravasation: If minor, puncture at another site, leaving the old needle in its place until end of procedure. If significant, stop procedure (see **3.** under **Complications**).
5. **Contrast.** 100–150 ml of iothalamate meglumine (Conray 43) (202 mg iodine/ml) or 50–100 ml of sodium diatrizoate meglumine (Renografin 60) (293 mg iodine/ml)—hand injection over 2 minutes.
6. Imaging
   a. Follow IV contrast column intermittently with fluoroscopy until contrast reaches the popliteal vein (50 ml).
   b. Obtain spot films especially of clot-filled veins of the calf or thigh.
   c. Obtain cut films of calf (anteroposterior [AP] and lateral [lat]), knee (AP and lat), thigh (AP, one oblique), pelvis (AP, obtained with patient tilted to supine position). (See Fig. 2-1.)
   d. Obtain kidney, ureter, bladder film [KUB] to check renal excretion of contrast.

COMMENTS

1. Preferential filling of superficial veins. With nonfilling of deep veins, apply tourniquet(s) at ankle or above knee, or both. Watch for compression artifact and incomplete filling of deep veins of calf. Tourniquet(s) may have to be released to avoid these problems.
2. To improve visualization of iliac vein and inferior vena cava (IVC) have patient compress femoral vein below inguinal ligament; compress calf and thigh (if no large clots are seen in large veins on fluoroscopy); raise leg or tilt table to horizontal position; and have patient release compression just prior to radiographic exposure of pelvis [6,7].

Postprocedure Management

1. Routine studies require no procedure-related management.
2. Encourage oral fluid intake for patients who can drink; IV fluids may be considered in hospitalized patients.
3. Wash out contrast at end of study by infusion of heparinized saline. This decreases incidence of postvenography thrombophlebitis [8] to about 3%, comparable to incidence

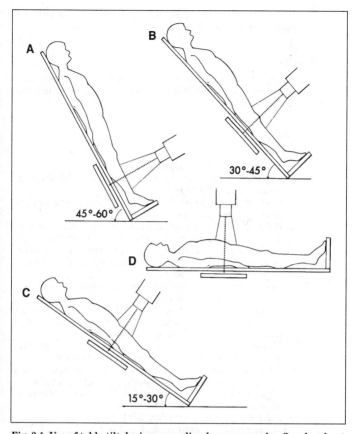

Fig. 2-1. Use of table tilt during ascending leg venography. Overhead cut films are then obtained as follows:

A. Below the knee with table tilted 45–60 degrees: AP and lat projections

B. Over the knee with table tilted 30–45 degrees: AP and lat projections

C. Over the thigh and groin with table tilted 15–30 degrees: AP projection

D. Supine frontal overhead film of pelvis and lower abdomen; opacification of the iliac veins and IVC is facilitated by the Valsalva maneuver during elevation of the examined leg. (From DS Kim and DE Orron. *Peripheral Vascular Imaging and Intervention.* St. Louis: Mosby–Year Book, 1992. P. 284.)

with nonionic media [5,8]; incidence reported with ionic contrast media is 30% [5,9] (see Complications).

Results

Sensitivity 100% for clots larger than 0.5 cm [2]. Specificity 95% using strict criterion of intraluminal filling defect in more than one view [2].

Complications

1. Infection (rare).
2. Postvenography thrombophlebitis
   a. Reported incidence using undiluted standard ionic contrast media: 30% [5,9,10].
   b. Peak incidence is at 24 hours, and symptoms appear to resolve without sequelae.
   c. Diluting ionic contrast medium, using a nonionic medium, reducing time of contact between contrast and endothelium, or flushing with heparin appears to reduce the incidence of postvenography thrombophlebitis to well under 10% [5,8].
3. Extravasation of contrast into subcutaneous tissue
   a. Stop infusion immediately.
   b. Assess size of extravasation: Less than 10 ml in a patient without peripheral arterial or venous disease is considered clinically insignificant [11–13].
   c. If minor extravasation occurs, puncture a new site, leaving old needle in place until end of study.
   d. Treat significant extravasation with analgesia and warm compresses for 24 hours; immediate local massage and leg elevation is useful [13]. The incidence of skin sloughing is rare [11,12].
   e. Inform referring physician of all occurrences.
4. **Adverse contrast reactions** [14,15]. See Table 28-2.
   a. Allergic: 5%.
   b. Death, probable: 0.006%.

Leg Descending Venography

Indications

Evaluation of valvular damage and incompetence in the post-thrombotic syndrome.

Relative Contraindications

See "Relative Contraindications" under "Leg Ascending Venography".

Preprocedure Preparation

See "Preprocedure Preparation" under "Leg Ascending Venography." The "Comments" do not apply here, however.

Procedure [16]

1. Access the common femoral vein in the standard aseptic fashion (see Chap. 1).
2. Place a Teflon sheath needle or a 4 Fr. dilator into the common femoral vein in an antegrade direction.
3. Place the patient in a 60-degree semi-upright position on a tilt table. Ask the patient to perform quiet respirations.
4. Inject 15 ml of 60% ionic high-osmolar contrast, or low-osmolar nonionic contrast with a concentration of 300 mg iodine per ml under fluoroscopic guidance.
5. Obtain spot films to document the degree of reflux as the contrast is slowly injected.
6. Repeat the procedure with the patient performing the Valsalva maneuver.
7. Bilateral injections are usually performed (unlike lower extremity ascending venography where only a single leg may need to be imaged). With both needles in place, injections of contrast are made simultaneously in order to demonstrate the iliac veins and lower IVC.

Postprocedure Management

1. Remove catheter and apply local pressure for 5–10 minutes.
2. Routine studies require no special postprocedure management.
3. Encourage oral fluid intake.
4. Watch the patient for about 30 minutes and then discharge.

Results [17]

1. Valvular incompetence is classified in the following manner:
   Grade 0—Competence, no reflux of contrast material.
   Grade 1—Minimal incompetence, reflux of contrast beyond the uppermost valve in the femoral vein but not beyond the proximal aspect of the thigh.
   Grade 2—Mild incompetence, reflux into the femoral vein to the level of the knee.
   Grade 3—Moderate incompetence, reflux to a level just below the knee.
   Grade 4—Severe incompetence, reflux into the paired calf veins at the level of the ankle.
   Grades 0 and 1 are considered normal.
2. Most patients will normally exhibit a degree of retrograde reflux of contrast while performing the Valsalva maneuver. The purpose of this maneuver is merely to identify the venous anatomy.

Complications

1. Contrast-related adverse reactions [14,15]. See Table 28-2.
2. Bleeding with hematoma formation (unusual in the absence of clotting disorders).

Arm Venography

Indications

1. To evaluate the upper extremity for the presence of superficial and DVT.
2. To evaluate the patient suspected of having superior vena cava (SVC) obstruction or stenosis.
3. To evaluate the patient suspected of having external compression of the axillary-subclavian vein secondary to clavicular fracture, thoracic outlet syndrome, neoplastic process, etc.
4. To determine the course and patency of upper extremity veins prior to the placement of a transvenous pacemaker or central venous catheter.
5. To evaluate the venous drainage proximal to a hemodialysis access site.
6. As part of the evaluation of a dysfunctional central venous catheter in the jugular or subclavian vein.

Relative Contraindications

1. Previous severe contrast reaction (premedicate if necessary).
2. Pregnancy (consider noninvasive US testing).
3. Renal insufficiency (see Chap. 30) or severely compromised cardiopulmonary status (consider noninvasive testing first).

Preprocedure Preparation

1. Upper extremity venography is routinely performed as an outpatient procedure.
2. Standard preparation consists of fluid restriction, checking renal function, and obtaining informed consent prior to IV contrast administration.
3. Obtain results of prior radionuclide venography, color-assisted Doppler US or previous contrast venograms.
4. Obtain the patient's vascular history, and understand the pertinent clinical questions to be answered by the venogram.
5. Establish venous access with a Butterfly or Teflon-type venous catheter of at least 22-gauge (preferably 18- or 20-gauge). Access may be on the dorsum of the hand or, if the area of interest is above the elbow, through a larger vein in the antecubital fossa.
6. Saline is injected by hand prior to contrast injection to establish that there is no swelling around the access site that would indicate fluid extravasation. A small amount of contrast is then injected while observing the needle tip under fluoroscopy to determine if there is extravasation of contrast material.

Procedure

1. The majority of upper extremity venography can be performed with digital subtraction technique. However, when there is nonoccluding thrombus, superior spacial resolution may be obtained from cut-film imaging. Newer, high-resolution digital units may make cut-film imaging obsolete.

2. **Injection parameters**
   a. **Digital subtraction imaging.** Injection rates of 2–4 ml/sec for a total injection volume of 8–20 ml of dilute contrast (contrast-saline ratio: 1 : 2 or 1 : 3) per view will give high-quality digital images. Power injection of these low volumes and rates may be used if confident that the venous access is stable. The access site is checked following each injection.
   b. **Cut-film imaging.** 20–40 ml of full-strength 60% ionic contrast media or 300 mg iodine/ml low-osmolar nonionic media, or 50–60 ml of iothalamate meglumine (Conray-43) (ionic: 202 mg iodine/ml).
   c. These injection and imaging parameters are guidelines. Very rapid or slow flow may require tailoring of the injection rates and volumes, as well as the filming sequence employed, to optimize the image and answer the clinical questions.

3. **Imaging.** One film per second should be adequate in most situations, using either digital or cut-film imaging. Cut-film imaging is carried out for 10–15 seconds. A delay may be programmed into the imaging sequence depending on the time of arrival of the contrast column into the field of view. This observation is made under fluoroscopy following a small test injection.

4. **Other considerations**
   a. It is essential that all venous channels be well-filled with contrast. A tourniquet just above the elbow may help to divert contrast to the basilic vein if injection is directly into a tributary of the cephalic vein.
   b. A small pillow or rolled towel placed behind the shoulder can help to "open" the thoracic outlet and prevent contrast from pooling in the axillary-subclavian vein region.
   c. In a few cases, when the axillary-subclavian vein does not empty easily into the brachiocephalic vein, it may be necessary to elevate the arm that is being injected to demonstrate that there is no mechanical stenosis preventing the flow of contrast.

Anatomy (see Appendix A)

1. The veins of the upper extremity, like the lower extremity, are grouped into a superficial and a deep system.
   Unlike the lower extremity, however, the superficial veins of the upper extremity are larger than the deep veins and carry most of the venous return.

    a. The superficial veins of the arm lie in the subcutane-
ous tissue.

      (1) Cephalic vein. Extends from the distal lateral fore-
arm, which forms from the dorsal venous system
of the hand, continues on the lateral aspect of the
arm, joining the axillary vein near the clavicle,
and communicates with the basilic vein at the
antecubital fossa by way of the median cubital
vein. The cephalic vein may be paired, can communicate with the internal jugular vein and anterior
jugular vein, and can function as a source of collaterals around an axillary-subclavian vein thrombosis.

      (2) Basilic vein. Extends from the medial aspect of
the distal forearm below the elbow, continues on
the medial aspect of the arm, and courses deep to
the subcutaneous fascia joining the brachial vein
to become the axillary vein.

      (3) Median antebrachial vein. Runs on the ventral as-
pect of the forearm and receives the drainage of the
palmar venous plexus.

      (4) Axillary vein. Begins at the lower border of the teres
major muscle. At the outer border of the first rib, it
becomes the subclavian vein. The subclavian vein
joins the internal jugular vein to become the
brachiocephalic (innominate) vein.

    b. The deep veins are small, paired, communicate with
each other, and accompany the arteries of the upper extremity. They are named for the arteries that they accompany and are called venae comitantes. They drain
into the axillary vein but are inconsistently opacified on
contrast venography.

Postprocedure Management

1. Allow all contrast material to wash out of the veins by
infusing heparinized saline (1000 units/liter) for several
minutes.

2. Encourage oral fluid intake for patients able to drink, or
prescribe IV fluid supplementation for patients unable to
drink.

3. Ensure adequate diuresis in patients with cardiovascular
compromise or previous episodes of CHF by prescribing diuretics as necessary.

4. Monitor Cr and BUN in patients with renal insufficiency to
evaluate for deterioration of renal function.

Results

1. Upper extremity venous thrombosis is not common and has
an incidence of 1–2% that of DVT of the leg [18,19]. Studies
show that thrombosis occurs in 28% of patients with subclavian catheters, often without symptoms [18–21]. Also, 12%
of patients with upper extremity venous thrombosis had
pulmonary emboli [20]. One study suggests that the inci-

dence of pulmonary embolism in upper-extremity deep venous thrombosis may be underestimated [21].

2. The venogram in acute upper extremity venous thrombosis shows an intraluminal defect within the vein without extensive collaterals being opacified. Chronic venous obstruction is demonstrated on venograms by an extensive collateral network bypassing the site of obstruction.

3. Major collateral pathways for axillary-subclavian vein obstruction [22]:

   a. Azygous system via the ascending lumbar veins or intercostal veins.

   b. Thoracoepigastric vein—external iliac vein.

   c. Vertebral veins with communication between the superior and inferior vena cava via the intercostal, lumbar, and sacral veins.

   d. Internal jugular-endocranial transverse sinuses.

   e. Suprascapularis, subscapularis, circumflex humeral, transverse cervical, and long thoracic veins.

4. Beware of false-positive results that may occur with:

   a. Underfilling of the vein with failure to opacify a segment creating a pseudothrombus.

   b. Inadvertent injection of air creating a filling defect.

   c. Extrinsic defects created by normal structures such as the pectoralis minor muscle and the humeral head with the patient's arm in hyperabduction. Obese individuals may fail to opacify a segment of the axillary vein in adduction—placing the arm in abduction should permit opacification of this segment [23].

Complications

See "Complications" under "Leg Ascending Venography."

Renal Venography

Indications

1. To evaluate the renal vein for tumor extension from renal cell carcinoma or external compression from tumors of nonrenal origin.

2. To evaluate the renal vein and intrarenal venous network in the workup of painless gross hematuria in the absence of a demonstrable neoplasm.

3. To confirm the diagnosis of renal vein thrombosis.

4. To define the anatomy of venous drainage in transplant donors when the vein is not opacified on the delayed phase of arteriography (particularly if the patient to receive the kidney is a child) or if there is a suspicion of an obstructive lesion.

5. Prior to retroperitoneal surgery, to better define the anatomy in cases of an anomalous number or orientation of the renal veins previously diagnosed by CT or MRI.

6. To relieve portal hypertension preoperatively, before the creation of a splenorenal shunt.

Relative Contraindications

1. Same as for leg and arm venography.
2. IVC thrombosis or obstruction by an IVC filter that would impede catheter advancement from either a femoral or antecubital approach.

Preprocedure Preparation

1. Renal venography is routinely performed as an outpatient procedure.
2. Standard preparation consists of restricting fluids, checking renal function, and obtaining informed consent prior to IV contrast administration.
3. IV sedation is achieved with midazolam (Versed) and analgesia with fentanyl (Sublimaze) (see Chaps. 38, 39, and 40), both administered in the standard manner with automated monitoring of pulse oximetry, ECG, and blood pressure.

Procedure

1. Access may be from either the femoral vein or jugular vein/antecubital vein approach.
   a. Femoral approach
      (1) Access is made to the common femoral vein, preferably on the right, in the standard aseptic fashion (see Chap. 1).
      (2) For the femoral approach a 5 Fr. or 6.5 Fr., 60-cm long Cobra-2, Levin-2, Simmons-1, or visceral-hook catheter with one or two side-holes created near the tip is chosen. The catheter is advanced over the guidewire to the level of the diaphragm, the guidewire removed, and the catheter flushed. The ostium of the renal vein is engaged with the catheter, and the guidewire is reintroduced and advanced into the vein a sufficient distance to allow the catheter to be advanced several centimeters to a point near the hilum of the kidney.
   b. Jugular vein/antecubital vein approach
      (1) Access is made to the internal jugular vein in the standard aseptic fashion (see Fig. 2-2 for anatomy). An anterior approach to the right internal jugular vein may be made as follows:
         (a) Use two fingers of left hand to palpate and retract the right carotid artery medially away from the anterior border of the sternocleidomastoid (SCM) muscle.
         (b) Choose a site approximately at the midpoint of the anterior border of the SCM muscle for needle introduction (about equidistant from the clavicle and the angle of the mandible).
         (c) Direct the needle caudally toward the ipsilateral nipple while angling it 45 degrees posteriorly with respect to the coronal plane. Alternatively, and equally effectively (with less

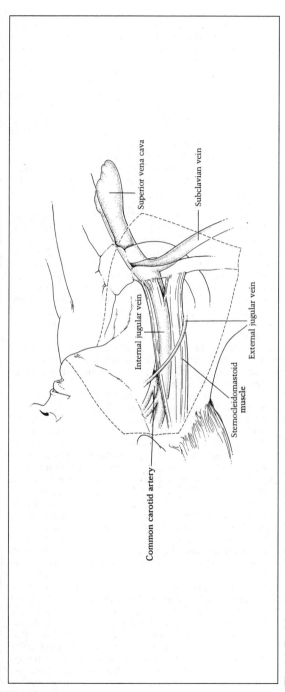

Fig. 2-2. Position, prep, and drape for right internal jugular vein puncture. (From TJ Vander Salm, BS Cutler, and HB Wheeler. *Atlas of Bedside Procedures* [2nd ed.]. Boston, 1988. P. 68. Published by Little, Brown and Company.)

morbidity), catheterize a large antecubital vein with a standard 19-gauge angiocath or a Microvascular Access Set (Cook, Inc., Bloomington, IN).

(2) A 0.035-in. straight hydrophilic coated guidewire (Glidewire; Terumo/MediTech, Watertown, MA) can then be advanced into the SVC. From this approach a multipurpose curved catheter (6.3 Fr.) or a Berenstein tapered catheter (5 Fr. or 6 Fr.) can be advanced behind the guidewire into the IVC to select the ostia of the renal veins.

(3) Occasionally, especially in young patients, venospasm will prevent advancement of the catheter. Starting a saline drip through the catheter and waiting 5–10 minutes usually will result in resolution of the spasm. Rarely, IV nitroglycerin (NTG) will be necessary. The patient should be warned that NTG may produce a headache that can be easily treated with acetaminophen.

2. Since most renal venography is performed to confirm the presence of renal vein thrombus, the catheter must be advanced with care into the renal vein. Once positioned within the renal vein, a gentle hand injection of approximately 5 ml of contrast is performed to detect the presence of thrombus in the main renal vein. Digital imaging or single-exposure spot filming may be used to document the thrombus.

3. In order to evenly opacify the renal venous network some type of flow reduction should be employed. Simply injecting the renal vein will not result in complete opacification of all venous channels. The exception will be in cases of mechanical flow reduction by renal artery stenosis.

4. Two methods of flow reduction have been described:

   a. Epinephrine, injected into the renal artery, has traditionally been used to cause arteriolar constriction and to decrease flow velocity in order to perform renal venography (see Chap. 40). The solution is made up by diluting 1 ml of 1 : 1000 epinephrine in 500 ml D5W (2 µg/ml). The usual dose is 8–10 µg (4–5 ml), which is diluted with D5W to a total volume of 20 ml and administered over 20–30 seconds through a catheter placed into the renal artery of the kidney being studied. Contrast is then immediately injected into the renal vein. The possibility that epinephrine may be toxic to the kidney when used for venograpy has been raised [24]; however, we have not found this to be the case.

   b. Partial balloon occlusion of the renal artery has been described to slow arterial flow [25]. A balloon-tipped catheter is inflated with dilute contrast media in the proximal renal artery to significantly slow inflow. Injection of 1000 to 2000 units of heparin into the renal artery follows. The venogram is then performed, after which the balloon is immediately deflated. Although this method appears somewhat involved, it may be useful in older patients with severe coronary artery

disease, in whom the use of epinephrine is relatively contraindicated.
5. Inject 76% diatrizoate meglumine sodium or nonionic low-osmolar contrast with an iodine concentration of 350 mg/ml at a rate of between 15–20 ml/sec. A total volume of 30–40 ml is injected.
6. Filming technique
    a. Digital subtraction imaging: 3 frames/second for approximately 10 seconds.
    b. Cut-film imaging: 3 films/second for 4 seconds, 2 films/second for 2 seconds, and 1 film/second for 4 seconds.

Postprocedure Management (see also Leg Ascending Venography)

1. Remove catheter and apply local pressure to the puncture site for 5–10 minutes to achieve hemostasis.
2. For outpatient exam, the patient may be discharged in 2–3 hours if there are no complications.
3. Routine studies require no special postprocedure management.

Complications

1. Embolization of thrombus from the renal vein.
2. Coronary artery spasm due to the use of epinephrine with resulting myocardial ischemia or dysrythmia.
3. Thrombus formation in the renal artery from arterial spasm in response to partial balloon occlusion.

Results

1. Complete renal vein thrombosis can be determined from the small volume hand injection of contrast. The contrast will collect within the interstices of the thrombus, and appears stationary or exhibits very slow washout.
2. With incomplete renal vein thrombosis, the contrast outlines the thrombus in the vessel and the thrombus appears as a filling defect. The thrombus may extend out of the renal vein into the IVC and may be seen to reach the right atrium.
3. Compression of the left renal vein as it passes between the angle created by the SMA and the aorta (the "nutcracker" phenomenon) has been described as a cause of left renal venous hypertension with resulting hematuria [26]. Other causes of left renal vein compression are retroperitoneal tumors, pancreatic body and tail tumors, and lymphadenopathy [27]. In cases of hemodynamically significant compression of the left renal vein, a pressure gradient can be measured between the renal vein and the IVC (normal gradient is < 2 cm water).
4. Renal vein varices are an unusual cause of gross hematuria that can be detected with renal venography [28].
5. In difficult cases, renal venography may be useful to differentiate between the congenitally absent and small contracted kidney [29]. Renal agenesis on the right shows

absence of the renal artery and vein. On the left side, even if the kidney does not develop, the dorsal segment of the renal collar does form a vein (ventral to the aorta) into which the left suprarenal and genital veins drain. In cases of renal dysplasia, a renal vein without any orderly segmental drainage can be demonstrated.

References

1. Hull R, et al. Cost effectiveness of clinical diagnosis, venography and non-invasive testing in patients with symptomatic deep-vein thrombosis. *N Engl J Med* 304:1561–1567, 1981.
2. Bettmann MA. Acute Leg Pain of Suspected Vascular Origin. In BJ McNeil, HL Abrams (eds.), *Brigham and Women's Handbook of Diagnostic Radiology.* Boston: Little, Brown, 1986. Pp. 225–229.
3. Spring DB, Akin JR, Margulis AR. Informed consent for intravenous contrast-enhanced radiography: A national survey of practice and opinion. *Radiology* 152:609–613, 1984.
4. Ockelford PA, et al. Lidocaine and the reduction of post-venographic pain. *Aust N Z J Med* 14:622–625, 1984.
5. Bettmann MA, et al. Contrast venography of the leg: Diagnostic efficacy, tolerance, and complication rates with ionic and nonionic contrast media. *Radiology* 165:113–116, 1987.
6. Smith TP, et al. Lower-extremity venography: Value of femoral-vein compression. *AJR* 147:1025–1026, 1986.
7. Dure-Smith P, Tison JB. Ilio-femoral segment and inferior vena cava visualization using a non-catheter technique: An adjunct of leg phlebography. *Radiology* 153:251–252, 1984.
8. Minar E, et al. Prevention of postvenographic thrombosis by heparin flush: Fibrinogen uptake measurements. *AJR* 143:629–632, 1984.
9. Albrechtsson U, et al. Double blind comparison between Iohexol and metrizoate in phlebography of lower limb. *Acta Radiol* (Suppl) 366:58–64, 1983.
10. Thomas ML, Briggs CM, Kuan BB. Contrast agent-induced thrombophlebitis following leg phlebography: Meglumine ioxaglate versus meglumine iothalamate. *Radiology* 147:399–400, 1983.
11. Spigos DG, Thane TT, Capek V. Skin necrosis following extravasation during peripheral phlebography. *Radiology* 123:605–606, 1977.
12. Gordon IJ. Evaluation of suspected deep venous thrombosis in the arteriosclerotic patient. *AJR* 131:531–533, 1978.
13. Kadir S. Venography. In S Kadir (ed.), *Diagnostic Angiography.* Philadelphia: Saunders, 1986. P. 555.
14. Rose JS. Invasive Radiology—Risks and Patient Care. Chicago: Yearbook, 1983. P. 53.
15. Goldberg M. Systemic reactions to intravascular contrast media. *Anesthesiology* 60:46–56, 1984.
16. Neiman HL. Techniques of Angiography. In HL Neiman, JST Yao (eds.), *Angiography of Vascular Disease.* New York: Churchill Livingstone, 1985. P. 21.
17. Herman, RJ, et al. Descending venography: A method of evaluating lower extremity venous valvular function. *Radiology* 137:63–69, 1980.
18. Coon WW, Willis PW. Thrombosis of axillary and subclavian veins. *Arch Surg* 94:657–663, 1966.

19. Adams JT, McEvoy RK, DeWeese JA. Primary deep venous thrombosis of upper extremity. *Arch Surg* 91:29–42, 1965.
20. Horattas MC, et al. Changing concepts of deep venous thrombosis of the upper-extremity—Report of a series and review of the literature. *Surgery* 104:561–567, 1988.
21. Monreal M, et al. Upper-extremity deep venous thrombosis and pulmonary embolism. *Chest* 99:280–283, 1991.
22. Neiman HL, Yao JS (eds.). *Angiography of Vascular Disease.* New York: Churchill Livingstone, 1985. P. 486.
23. Hewitt RL. Acute axillary vein obstruction by the pectoralis minor muscle. *N Engl J Med* 279:595, 1968.
24. Cochran ST, et al. Nephrotoxicity of epinephrine assisted venography. *Invest Radiol* 17:583–592, 1982.
25. Kadir S. Balloon occlusion technique for renal venography. *Fortschr Geb Rontgenstr* Nuklearmed Erganzungsbd 131:185–186, 1979.
26. Sacks BA, et al. Left renal venous hypertension in association with the nutcracker phenomenon. *Cardiovasc Intervent Radiol* 4:253–255, 1981.
27. Cope C, Isard HJ. Left renal vein entrapment. A new diagnostic finding in retroperitoneal disease. *Radiology* 92:867–872, 1969.
28. Mitty HA, Goldman H. Angiography in unilateral renal bleeding with a negative urogram. *AJR* 121:508–517, 1974.
29. Athanasoulis CA, Brown B. Baum S. Selective renal venography in differentiation between congenitally absent and small contracted kidney. *Radiology* 108:301–305, 1973.

Pulmonary Angiography

Krishna Kandarpa

Indications [1–6]

1. To reconcile a discrepancy between the clinical index of suspicion for a pulmonary embolism (PE) and the assessment of its probability on a radionuclide ventilation-perfusion ($\dot{V}/\dot{Q}$) scan. For example, for patients in whom the clinical index of suspicion for PE is high, but the probability by $\dot{V}/\dot{Q}$ scan is low. In the PIOPED (Prospective Investigation of Pulmonary Embolism Detection) study, 40% of such patients had angiographically proven emboli [7]. Only a clear concordance between clinical evaluation and $\dot{V}/\dot{Q}$ scan interpretation can confidently diagnose or exclude PE [7].

2. When the $\dot{V}/\dot{Q}$ scan is interpreted as [7–9]*:

   a. **Intermediate** (or moderate—may include "indeterminate" studies) probability for pulmonary embolism. In the PIOPED study, 30% of these patients had angiographically proven PE. If in addition, the index of clinical suspicion was intermediate (20–79% probability) or high (80–100% probability), the angiograms were positive in 28% and 66% of patients, respectively.

   b. **High-probability** scan in a patient for whom anticoagulation or thrombolytic therapy carries a high risk (angiography is useful for ruling out clinical mimics of PE). In the PIOPED study, angiograms were positive in 87% of all patients with high-probability scans. Most important in the present context, 56% of patients with a low (0–19% probability) clinical index of suspicion and a high $\dot{V}/\dot{Q}$ scan probability for PE, had positive angiograms [7].

3. Prior to inferior vena cava (IVC)-filter placement, if extremity deep vein thrombosis (DVT) or renal vein thrombosis could not be documented as a source for emboli [11].

4. Suspicion of massive PE causing hemodynamic compromise in a patient who may benefit from emergency percutaneous or surgical thromboembolectomy [6]. Echocardiography and IV digital subtraction angiography may have a diagnostic role in this setting [12].

5. Evaluation of chronic thromboembolic disease in the central pulmonary arteries causing pulmonary hypertension in patients who are potential candidates for thromboembolectomy [13].

6. Evaluation of congenital abnormalities.

Relative Contraindications

A cardiology evaluation may be needed in certain cases.

1. Coexistent severe pulmonary hypertension (see **3.** under

---

*The correlation between angiography and $\dot{V}/\dot{Q}$ scan probability depends on the criteria used to interpret the $\dot{V}/\dot{Q}$ scan [10]; thus, slight variation in results may be noted between studies.

Procedure). Noninvasive assessment of pulmonary pressure/flow characteristics by echocardiography [14] (and perhaps in the future by magnetic resonance angiography (MRA) [15]) may be helpful.

2. Left bundle branch block on ECG. Place a transvenous pacing catheter to break complete heart block in the event that catheter-induced right bundle branch block (RBBB) occurs.

3. Ventricular irritability. Perform a pulmonary arteriogram only if the risk of anticoagulant or thrombolytic therapy is high, since objective evidence of PE is mandatory prior to therapy.

4. Other concomitant life-threatening illness (e.g., congestive heart failure [CHF]), should be evaluated and treated appropriately before the patient is subjected to an angiogram.

5. Severe prior documented contrast reaction (see Chaps. 1, 28, and 29).

Preprocedure Preparation

1. Standard preprocedure preparation for angiography (see Chap. 1).

2. Check cardiopulmonary status (history, physical exam, diagnostic tests, etc.). Although individual clinical and laboratory parameters may be nonspecific, a combination of significant manifestations suggestive of PE are valuable in selecting patients for further diagnostic studies [8].

3. Review
   a. **CXR.** Primarily serves to rule out clinical mimics of PE and aids in the interpretation of the $\dot{V}/\dot{Q}$ scan [16].
   b. **ECG.** Rule out acute myocardial infarction (AMI), assess arrhythmias, evaluate right ventricular strain (p-pulmonale, right-axis deviation, RBBB, or S1Q3T3).
   c. **$\dot{V}/\dot{Q}$ scan.** In conjunction with the clinical assessment, helps in selecting patients for arteriography, and also serves as a road map to tailor the pulmonary arteriogram.
   d. **Venous studies.** A cost-saving diagnostic strategy, which considers the results of the $\dot{V}/\dot{Q}$ scan in conjunction with lower extremity evaluation for DVT, and can obviate the need for pulmonary angiography in patients whose treatment would be the same whether they have a PE or DVT (e.g., anticoagulation) [9]. In the subgroup of patients with low- or intermediate-probability $\dot{V}/\dot{Q}$ scans, only those with normal bilateral lower extremity compression US examination may need further evaluation with pulmonary arteriography [17].
   e. **Right-sided hemodynamics** (if available from previously placed Swan-Ganz catheter). A pulmonary capillary wedge pressure (PCWP) is useful in ruling out left-sided failure; right ventricular end diastolic pressure (RVEDP) and PA pressure can determine the degree of pulmonary hypertension, if any, and serve to guide a tailored pulmonary angiogram.

4. Check serum electrolytes, BUN/Cr, coagulation param-

eters (PTT < 1.5 × control; PT < 15 seconds), platelets (> 75,000/dl).

5. Treat arrhythmias with prophylactic lidocaine 50–100 mg IV; obtain cardiology consult.

6. Study must be done with **continuous cardiac monitoring in all patients.** Prepare to place transvenous pacer, if the patient has a left bundle branch block.

Procedure

1. **Venous access.** 8–9 Fr. venous sheath is introduced by Seldinger technique into the femoral vein (preferably right) if there is no evidence of iliofemoral thrombosis. Up to 14% of patients undergoing pulmonary angiography can have thrombus in the IVC [18].

2. **Catheters**
   a. 7 Fr. or 8.3 Fr. Grollman catheter (or 7 Fr. pigtail catheter that can be manipulated with a tip-deflecting wire).
   b. 7 Fr. Swan-Ganz catheter for pressure measurements and possible subselective balloon occlusion injections. This catheter also may be exchanged over a wire for another diagnostic catheter, if necessary; this should be done expeditiously to avoid inducing arrhythmias when the endocardium is exposed to the bare wire.

3. **Measure right heart pressures.** About 30% of patients undergoing pulmonary angiography can have pulmonary hypertension [3].* RVEDP must be less than or equal to 20 mm Hg (and PA systolic pressure ≤ 70 mm Hg); if these pressures are greater, the mortality associated with pulmonary angiography is increased [19]. In such a case, use subselective injection (with balloon occlusion technique, if necessary) or nonionic contrast media, or both. These safety measures are even more important if cardiac output is determined to be below normal [6].

4. **Arteriographic technique**
   a. Contrast. Diatrizoate meglumine (Hypaque 76) or sodium diatrizoate meglumine (Renografin 76). In patients with elevated right-sided pressures, nonionic agents such as Iohexol 350, Iopamidol 370, or Hexabrix 320 should be considered.
   b. Injection
      (1) Selective. Right or left pulmonary artery: 40–50 ml at 20–25 ml/second.
      (2) Subselective. Use V̇/Q̇ scan as guide, especially in patients with pulmonary hypertension (RVEDP ≥ 20 mm Hg)—tailor rate and volume to size of region studied (5–15 ml/second for 2 seconds; with balloon occlusion, no more than 5–7 ml total volume) [20].
      (3) Main PA injection. 70 ml at 35 ml/second, for the anatomic evaluation of central pulmonary arteries with congenital anomalies [20].

*Classification of pulmonary hypertension: PA pressure of 30–40 mm Hg = mild; 40–70 mm Hg = moderate; greater than 70 mm Hg = severe.

c. Imaging. Use V̇/Q̇ scan as a road map; the demonstration of a single clot is usually all that is necessary to make a decision about therapy.

   (1) Always film with maximal inspiration (see Chap. 32 for filming program; obtain scout films to optimize inspiration, field of view, and radiographic technique).

   (2) Begin with ipsilateral anterior and posterior oblique (45–60 degrees) views of the side most suspected on V̇/Q̇ scan. Additional AP views may on occasion be needed.

   (3) Superselective magnified peripheral views may be needed, especially if the V̇/Q̇ scan suggests small peripheral emboli, which can be missed when injections are made centrally [6,7]. 76% of the PIOPED patients had only a single clot on the angiogram; of these 25% were located peripherally [6,7].

   (4) If a balloon catheter is used for subselective injection, make sure that it is never totally occlusive during the injections.

5. In the event of suspected cardiac trauma, stop the procedure immediately. Evaluate the patient for cardiac tamponade (pressures, ECG, emergency echocardiogram on the table).

Postprocedure Management

1. Standard postangiographic management.
2. **Cardiac trauma.** Discontinue anticoagulants; admit to cardiac intensive care unit.
3. **Frequent premature ventricular contractions (PVCs).** Bolus lidocaine 50 mg IV via catheter into RA (total up to 100 mg). For recurrent ventricular tachycardia (VT): bolus (as for frequent PVCs), and start drip at 2–4 mg/minute. Avoid rapid infusion, which may cause decreased cardiac contractility and possibly seizures.
4. If a patient with PE on angiography has a contraindication to anticoagulant or thrombolytic therapy, percutaneous placement of an IVC filter should be considered before the catheter is removed (see Chap. 15)

Results

SENSITIVITY

If done promptly and carefully, the sensitivity of pulmonary arteriography is extremely high [8,9]. A negative angiogram of high quality essentially rules out a clinically significant PE [6].

SPECIFICITY

Using the rigid criteria of unequivocal intraluminal filling defect or abrupt arterial cutoff, the specificity of pulmonary arteriography is almost 100% [9]. The false-negative rate of angiography (determined by follow-up surveillance) was 0.6% in the PIOPED study [21].

Comments

1. A pulmonary angiogram performed 24 hours after the acute episode may be falsely normal since fragmentation and partial lysis can occur within this period [20].
2. PE may resolve spontaneously within 10–14 days after the acute episode [5].
3. The only definitive angiographic sign of PE is unequivocal evidence of an intraluminal filling defect or abrupt arterial cutoff, or both [20]. An intraluminal filling defect is seen in 94% of positive angiograms [22].
4. In the PIOPED study, 3% of angiograms were nondiagnostic and 1% were incomplete (usually because of a complication) [21]. Consensus among independent readers decreased from 97% in the main and lobar branches to only 40% in the peripheral branches.
5. Careful interpretation of pulmonary angiograms in the setting of chronic pulmonary thromboembolic disease is essential for determining operability. The angiographic findings of chronic PE can be subtle [23]; they include pouching defects, webs, mural irregularities, luminal narrowing, and occlusion [13].
6. The V/Q scan has diagnostic value even in patients with chronic obstructive pulmonary disease and should not be bypassed for an arteriogram when an acute PE is suspected in these patients [24]. Although most scans show intermediate probability, high- or low-probability and normal scans are able to diagnose or exclude PE to the degree that further evaluation is seldom unnecessary.

Complications [18,19,21]

1. Death: 0.1–0.5% [3,18,21]. In a review of 1350 pulmonary angiograms, Mills et al. [19] reported a mortality rate of 0.2%; all of these patients had an RVEDP greater than 20 mm Hg.* Another study found that among patients with severe pulmonary hypertension and elevated RVEDP, death occurs in less than 0.5% [3].
2. In the PIOPED study (n = 1111 patients), the rates of nonfatal major and minor complications were 1% and 5%, respectively [21]. Specific complications reported elsewhere [19] are as follows:
   a. RV perforation: 1% (no sequelae).
   b. Endocardial stain: 0.4% (no sequelae).
   c. Significant symptomatic arrhythmia: 0.8%.
   d. Cardiopulmonary arrest: 0.4%.
   e. Renal dysfunction: 1%, usually in older patients [21].
   f. Contrast reaction: 0.8%.

*For comparison, untreated mortality from PE is estimated at 26% and treated mortality at 8% [18].

References

1. McNeil BJ. Ventilation-perfusion studies and the diagnosis of pulmonary embolism: Concise communication. *J Nucl Med* 21: 319–323, 1980.
2. Braun SD, et al. Ventilation-perfusion scanning and pulmonary angiography: Correlation in clinical high-probability pulmonary embolism. *AJR* 143:977–980, 1984.
3. Perlmutt LM, et al. Pulmonary arteriography in the high-risk patient. *Radiology* 162:187–189, 1987.
4. McNeil BJ. Pulmonary Embolism. In BJ McNeil, HL Abrams (eds), *Brigham and Women's Handbook of Diagnostic Imaging*. Boston: Little, Brown, 1986. Pp. 124–128.
5. Newman GE. Pulmonary angiography in pulmonary embolic disease. *J Thorac Imaging* 4:28–39, 1989.
6. Sostman HD, Newman GE. Evaluation of the Patient with Suspected Pulmonary Embolism. In DE Strandness, A van Breda (eds.), *Vascular Diseases: Surgical and Interventional Therapy* (1st ed.). New York: Churchill Livingstone, 1994. Pp. 913–929.
7. Value of the ventilation/perfusion scan in acute pulmonary embolism. Results of the prospective investigation of pulmonary embolism diagnosis (PIOPED). The PIOPED Investigators. *JAMA* 263:2753–2759, 1990.
8. Stein PD, et al. Clinical, laboratory, roentgenographic, and electrocardiographic findings in patients with acute pulmonary embolism and no pre-existing cardiac or pulmonary disease. *Chest* 100:598–603, 1991.
9. Stein PD, et al. Strategy for diagnosis of patients with suspected acute pulmonary embolism. *Chest* 103:1553–1559, 1993.
10. Webber MM, et al. Comparison of Biello, McNeil, and PIOPED criteria for the diagnosis of pulmonary emboli on lung scans. *AJR* 154:975–981, 1990.
11. Ferris EJ, George W. Holmes Lecture. Deep venous thrombosis and pulmonary embolism: Correlative evaluation and therapeutic implications. *AJR* 159:1149–1155, 1992.
12. Musset D, et al. Acute pulmonary embolism: Diagnostic value of digital subtraction angiography. *Radiology* 166:455–459, 1988.
13. Auger WR, et al. Chronic major-vessel thromboembolic pulmonary artery obstruction: Appearance at angiography. *Radiology* 182: 393–398, 1992.
14. Himelman RB, et al. Noninvasive evaluation of pulmonary artery pressure during exercise by saline-enhanced Doppler echocardiography in chronic pulmonary disease. *Circulation* 79:863–871, 1989.
15. Kondo C, et al. Pulmonary hypertension: Pulmonary flow quantification and flow profile analysis with velocity-encoded cine MR imaging. *Radiology* 183:751–758, 1992.
16. Worsley DF, et al. Chest radiographic findings in patients with acute pulmonary embolism: Observations from the PIOPED Study. *Radiology* 189:133–136, 1993.
17. Beecham RP, et al. Is bilateral lower extremity compression sonography useful and cost-effective in the evaluation of suspected pulmonary embolism. *AJR* 161:1289–1292, 1993.
18. Ferris EJ, Athanasoulis CA, Clapp PC. Inferior vena cavography correlated with pulmonary angiography. *Chest* 59:651–653, 1971.

19. Mills SR, et al. The incidence, etiologies, and avoidance of complications of pulmonary angiography in a large series. *Radiology* 136:295–299, 1980.
20. Kadir S. Pulmonary Angiography. In S Kadir (ed.), *Diagnostic Angiography* Philadelphia: Saunders, 1986. Pp. 598–605.
21. Stein PD, et al. Complications and validity of pulmonary angiography in acute pulmonary embolism. *Circulation* 85:462–468, 1992.
22. Hull RD, et al. Pulmonary angiography, ventilation lung scanning, and venography for suspected pulmonary embolism and abnormal perfusion lung scan. *Ann Intern Med* 98:891–899, 1983.
23. Brown KT, Bach AM. Paucity of angiographic findings despite extensive organized thrombus in chronic thromboembolic pulmonary hypertension. *J Vasc Interv Radiol* 3:99–102, 1992.
24. Lesser BA, et al. The diagnosis of acute pulmonary embolism in patients with chronic obstructive pulmonary disease. *Chest* 102:17–22, 1992.

Cardiac Catheterization and Angiography

Krishna Kandarpa

Indications [1–4]

1. Unstable angina unresponsive to appropriate medical management.
2. Prinzmetal's angina (due to spasm).
3. Patient with major complication after acute myocardial infarction (MI; e.g., shock, congestive heart failure [CHF] due to resectable ventricular aneurysm, mitral regurgitation due to ruptured papillary muscle, ventricular septal defect).
4. Highly positive exercise tolerance test with ischemic changes and hypotension (to rule out left main coronary artery stenosis).
5. Recurrent symptoms in patients who have undergone coronary artery bypass surgery.
6. Chest pain of uncertain etiology (or patient's "need to know").
7. Asymptomatic patient with positive routine exercise tolerance test (50% have significant coronary artery disease [CAD]).
8. Patients in certain occupations (e.g., airline pilots) whose routine resting electrocardiograms (ECGs) show new ischemic changes.
9. Nonatherosclerotic lesions
   a. Aortic stenosis with associated chest pain (also patients older than 50 without chest pain).
   b. Signs and symptoms secondary to coronary anomalies.
   c. Cardiomyopathy.

Relative Contraindications [1–6]

1. Recent MI, unless therapeutic intervention is contemplated.
2. Very poor left ventricular function.
3. Correctable problems, such as:
   a. Ventricular irritability.
   b. Uncontrolled hypertension.
   c. Anticoagulant therapy.
   d. Anemia.
   e. Digitalis toxicity.
   f. Febrile illness.
   g. Electrolyte abnormalities (e.g., hypokalemia).

Preprocedure Preparation

1. Evaluate history and physical examination, and document the appropriateness of performing the procedure.
2. Obtain informed consent.
3. Check laboratory results: BUN, Cr, PT, PTT, platelets, etc.

4. Limit oral intake to *clear liquids only* after midnight preceding the day of the examination or 8 hours prior to angiogram. Oral medications may be continued.
5. Start IV hydration on night before study, adjusting for patient's cardiovascular and renal status.
6. Oral anticoagulants: Stop 1 day prior to admission and start IV heparin on admission. Discontinue IV heparin 4 hours before puncture. (See Comments under Preprocedure preparation in Chap. 1).
7. On-call orders for the floor
   a. Diazepam (Valium) 5–10 mg PO and diphenhydramine hydrochloride (Benadryl) 25–50 mg PO 30 minutes prior to catheterization.
   b. For unusual anxiety, add meperidine hydrochloride (Demerol) 25–100 mg IM (adjust for body weight).
   c. Record vital signs prior to leaving floor; patient must void urine.
   d. Transfer patient to angiography suite with identification plate, chart, and latest laboratory values.
8. Preangiography preparation: Puncture-site preparation, sterile drapes, etc. (see Chap. 1).

Procedure [1,2]

1. Right heart catheterization (optional, but recommended for most cases)
   a. Place 6 Fr. venous sheath in femoral vein.
   b. Swan-Ganz catheter for pressure measurements.
   c. Right atrial pacing catheter, for patients with left bundle branch block.
2. Left heart catheterization
   a. Place 5–7 Fr. arterial sheath in femoral artery. Smaller caliber catheters cause fewer puncture-site complications; however, they may be technically more difficult to use and may compromise the diagnostic quality of the angiogram on occasion [7–11].
   b. Pigtail catheter for ventriculogram.
   c. Judkins/Amplatz catheters for coronary injection.
   d. On occasion, antecubital cutdown is used, if femoral approach is not possible. Alternatively, direct percutaneous puncture of the brachial artery can be safely used [7,12].
3. Administer IV heparin 5000 units prior to coronary arteriography, before any catheter is advanced around the aortic arch [13].
4. Administer sublingual nitroglycerin (to dilate vessels) and IV atropine 0.4–0.6 mg (to prevent bradycardia) prior to coronary angiography.
5. Contrast media. Nonionic low-osmolar contrast agents (e.g., iopamidol) cause fewer adverse reactions and untoward physiologic changes during coronary angiography than do conventional high-osmolar or ionic low-osmolar (e.g., ioxaglate) agents [14–16].
6. Imaging. Image intensifier (II) above patient; angles refer to position of II

    a. Best projections for coronary arteries [1]
- **(1)** Left main coronary artery: anteroposterior (AP).
- **(2)** Bifurcation of left main coronary artery and proximal left anterior descending (LAD) and circumflex (CFX) arteries: 45–60-degree left anterior oblique (LAO) with 30-degree cranial angulation.
- **(3)** Proximal left CFX and proximal LAD artery: 45–60-degree LAO with 30-degree caudal angulation (spider view).
- **(4)** Entire LAD and proximal CFX: 30–45-degree right anterior oblique (RAO).
- **(5)** Proximal left CFX, obtuse marginal branches and diagonals: 30–45-degree RAO with 20–30-degree caudal angulation.
- **(6)** Proximal LAD and proximal diagonal branches: 30–45-degree RAO with 20–30-degree cranial angulation.
- **(7)** Right coronary artery: 30–45-degree RAO, and 45–60-degree LAO with 5–10-degree cranial angulation to open up the origin of the posterior descending artery.

    b. Best projections for left ventriculogram: 30–45-degree RAO (for anterior, apical, and inferior walls), and 45–60-degree LAO with 20–30-degree cranial angulation (for septum, apical, and posterolateral walls).

Postprocedure Management

1. In uncomplicated cases, routine postangiography management (see Chap. 1) with special attention to
   - **a.** Reverse heparin with slow IV protamine sulfate [17] 10 mg/1000 units of heparin (administered only if the patient is not on NPH [neutral protamine hagedorn] insulin) [18].
   - **b.** Check cardiac status and ECG.
   - **c.** Resume previous medications.
   - **d.** Check blood pressure, pulse, and groin q15min × 1 hour, then qh × 4 hours, then q4h × 16 hours.
   - **e.** Encourage oral fluids, 2–3 liters over 6–8 hours.
   - **f.** Bed rest for 6 hours (arm case); until next morning for percutaneous femoral procedure.
   - **g.** Check cardiac enzymes the following morning [2].
2. In cases with cardiac complications: Admit patient to cardiac intensive care unit.

Results

Excellent for defining preoperative anatomy (i.e., percutaneous transluminal coronary angioplasty [PTCA] or bypass surgery) and extent of disease. However, there is no correlation between morphologic severity assessed visually and the true hemodynamic severity of a focal lesion [19–21]. Qualitative descriptions of lesions are important for determining a lesion's stability and its relation to clinical ischemic syndromes [4]. Quantitative coronary arteriography must be used for any clinical research on the natural history or treatment of CAD [19–23]. Magnetic resonance angiography [24] and spiral (helical) CT [25] are presently being evaluated as alternative noninvasive imaging modalities for the assessment of the proximal coronary circulation. Similarly, left ventricular function and anatomy are also being studied with these modalities [26,27].

Complications [2,5,6]

1. Risk of serious complications (stroke, MI, death) is less than 1%
    a. Overall mortality of cardiac catheterization and angiography: 0.1–0.4% [5,6].
    b. Mortality, coronary angiography: 0.24%.
    c. MI after cardiac catheterization: 0.2%.
    d. Ventricular fibrillation: under 0.6%.
    e. Cerebrovascular compromise: 0.13%.
2. Factors predisposing to serious complications
    a. Unstable angina.
    b. Subendocardial MI.
    c. Insulin-dependent diabetes mellitus.
3. Risk factors for death
    a. Left main CAD.
    b. Severe left ventricular dysfunction: left ventricular ejection fraction less than 30% [6]; mean pulmonary capillary wedge pressure (PCWP) more than 30 mm Hg.
    c. Age greater than 60 years.
    d. New York Heart Association (NYHA) Class IV function.
    e. Other
        (1) Valvular disease (e.g., aortic stenosis).
        (2) Extensive MI.
        (3) Cardiomyopathy.

References

1. Levin DC. Technique of Coronary Arteriography. In HL Abrams (ed.), *Abrams' Angiography: Vascular and Interventional Radiology* (3rd ed.). Boston: Little, Brown, 1983. Pp. 485–502.
2. Grossman W. *Cardiac Catheterization and Coronary Angiography* (2nd ed.). Philadelphia: Lea and Febiger, 1980.
3. Abrams HL, Kandarpa K. Angiography in Coronary Disease. In S Baum (ed.), *Abrams' Angiography: Vascular and Interventional Radiology* (4th ed.). Boston: Little, Brown. In press.
4. Fuster V, et al. The pathogenesis of coronary artery disease and the acute coronary syndromes. *N Engl J Med* 326:242–250, 1992.
5. Abrams HL, Aruny JE. Complications of Coronary Arteriography. In HL Abrams (ed.), *Abrams' Angiography: Vascular and Interventional Radiology* (4th ed.). Boston: Little, Brown. In press.
6. Lozner EC, et al. Coronary arteriography 1984–1987: A report of the Registry of the Society for Cardiac Angiography and Interventions. II. An analysis of 218 deaths related to coronary arteriography. *Cathet Cardiovasc Diagn* 17:11–14, 1989.
7. Lupon-Roses J, et al. Percutaneous right brachial artery approach with 5F catheters for studying coronary artery disease. *Cathet Cardiovasc Diagn* 22:47–51, 1991.

8. Brown RI, MacDonald AC. Use of 5 French catheters for cardiac catheterization and coronary angiography: A critical review. *Cathet Cardiovasc Diagn* 13:214–217, 1987.

9. Colle JP, et al. Nondiagnosed left main ostial stenosis partly due to the use of 5 French coronary angiographic catheters. *Cathet Cardiovasc Diagn* 22:180–183, 1991.

10. Ellis SG, et al. Accuracy and reproducibility of quantitative coronary arteriography using 6 and 8 French catheters with cine angiographic acquisition. *Cathet Cardiovasc Diagn* 22:52–55, 1991.

11. Kohli RS, et al. Study of the performance of 5 French and 7 French catheters in coronary angiography: a functional comparison. *Cathet Cardiovasc Diagn* 18:131–135, 1989.

12. Mills RM, et al. Clinical experience with percutaneous brachial coronary angiography in a "Judkins" laboratory. *Cathet Cardiovasc Diagn* 19:286–288, 1990.

13. Antonovic R, Rosch J, Dotter CT. The value of systemic arterial heparinization in transfemoral angiography: A prospective study. *AJR* 127:223–225, 1976.

14. Gertz EW, et al. Adverse reactions of low osmolality contrast media during cardiac angiography: A prospective randomized multicenter study. *J Am Coll Cardiol* 19:899–906, 1992.

15. Missri J, Jeresaty RM. Ventricular fibrillation during coronary angiography: Reduced incidence with nonionic contrast media. *Cathet Cardiovasc Diagn* 19:4–7, 1990.

16. Vik-Mo H, et al. Influence of low osmolality contrast media on electrophysiology and hemodynamics in coronary angiography: Differences between an ionic (ioxaglate) and a nonionic (iohexol) agent. *Cathet Cardiovasc Diagn* 21:221–226, 1990.

17. Dotter CT, et al. The value of protamine following heparin covered angiography: Double blind placebo-controlled study. *Radiology* 135:299, 1980.

18. Stewart WJ, et al. Increased risk of severe protamine reactions in NPH insulin-dependent diabetics undergoing cardiac catheterization. *Circulation* 70:782–792, 1984.

19. Hermiller JB, et al. Quantitative and qualitative coronary angiographic analysis: Review of methods, utility, and limitations. *Cathet Cardiovasc Diagn* 25:110–131, 1992.

20. Gould KL. Percent coronary stenosis: battered gold standard, pernicious relic or clinical practicality? *J Am Coll Cardiol* 11:886–888, 1988.

21. Beauman GJ, Vogel RA. Accuracy of individual and panel visual interpretations of coronary arteriograms: implications for clinical decisions. *J Am Coll Cardiol* 16:108–113, 1990.

22. Marcus ML, et al. Visual estimates of percent diameter coronary stenosis: " A battered gold standard." *J Am Coll Cardiol* 11:882–885, 1988.

23. Gould KL, Kirkeeide RL, Buchi M. Coronary flow reserve as a physiologic measure of stenosis severity. *J Am Coll Cardiol* 15:459–474, 1990.

24. Manning WJ, Li W, Edelman RR. A preliminary report comparing magnetic resonance coronary angiography with conventional angiography. *N Engl J Med* 328:828–832, 1993.

25. Tello R, et al. Spiral CT evaluation of coronary artery bypass graft patency. *J Comput Assist Tomogr* 17:253–259, 1993.

26. Sechtem U, et al. Regional left ventricular wall thickening by magnetic resonance imaging: Evaluation in normal persons and

patients with global and regional dysfunction. *Am J Cardiol* 59:145–151, 1987.

27. Sechtem U, et al. Diagnosis of left ventricular thrombi by magnetic resonance imaging and comparison with angiocardiography, computed tomography and echocardiography. *Am J Cardiol* 64:1195–1199, 1989.

Vascular Interventional Procedures

Percutaneous Intraarterial Procedures

Regional Intraarterial Thrombolysis

Krishna Kandarpa

The **purpose** of intraarterial thrombolysis is to rapidly restore blood flow to the ischemic limb and to identify underlying lesions for treatment by surgical and/or percutaneous techniques.

Indication

Thrombotic or embolic occlusion of a native artery or bypass graft causing new-onset claudication or limb-threatening ischemia [1–5].

Contraindications

ABSOLUTE [1–4]

1. Active internal bleeding.
2. Irreversible limb ischemia (severe sensorimotor deficits, muscle rigor).
3. Recent stroke (arbitrary guideline: transient ischemic attack [TIA] within 2 months; or cerebrovascular accident [CVA] within 6 months; some prefer to wait up to 12 months).
4. Intracranial neoplasm or recent (within 2 months) craniotomy.
5. Protruding mobile left heart thrombus.

RELATIVE [6]

The consideration for thrombolysis in this group of patients should be rare, and the need should far outweigh the risk of treatment. Careful clinical evaluation and sound judgment in patient selection are essential. Prophylactic measures should be taken to minimize risk.

1. History of gastrointestinal bleeding.
2. Recent major surgery (10 days), including biopsy.
3. Recent trauma.
4. Recent CPR.
5. Severe uncontrolled high blood pressure (diastolic BP $\geq$ 125 mm Hg).
6. Emboli from cardiac source (obtain echocardiogram if suspected).
7. Subacute bacterial endocarditis.
8. Coagulopathy.
9. Pregnancy and postpartum period (< 10 days).
10. Severe cerebrovascular disease.
11. Diabetic hemorrhagic retinopathy.

Preprocedure Preparation

1. Routine preangiography workup, including informed consent.

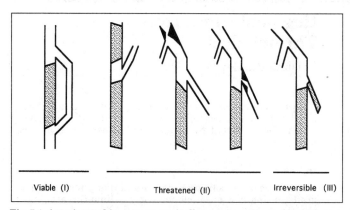

Viable (I)   Threatened (II)   Irreversible (III)

Fig. 5-1. Arteriographic patterns typically corresponding to clinical acute ischemia categories: (I) viable limbs often show a single segmental occlusion with patent collaterals and reconstitution of calf runoff vessels; (II) threatened limbs can have tandem lesions in series or in parallel with patent collaterals and reconstitution of calf runoff vessels; and (III) irreversible ischemic limbs have extensive parallel thrombotic occlusions, occluded collaterals, and no distal reconstitution of runoff vessels. (After TO McNamara, Thrombolysis as an alternative initial therapy for the acutely ischemic limb. *Semin Vasc Surg* 5:89–98, 1992.)

2. **Laboratory evaluation:** Hct/Hgb (> 10/30); platelet count (> 100K); baseline BUN/Cr; PT/PTT or, alternatively, activated clotting time (ACT); fibrinogen levels (optional).
3. Review of previous angiograms and noninvasive vascular studies can be useful for **planning the access site.** The selected puncture site should provide the most direct route possible to the thrombus in order to facilitate catheter manipulation and potential angioplasty and/or atherectomy. Careful direct puncture of a graft is usually risk-free; however, axillary artery puncture should be avoided when thrombolysis is planned.

Procedure

1. Perform a **baseline arteriogram** to document the extent of thrombus and disease (Fig. 5-1).
2. Place an intraarterial (IA) sheath (highly recommended); it will facilitate catheter exchanges and minimize trauma at the puncture site (Fig. 5-2).
3. Introduce the infusion catheter and wire coaxially through the sheath. Cross the entire length of thrombus with an 0.035–0.038-in. straight flexible-tip wire, a hydrophilic-polymer-coated wire or equivalent. A thrombus that is resistant to guidewire passage (**guidewire traversal test**) is probably chronic and may be difficult to lyse [7]. However, chronic thrombi per se should not discourage an attempt at thrombolysis [8]. If the thrombus is crossed successfully, gently macerate thrombus with a J-wire

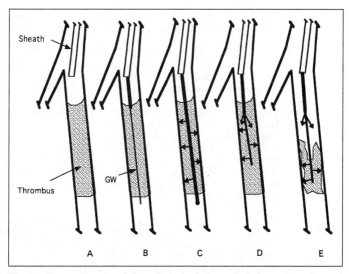

Fig. 5-2. Stages of regional thrombolysis. A. An occluded segment of vessel is demonstrated arteriographically. B. A coaxial catheter is introduced through the IA sheath and advanced into the proximal thrombus, and a guidewire is then advanced to the distal end of the thrombus (GW traversal test). C. A tip-occluded multiside-orifice catheter is advanced into the entire thrombus, which is saturated with a bolus dose of lytic agent deposited by rapid pulse-spray infusion. (Alternatively, an end-hole catheter or a catheter with fewer distal side-holes is advanced distally and then retracted proximally while depositing small doses of lytic agent at each station.) D. Continuous infusion is administered with an end-hole catheter with its tip in the proximal thrombus and a smaller side-hole catheter which is advanced much farther into the clot. (A distal untreated segment of thrombus is shown here, but a side-hole catheter, with its tip occluded, may be advanced so as to bathe the thrombus with lytic agent throughout its length.) E. As thrombolysis progresses, both catheters may be advanced, but with this configuration the inner catheter alone may be advanced into the receding thrombus front. This is continued until the entire thrombus is dissolved and an underlying obstructing lesion is uncovered for treatment by angioplasty or surgery.

(avoid excessive intimal damage, which can result in further thrombosis). If the guidewire fails to cross the thrombus, a short trial of thrombolysis with the catheter just proximal to the thrombus is still appropriate.

4. **Catheter selection.** A variety of infusion catheters are currently available (see Table 31-5). Many of these "infusion systems" can be used for both conventional slow-infusion and newer pulsed-infusion methods. Most of these catheters have side orifices distributed over different lengths to match thrombus length. These include:

   a. Angiodynamics (Glens Falls, NY) pulse-spray system (with pressure responsive slit orifices, 4–5 Fr.). Requires a 0.035-in.-tip occluding wire for pulse-spray. The wire may have to be removed for slow infusion. This is the only system designed for high-pressure infusion.

   b. The EDM (Advanced Cardiovascular Systems [ACS],
   Temecula, CA) multilumen, multi-sidehole catheter
   (4.7 Fr.).

   c. The McNamara coaxial catheter infusion set (Cook,
   Inc., Indianapolis, IN). Allows the infusion length to
   be varied (via the inner 3 Fr. catheter) as thrombolysis
   progresses without having to exchange the outer (5.5
   Fr.) catheter.

   d. The Cook multisideport catheter (5 Fr.) infusion set.
   Requires a (ball) tip occluding wire.

   e. The Mewissen multi-sidehole over-the-wire infusion
   catheter (5 Fr.) which can be used either alone or in
   combination with a coaxially placed 0.035-in. Katzen Infusion Wire (both by MediTech/Boston Scientific,
   Watertown, MA), thereby emulating the advantages of
   the McNamara catheter. Both of these catheters can
   be used for pulse spraying.

   f. There are at least two 3 Fr.-endhole catheters: T3
   (Cook, Inc.) and the Cragg Convertible Wire (Medi-
   Tech) which can be used coaxially (via outer catheter
   with 0.038-in. ID) for distal infusion.

5. Thrombolytic agents (Table 5-1). Although **urokinase**
(UK) is a more expensive lytic agent (per vial) than **streptokinase** (SK), there appears to be general consensus that
it is the safer and more cost-effective drug for peripheral
arterial thrombolysis [9–12]. **Recombinant tissue plasminogen activator** (rt-PA) causes rapid early lysis
[13,14], but it is more expensive than UK. A recent clinical
study randomized patients to either rt-PA or to UK for
peripheral arterial thrombolysis and confirmed the early
rapid effect. However, this study also showed that rt-PA
caused greater suppression of fibrinogen levels and that
between the two agents there was no significant difference
in success of complication rates, in the number of patients
achieving lysis at 24 hours, or in the 30-day clinical outcome [15]. Although none of these agents is approved by
the Food and Drug Administration for peripheral arterial
thrombolysis, UK is presently the most commonly used
lytic agent in the United States.

**Table 5-1. Comparative results and complications of regional
peripheral arterial thrombolytic therapy** (%)

	UK	rt-PA	SK
Clinical success	~ 95	~ 90	~ 60
Amputation[a]	8–11	15–20	16
Major bleeding[b]	3–6	10–20	10–30
Death	0–1.6	2–10	2–4

[a]Usually as a consequence of the preexisting severity of ischemia, rather
than of thrombolytic therapy.
[b]For example, puncture site or retroperitoneal hematoma needing
intervention.
Source: Range of results compiled from references [1–7,9–16,25–28].

a. **Transthrombus bolus.** It has been suggested that high-dose transthrombus bolusing of UK significantly decreases the time for completion of lysis, total UK dose, and complication rates [16]. Bolusing is accomplished by depositing approximately 10–25K IU of concentrated urokinase (10–25K IU/ml) per 10 cm of thrombus, preferably using a catheter with **multiple side orifices** and **pulsed-spray technique** [17–19] in order to saturate the thrombus. The bolusing should start distally, and the catheter should be progressively retracted proximally. Some workers [18] advocate leaving a distal plug of thrombus in place in order to avoid possible embolization caused by forced infusion (pulse-spray). Others bolus the entire thrombus in order to reestablish flow quickly. Small distal emboli of thrombus usually dissolve with continued infusion of the lytic agent [18,19].

b. **Continuous IA infusion.** Several options are available here. Conventionally, continuous UK infusion is started with a volumetric infusion pump and with either a coaxial 3 Fr. end-hole catheter or an outer 5 Fr. catheter embedded in the proximal portion of the thrombus [1]. The catheter is advanced distally as lysis progresses. Currently, the infusion systems described previously allow various options for bathing the thrombus with lytic agents. By selecting the proper system, the entire thrombus or any segment(s) of it can be infused with lytic agent, and catheter manipulations can be minimized. The selected dose of lytic agent may be divided between the proximal and distal catheters as desired. Since blood flow to the ischemic limb must be restored as soon as possible, the selected catheter(s) should be nonobstructively positioned, and patients should be systemically heparinized.

> **Urokinase Infusion Protocol***
> **Urokinase concentration:** 3000 IU/ml
> **Transthrombus bolus:** 150–250 K IU
> **Continuous infusion:** 4000 IU/min for 2 hours,
> *then*
> 2000 IU/min for 2 hours,
> *then*
> 1000 IU/min for the duration

c. **Intravenous anticoagulation.** Bolus IV **heparin** (70 units/kg), and start continuous IV infusion at 600–1200 units/hour [1–4] to prevent thrombus formation around the catheter. This may be initiated as soon as the thrombus is crossed with a wire. Heparin should be adjusted to maintain either PTT or ACT [20] at therapeutic range as described in the next section. Recent studies suggest that smaller doses (100 units/hour)

*Brigham and Women's Hospital.

through the IA sheath may be sufficient to prevent pericatheter thrombus [21].

Postprocedure Management

1. **Pressure bandage** at site of catheter entry; **check puncture site** q30min × 4 hours, then q2h during infusion.
2. Transfer patient to **intensive care unit.** Monitor **vital signs** frequently per ICU protocol. Check extremity for **pulses** (palpation/Doppler) q4h or more frequently as clinically dictated.
3. **Laboratory monitoring**
   a. Check **Hct; PT and PTT or ACT** q2h × 2, then as needed.
   b. Desired PTT is 2.0–2.5 times control level (with a control level of 35 seconds, target **PTT** would be **70–90 seconds**). The **ACT** should be around **300 seconds** during lytic therapy.
4. Monitor fluid input/output, Cr daily.
5. Avoid IM injections.
6. Infuse heparinized saline (1500 units heparin in 500 ml NS) via outer coaxial catheter (at KVO rate), if this catheter is not being used for lytic agent.
7. In case of fever, acetaminophen (Tylenol) is suggested; however, acetylsalicylic acid (aspirin), which has antiplatelet activity, is not necessarily detrimental in most cases.
8. Return for **repeat angiogram** in 4–12 hours for progress check or as deemed necessary clinically.
9. **Terminate lysis** on evidence of successful recanalization (clinical improvement, return of Doppler signals), complication, or failure.
   a. Discontinue UK and heparin simultaneously; remove inner catheter and pull back outer catheter, leaving only a short segment of it within the artery. If an arterial sheath is employed, the infusion catheters may be removed from the patient. Continue heparinized saline infusion via the outer catheter or IA sheath.
   b. Treat underlying stenotic or occlusive lesion(s) by prompt percutaneous transluminal angioplasty (PTA), atherectomy, or surgical revascularization [3,5,7].
   c. Remove catheter/sheath 4 hours later. For earlier removal (1–2 hours), if PTT or ACT are elevated, protamine sulfate 30 mg slow IV infusion may be given (barring other contraindications).
   d. Restart IV anticoagulation in 4–6 hours (after removal of IA sheath and successful groin compression), if peripheral thrombus was from an *embolic* source or if anticoagulation is otherwise indicated.

Results (see Table 5-1)

Cumulative results [5,9,14] from published series on thrombolysis with UK for acutely ischemic limbs: positive thrombolytic outcome 85–95%; mean duration of infusion, approximately 24 hours. A rapid early (< 2 hours) response to throm-

Table 5-2. Overall incidence of complications of peripheral arterial thrombolysis

Complication	Incidence (%)
Major bleeding	6.6
Intracranial hemorrhage	0.5
Retroperitoneal hemorrhage	0.3
Minor bleeding	6.3
Limb-related complications	
Distal embolization	5.2
Amputation	
Due to distal embolization	0.8
Due to preexisting severe ischemia	8.0
Reperfusion syndrome	0.7
Compartment syndrome	2.0
Concurrent rethrombosis	3.0
Local arterial dissection	0.6
Systemic complications	
Acute renal failure	0.3
Acute myocardial infarction	0.2
Other	
Nonhemorrhagic stroke	<1.0
Death	0.8

Source: Compiled from two reviews of the literature on regional thrombolysis for peripheral arterial occlusions by Gardiner et al. [29] (n = 1787 cases) and McNamara et al. [30] (n = 1000 cases).

bolysis is associated with improved initial success [1]. Durations of infusion are generally reported to be shorter with rt-PA [13,14] and much longer with SK [1,2,9]. Duration of treatment may vary with the doses and rates of infusion used [15,22]. The lower success rates and higher complication rates of SK relative to UK are most likely related to the greater plasminogen and fibrinogen depletion caused by the former agent [23]. Long-term patency is improved if the underlying lesions are treated promptly by percutaneous and/or surgical techniques [3,5,7,24]. Long-term patency is generally better for successfully treated suprainguinal occlusions (versus infrainguinal occlusions) [7,24] and vein grafts (versus synthetic grafts) [3]. If thrombolysis fails, simple thrombectomy and/or graft revision also tend to fair poorly [2].

Complications (Table 5-2)

Sullivan et al. [16] showed that the probability of a major complication increases dramatically with the duration of thrombolysis. Reported incidences of major complications for the three commonly used agents are compared in Tables 5-1 and 5-2 [1–7,9–16,25–30]. The incidence of a major allergic reaction with SK or rt-PA is under 0.5%, and 0% with UK; intracranial hemorrhage is less than 1% with SK and rt-PA, and 0% with UK; total stroke is about 1% with SK, under 1.4% with rt-PA, and 0% with UK [27]. Other reported incidences of complications of thrombolysis are as follows: peripheral embolization, 5–15% [1,4,25,29,30]; pericatheter thrombus formation (with IV heparinization), 3–5% [1,4,29,30]; compartment syndrome, about 2% [28–30]; sepsis or renal failure, under 1% [29,30]; and pseudoaneurysm formation at the puncture site, under 1% [1].

Management of Complications During Lytic Agent Infusion

1. Severe bleeding
   a. Discontinue thrombolytic agent and IV heparin.
   b. Consider transfusion of whole fresh blood, packed red blood cells (PRBC), fresh frozen plasma (FFP) (2–4 units may be needed).
   c. For severe continuing hemorrhage, consider aminocaproic acid (Amicar 5 gm PO or slow IV infusion; then 1 gm/hour for 2–4 hours).
   d. Avoid dextran [6].
   e. Find source of internal bleeding to take specific corrective measures (e.g., CT scan for occult retroperitoneal hemorrhage).
2. Distal embolization of thrombus. Occurs in about 10% of cases. Usually resolves with continued lytic therapy. Embolectomy is rarely needed.
3. Allergic reaction
   a. Rare with UK; more frequently associated with SK and rt-PA.
   b. Rare episodes of mild bronchospasm, skin rash, and transient fever are reported with UK.
   c. Recently, there have been reports of chills and rigors following large boluses of UK (e.g., 500K IU given for thrombolysis of dialysis fistulas). This is most likely related to the current manufacturing process for UK (Abbokinase; Abbot Laboratories, Chicago, IL). These symptoms may be treated prophylactically with acetaminophen 1 gm PO and diphenhydramine hydrochloride (Benadryl) 50 mg PO, given 30–60 minutes prior to UK infusion. If a reaction occurs once UK infusion has started, symptoms may be treated with meperidine hydrochloride (Demerol) 50 mg IV or cimetidine 300 mg IV.

References

1. McNamara TO, Fischer JR. Thrombolysis in peripheral arterial and graft occlusions: Improved results using high dose urokinase. *AJR* 144:764–775, 1985.
2. Gardiner GA, et al: Thrombolysis of occluded femoropopliteal grafts. *AJR* 147:621–626, 1986.
3. Sullivan KL, et al. Efficacy of thrombolysis in infrainguinal bypass grafts. *Circulation* 83(Suppl I):I-99–I-105, 1991.
4. Belkin M, et al: Intra-arterial fibrinolytic therapy. *Arch Surg* 121:769–773, 1986.
5. McNamara TO. Thrombolysis as an alternative initial therapy for the acutely ischemic limb. *Semin Vasc Surg* 5:89–98, 1992.

6. *Physicians' Desk Reference* (49th ed.). Oradell, NJ: Medical Economics Company, 1995.
7. McNamara TO, Bomberger RA. Factors affecting initial and six month patency rates after intra-arterial thrombolysis with high dose urokinase. *Am J Surg* 152:709–712, 1986.
8. Luppatelli L, et al. Selective thrombolysis with low-dose urokinase in chronic arteriosclerotic occlusions. *Cardiovasc Intervent Radiol* 11:123–126, 1988.
9. Van Breda A, et al. Relative cost-effectiveness of urokinase versus streptokinase in the treatment of peripheral vascular disease. *J Vasc Interv Radiol* 2:77–87, 1991.
10. Janosik JE, et al. Therapeutic alternatives for subacute peripheral arterial occlusion: Comparison by outcome, length of stay, and hospital charges. *Invest Radiol* 26:921–925, 1991.
11. Traughber PD, et al. Intraarterial fibrinolytic therapy for popliteal and tibial artery obstruction: Comparison of streptokinase to urokinase. *AJR* 149:543–456, 1987.
12. Belkin M, et al. Intra-arterial fibrinolytic therapy: Efficacy of streptokinase vs. urokinase. *Arch Surg* 121:769–773, 1986.
13. Graor RA, et al. Thrombolysis with recombinant human tissue-type plasminogen activator in patients with peripheral artery and bypass graft occlusions. *Circulation* 74(Suppl I):I-15–I-20, 1986.
14. Graor RA, et al. Efficacy and safety of intraarterial local infusion of streptokinase, urokinase, or tissue plasminogen activator for peripheral arterial occlusion: A retrospective review. *J Vasc Med Biol* 2:310–315, 1990.
15. Meyerovitz MF, et al. Recombinant tissue-type plasminogen activator versus urokinase in peripheral arterial and graft occlusions: A randomized trial. *Radiology* 175:75–78, 1990.
16. Sullivan KL, et al. Acceleration of thrombolysis with a high-dose transthrombus bolus technique. *Radiology* 173:805–808, 1989.
17. Mewissen MW, et al. Symptomatic native arterial occlusions: Early experience with "over-the-wire" thrombolysis. *J Vasc Interv Radiol* 1:43–47, 1990.
18. Valji K, et al. Pulsed-spray Thrombolysis of arterial and bypass graft occlusions. *AJR* 156:617–621, 1991.
19. Kandarpa K, et al. Intraarterial thrombolysis of lower extremity occlusions: A prospective, randomized comparison of forced periodic infusion and conventional slow continuous infusion. *Radiology* 188:861–867, 1993.
20. Rath B, Bennett DH. Monitoring the effect of heparin by measurement of activated clotting time during and after PTCA. *Br Heart J* 63:18–21, 1990.
21. LeBlang SD, et al. Low-dose urokinase regimen for the treatment of lower extremity arterial and graft occlusions: Experience in 132 cases. *J Vasc Interv Radiol* 3:475–483, 1992.
22. Berridge DC, et al. Tissue plasminogen activator in peripheral arterial thrombolysis. *Br J Surg* 77:179–182, 1990.
23. Holden RW. Plasminogen activators: Pharmacology and therapy. *Radiology* 174:993–1001, 1990.
24. Durham JD, Rutherford RB. Assessment of long-term efficacy of fibrinolytic therapy in the ischemic extremity. *Semin Intervent Radiol* 9:166–173, 1992.
25. Kaufman JA, Bettmann MA. Thrombolysis of peripheral vascular occlusions with urokinase: A review of the clinical literature. *Semin Intervent Radiol* 9:159–165, 1992.

26. Palaskas C, Totty WG, Gilula LA. Complications of local intra-arterial fibrinolytic therapy. *Semin Intervent Radiol* 2:396–404, 1985.

27. Woo KS, White HD. Comparative tolerability profiles of thrombolytic agents: a review. *Drug Safety* 8:19–29, 1993.

28. Koltun WA, et al. Thrombolysis in the treatment of peripheral vascular occlusions. *Arch Surg* 122:901–905, 1987.

29. Gardiner GA, Sullivan KL. Complications of Regional Thrombolytic Therapy. In S Kadir (ed.), *Current Practice of Interventional Radiology*. Philadelphia: BC Decker, 1991. Pp. 87–91.

30. McNamara TO, Goodwin SC, Kandarpa K. Complications associated with thrombolysis. *Semin Intervent Radiol* 2:134–144, 1994.

Extremity Balloon Angioplasty

Maria G. M. Hunink
Krishna Kandarpa

Balloon angioplasty increases the luminal diameter of a stenotic artery by causing plaque fracture, often with accompanying local intimal-medial dissection [1,2].

Indications

1. Lifestyle-limiting claudication.
2. Critical ischemia (rest pain, ulcer, gangrene).
3. To increase inflow or outflow prior to or after bypass surgery.
4. Bypass graft stenosis.

Indications Despite Unfavorable Anatomy [1]

1. Saphenous vein is unavailable or inadequate for a bypass.
2. Amputation is expected; PTA may move the level distally.
3. Patient has a high surgical risk.
4. Patient has a short life expectancy.

Contraindications

ABSOLUTE

1. Patient is medically unstable.
2. Stenosis is not hemodynamically significant.
3. Stenosis is immediately adjacent to an aneurysm [2].
4. Ulcerative disease with evidence of distal embolization is present [1].

RELATIVE (unfavorable anatomy)

1. Long-segment, multifocal stenoses.
2. Long-segment occlusion, unless converted to discrete stenosis with thrombolysis.
3. Stenosis has a large amount of adjacent acute or subacute thrombus (likely if symptoms presented suddenly or worsening occurred within less than 6–8 weeks), unless treatment with thrombolysis is available and successful [1].
4. Long-segment, multifocal infrapopliteal disease, if there is a large vessel at the ankle suitable for bypass [1].
5. Heavy calcification, particularly if eccentric.
6. Lesion in essential collateral vessel.

Preprocedure Preparation

1. Standard preangiography preparation. Double-check renal function if diagnostic arteriography has recently been performed.
2. Check noninvasive studies (segmental Doppler pressures, ankle/brachial indices [ABI], duplex Doppler) and prior arteriograms.

3. Obtain baseline preprocedure Doppler study including ABI.
4. Premedication. Aspirin 325 mg PO the night before or the morning of the PTA. Nifedipine 10 mg sublingual 15–30 minutes prior to PTA (unless the patient is already on verapamil or diltiazem); duration of action is 4–6 hours.

Procedure (Fig. 6-1)

1. Document the lesion (on two views) and distal runoff with angiography. Intraarterial digital subtraction angiography and **road-mapping** techniques are very useful for rapid imaging guidance during the procedure. Intraarterial infusion of 100 μg nitroglycerin is recommended if an apparent severe stenosis is to be distinguished from **vasospasm** [1].
2. If the **hemodynamic significance** is questioned, measure the pressure gradient across the stenosis. Any peak-to-peak systolic or mean pressure gradient at rest in the arteries is abnormal [1]; however, a gradient < 20 mm Hg in the iliac arteries is considered to be nonsignificant [3]. Following flow augmentation with IA infusion of 15–25 mg tolazoline or 100 μg nitroglycerin, a gradient of 15–20 mm Hg above rest is considered significant [1,3]. One should not rely completely on "an absolute value" for a significant gradient (e.g., 20 mm Hg), since the pressure gradient is determined by, among other parameters, the blood flow rate within the vessel at the time the measurement is made [4]. If the catheter used to measure the gradient is nearly of the same caliber as the stenosis, the measurement is unreliable. Correlation with clinical symptoms and noninvasive studies should be used to determine the true physiological significance of a lesion.
3. Recommended **access** for PTA
   a. For aortic and aortic-bifurcation PTA: bilateral retrograde femoral arteries.
   b. For common and external iliac PTA: ipsilateral retrograde femoral artery.
   c. For common femoral, proximal superficial, and proximal deep femoral PTA: contralateral retrograde femoral artery.
   d. For superficial femoral, deep femoral, and infrapopliteal PTA: ipsilateral antegrade femoral artery.
4. Use an **arterial sheath** to facilitate
   a. Multiple exchanges.
   b. Measuring pressures.
   c. Injection of contrast and needed pharmaceuticals, *and*
   d. To minimize entry-site trauma. Oversize sheath by 1 Fr. (for very large balloons, 2 Fr.) and check that the balloon passes easily through the sheath.
5. After successfully crossing the lesion 2500–5000 units (or 70 units/kg for adults) **IV heparin** (or IA) should be given for both its anticoagulant and antispasmodic effects. Determining the activated clotting time (ACT) during the procedure is useful for optimizing the duration of drug effect to only what is necessary.

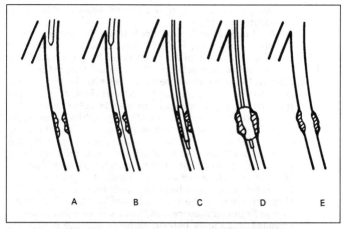

Fig. 6-1. Stages of angioplasty. A. A focal stenosis in the superficial femoral artery. B. The lesion is crossed with one of various catheter-guidewire combinations (see text). C. Real-time DNA road-mapping or external metallic markers are used to localize the lesion fluoroscopically and the balloon is advanced to bridge the lesion. D. Several 30–45-second inflations are performed; with the deflated balloon still across the lesion, a 0.025-in. (or smaller) guidewire is placed distal to the lesion through a Y-connector arrangement proximally. This connector allows one to inject contrast through the lumen or to make pressure gradient measurements while the balloon catheter is retracted over the smaller guidewire. E. Shows the final angiographic result. Circumferential fibers in the vessel wall rupture, increasing lumen area—the plaque itself is incompressible.

6. Choose the PTA **balloon catheter**
   a. **Size.** The balloon diameter should be equal to the adjacent normal vessel diameter measured on cut-film arteriography. This will generally oversize the balloon by 10–20%, which is desirable. Balloons come in sizes 2–20 mm diameter, and 2–10 cm length on 3.8–9.0 Fr. catheters, and can take 4–17 atmospheres pressure. Commonly used initial balloon diameters are 8 mm in the common iliac, 6–7 mm in the external iliac, 5 mm in the superficial femoral, 4 mm in the popliteal, and 3.0–3.5 mm in the infrapopliteal arteries [5].
   b. High-pressure irradiated polyethylene balloons (**noncompliant materials**) can avoid overdistention and balloon rupture [1].
   c. **Low-profile** balloons
      (1) Help minimize entry-site complications, especially if a sheath is not used.
      (2) Aid in negotiating severe stenoses.
      (3) Are necessary for PTA of infrapopliteal vessels [2].
   d. **Trackability** (i.e., the tendency of a catheter to follow a wire placed in the desired position) is important if the lesion is peripheral or on the contralateral side to

the puncture site, or if tortuous vessels have to be negotiated [2].

   e. A **"kissing balloon" technique** is recommended when performing PTA of bifurcations (e.g., to perform PTA of the aortoiliac bifurcation by positioning one balloon at each origin of the common iliac artery).

7. **Lesion location relative to access site.** If the lesion is close to the access site and easily reached, the crossing guidewire and balloon catheter may be introduced coaxially together through the sheath (e.g, a Wholey steerable wire [Advanced Cardiovascular Systems; ACS], which has a flexible tip that can be shaped, with a torquable stiff shaft; or TAD wire [ACS], which has a tapered flexible tip of variable length that can be shaped, with a stiff shaft). If the stenosis is severe or can be reached only after negotiation of curves, it may be necessary to first use a guidewire that can pass by the tortuosity and/or the lesion (high-torque floppy, glidewire, etc.) but must be upsized or exchanged to support balloon catheter passage across the stenosis. To do this, advance the diagnostic catheter coaxially past the lesion and exchange for a stiffer guidewire (e.g., Rosen wire; Cook, Bloomington, IN).

8. Having marked the lesion with real-time DSA road-mapping or external metallic markers, cross the lesion carefully, avoiding excessive force. The following **guidewires** may be used.

   a. For **large vessels:** 0.035–0.038-in. 15 mm J, floppy straight tip, long floppy Bentson, long tapered straight, Wholey steerable (ACS, Temecula, CA), movable core J-tip, tight 1.5 mm J, high-torque floppy, or a glidewire (straight, angled or long tapered) (Terumo; Meditech, Watertown, MA).

   b. For **small vessels**: 0.014–0.018-in. floppy (steerable) guidewire, 0.018–0.025-in. small vessel Glidewire (Meditech), or Flex-T (ACS).

   c. For recanalization of **occlusions:** Rosen wire, 1.5 mm tight J, or glidewire.

   d. **Wire technique.** Extra care must be taken with the Glidewire, and other similar smooth-surfaced wires, to avoid dissection. Avoid advancing the catheter too close to the lesion. Like most wires, the smooth surface guidewires need some room in order to keep the tip flexible and to avoid dissection and perforation. Unlike other wires, however, the smooth "slippery" surface predisposes to easy subintimal passage of the tip. A torque device is very helpful for maneuvering the wire through the lumen. Occasionally, a preshaped catheter may be helpful in crossing certain lesions (e.g., Simmons, or Sos-Omni [AngioDynamics, Glens Falls, NY]). For a bifurcation stenosis, guidewires are positioned in both vessels and PTA is performed simultaneously (for the aortic bifurcation: "kissing balloon" technique) or sequentially (for popliteal artery branches).

9. **Vasospasm** can be prevented and treated, especially when performing PTA of small vessels or if flow distally is poor, with the vasodilators listed below. Careful BP

monitoring is required when administering vasodilator drugs.

   a. Nifedipine 10 mg sublingual 15–30 minutes prior to PTA (unless the patient is already on verapamil or diltiazem).

   b. Nitroglycerin 100–200 μg IA bolus before crossing the lesion, distally after crossing, and repeat if vasospasm is observed [2,5]. Transdermal nitroglycerin patches also may be useful. Because nitroglycerin is absorbed by plastic, glass syringes should be used [5].

   c. Verapamil 2.5 mg IV. (Contraindicated in patients with cardiac conduction abnormalities, ventricular dysfunction, or hypotension.)

10. Leave the guidewire well distal to the site and fix the tip so that it does not move at all. Then **advance the balloon across the lesion** using digital subtraction angiography (DSA) road-mapping or external metallic markers to localize the lesion. With multiple stenoses, start with the most distal one, except if stenoses in both the femoral-popliteal and infrapopliteal arteries are to be treated, in which case the femoral-popliteal lesion is dilated first.

11. **Inflate** the balloon using a pressure gauge—being careful not to exceed the maximum specified pressure—for 30–120 seconds, 1 to 3 times. Use contrast 1 : 3 diluted to inflate and visualize the balloon. Effacement of a "waist" where the plaque is being compressed is a sign of effective PTA. Mild to moderate pain in an alert patient is a sign of effective dilatation; very severe persistent pain is suggestive of rupture. Deflate the balloon with a large-bore syringe immediately and completely to avoid thrombus formation around it.

12. **Retract the balloon catheter** over the guidewire, leaving the wire across the lesion. Before and during removal of the balloon catheter, suctioning with a large-bore syringe helps to keep the balloon completely deflated. Some balloons require clockwise (or counterclockwise, depending on the design) rotation to wrap the "wings" around the balloon. Obtain a **"check" angiogram** with the guidewire across the lesion. Contrast may be injected through the side-arm of the sheath, via a side-arm adapter, through the catheter, or by exchanging for a diagnostic catheter in the case of aorto-, iliac-, or common-femoral PTA. Avoid injection through an end-hole catheter close to the PTA site as this may cause or propagate a dissection [1]. If necessary, measure pressures across the site. A residual stenosis of > 40–50% should be **redilated** with a balloon 0.5–1.0 mm larger in diameter than the one just used.

13. If the check angiogram and pressures are satisfactory, remove the wire and perform a **final post-PTA angiogram**.

14. **Avoid recrossing the PTA site** with a guidewire immediately after dilatation. If this is absolutely necessary (i.e., in cases of threatening occlusion), do so *very* carefully.

15. A post-PTA intimal cleft is normal and usually resolves within 3 months.

Postprocedure Management

1. Allow the heparin to wear off in 2–4 hours after administration before removing the sheath. The plasma half-life of heparin is between 1 and 2 hours. Determining the ACT (< 180 seconds) before attempting **sheath removal and groin compression** is useful, and may avoid groin complications. Some authors prefer reversing the heparin with 10 mg protamine sulfate/1000 units of active heparin after PTA of large vessel lesions [1]. Compress for 20–30 minutes.
2. Standard postangiography management.
3. **Continued IV heparinization**
   a. May be indicated if:
      (1) PTA was performed on an infrapopliteal or small femoral-popliteal vessel. Some authors recommend always giving heparin after femoral-popliteal PTA [6].
      (2) There is a dissection extending beyond the PTA site.
      (3) There is poor distal runoff.
      (4) There is a low-flow state.
   b. **Suggested protocol.** To achieve the benefit of anticoagulation without bleeding, IV heparin may be started promptly after hemostasis is achieved at 1000 units/ hour, without giving another bolus. Heparinization may be continued for 24–48 hours, while maintaining the PTT at 1.5–2.5 times the baseline value and monitoring closely for complications.
4. Obtain postprocedure Doppler pulses, including ABI; repeat 24–48 hours post-PTA.
5. Encourage exercise (after 48 hours) and discourage smoking.
6. Antiplatelet therapy [1]: Aspirin 80–325 mg PO/day for at least 6 months is recommended. Dipyridamole 50–75 mg PO tid may be added. Long-term benefit of this adjunctive treatment is unproved.
7. Follow-up: at 1 day; 1, 3, 6, and 12 months; and every year thereafter. Perform a history (symptoms at rest; claudicating and maximum walking distance, smoking and exercise history), physical examination (pulses; examine extremity for ischemic changes), and Doppler pulses including ABI.

Patency Results (see Tables 6-1, 6-2)

REPORTING PATENCY RESULTS

1. An improvement of ABI of > 0.10 with relief of symptoms is considered a success [7]. During follow-up a decrease in ABI of > 0.15 compared with the maximum early post-PTA ABI, and/or recurrence of symptoms, is considered a failure. The thigh/brachial index is probably a more reliable index for aortoiliac disease [7].
2. The initial success rate should be reported and initial failures are usually included in the patency analysis [7,8].

If initial failures are included in the results, the patency among patients with an initially successful angioplasty may be derived by dividing by the initial success rate.

3. Primary patency refers to those vessels or bypass grafts that remain patent without any further intervention. Secondary patency refers to all vessels or bypass grafts that remain patent, with or without additional procedures. Primary revised patency is used in the surgical literature and implies patency with limited intervention to maintain patency of a bypass graft [7,8].

4. Patency results should be analyzed and reported using actuarial life table or Kaplan-Meier analysis, reporting the number of limbs at risk in each interval during follow-up [7,8].

5. Thirty-day mortality should be reported to make results comparable to surgical data.

PTA VERSUS SUPERVISED EXERCISE AND BYPASS

1. There are only two published randomized controlled trials comparing PTA with supervised exercise and bypass.
   a. **PTA and supervised exercise** [9]. Thirty-six patients with unilateral claudication were randomized. Significantly more patients undergoing supervised exercise stopped smoking, confounding the results. The ABI increase after 3–9 months was 0.21 with PTA, and 0 with exercise. However, with exercise, the claudicating and maximum walking distance increased progressively, while in all PTA patients this was limited at 12 months by contralateral disease. Note that exercise also prevented and treated contralateral disease while PTA was performed unilaterally in this trial.
   b. **PTA and bypass** [10]. Two hundred and ninety-two patients were randomized. Aortoiliac PTA had a 5-year primary patency of 62%, and bypass, 81%. No difference was demonstrated between femoral-popliteal PTA and bypass, with 5-year primary patencies of 59% and 55%, respectively. A recent update of this study reported no significant differences in outcome between PTA and bypass surgery (median follow-up period of 4 years), with both groups attaining an immediate and sustained improvement in hemodynamics and quality of life [11].

2. The case-mix of the study population influences the results. In multivariate analysis, **factors predictive of PTA failure** are: site distal to the common iliac artery, occlusion, critical ischemia, and poor distal runoff (Table 6-1).

3. Repeat PTA has equivalent results to primary PTA [12].

4. Factors predictive of failure after bypass surgery are critical ischemia and synthetic graft material; and in the case of a synthetic graft, the site of the distal anastomosis (Table 6-2).

Table 6-1. Summary of primary patency results for angioplasty in the treatment of peripheral arterial disease, adjusted to include initial failures

Site, indication, lesion type, runoff, reference	Initial[a]	1-yr	3-yr	5-yr
Aortoiliac [12–15]	92	82	76	70
Stenosis and claudication	93	86	84	83
Stenosis and ischemia	88	73	58	50
Occlusion and claudication	85	65	50	41
Occlusion and ischemia	83	55	35	26
Femoral-popliteal [13,15–23]	89	59	52	45
Stenosis and claudication	95	79	74	68
Stenosis and ischemia	90	62	54	47
Occlusion and claudication	87	52	43	35
Occlusion and ischemia	75	26	18	12
Infrapopliteal [24]	93[b]	80[b]	65[b]	—
Bypass graft [25]	70	42	25	18
Single lesion	77	59	59	—
Multiple lesions	67	32	6	—

Claudication = disabling claudication; ischemia = critical ischemia;
RF = risk factor predictive of long-term failure.
[a]Initial technical and clinical success. To calculate the patency among those patients who had an initial successful angioplasty, divide by the initial success rate.
[b]Secondary patency, primary not reported.

Table 6-2. Summary of primary patency results for bypass surgery in the treatment of peripheral arterial disease

Site, material, and indication	1-yr	3-yr	5-yr
Aortoiliofemoral [26,27]	95	89	85
No femoral-popliteal disease	98	94	89
With femoral-popliteal disease	95	82	74
Femoral-popliteal [16,28–32]			
VEIN claudication	91	86	80
VEIN ischemia	84	76	66
PTFE-AK claudication	90	81	75
PTFE-BK claudication	85	73	65
PTFE-AK ischemia	76	58	47
PTFE-BK ischemia	66	44	33
Femoral-infrapopliteal [28–32]			
VEIN ischemia	70	66	60
PTFE ischemia	45	26	12

Claudication = disabling claudication; ischemia = critical ischemia;
VEIN = in situ or reversed saphenous vein bypass; PTFE = polytetrafluoroethylene (synthetic) graft; AK = above-knee distal anastomosis; BK = below-knee distal anastomosis.

Complications

1. **Overall** incidence of complications is 9–10% [2,5,33]. Complications **requiring treatment** occur in 2.0–2.5% of procedures performed [2].

   a. **Procedure-related mortality** is generally 0.1–0.5% [2,13]. Thirty-day mortality is higher (0.9%), and in elderly patients with critical ischemia, mortality may be as high as 6% [35].

   b. **Systemic complications** include sepsis (0.2%), transient acute tubular necrosis (0.3–1.0%), and cardiac or pulmonary problems (0.4%) [2,5,34].

   c. **Major local complications** include thrombotic occlusion (2%), distal embolization (2%), false aneurysm (0.3–2.0%), AV fistula (0.1–0.3%), arterial rupture (0.3%–3.0%), and amputation (0.2%) [2,5,33]. Arterial rupture is usually due to an oversized balloon. Factors predisposing to arterial rupture are steroid medication and underlying vascular abnormalities [5].

   d. **Minor local complications** include hematoma (2–4%), guidewire perforation without bleeding (0.3%), dissection extending beyond the PTA site (1–4%), and balloon rupture [2,5,33].

2. For comparison, statistics for **morbidity and mortality of bypass surgery** follow.

   a. Thirty-day operative mortality increases with age [35]:

	< **75 yr**	≥ **75 yr**
Aortoiliac/aortofemoral (for occlusive disease)	2.9%	12.3%
Femoral-popliteal/ femorotibial	2.2%	6.7%

   b. Overall complications range from 11–23%, major complications occur in 7–15% [26,28,29].

   c. Preoperative ischemia on Holter monitoring is the major predictor of a postoperative cardiac event (sensitivity 88%, specificity 91%) [36].

3. Management

   a. **Acute occlusion.** This may be due to vasospasm, an obstructing dissection, or thrombosis [5]. Give 1000–2000 units IV heparin and 100–200 µg IA nitroglycerin. If vasospasm is the cause, this will restore flow; if not, an intimal flap may be the problem and repeating PTA to "tack down" the flap may work. Alternatively, atherectomy or stent placement may be performed. If occlusion persists, local thrombolysis (UK 4000 units/minute for 2–3 hours) can be performed [6] before further intervention.

   b. **Distal embolization.** If small and insignificant, systemic heparinization is acceptable. If large, aspiration with a large-bore nontapered catheter, percutaneous or surgical embolectomy, or thrombolysis should be considered. If acute ischemia develops, urgent surgical removal is necessary to avoid compartment syndrome and/or limb loss.

   c. **False aneurysm/arteriovenous (AV) fistula at puncture site.** Ultrasound-guided compression, with adequate sedation and pain control. If unsuccessful, surgical intervention is required [37].

   d. **Arterial rupture with extravasation.** The PTA procedure should be stopped. Occlude the rupture site with the PTA balloon (or "stack" distal perfusion balloon), maintaining distal flow, for 20 minutes [5]. Alert the vascular surgeon and type and cross-match for packed red blood cells (PRBCs). If extravasation persists, reinflate the balloon. If control of bleeding is not obtained, urgent surgical intervention is necessary. If necessary, a repeat attempt at PTA may be made 2–4 weeks later.

   e. **Extensive dissection beyond PTA site.** The PTA procedure should be stopped and, if necessary, repeated 2–4 weeks later. IV heparin should be given postprocedure as discussed above.

   f. **Balloon rupture.** Remove the balloon catheter through a sheath. If no injury has occurred at the PTA site, as is usually the case, continue PTA with a new balloon.

Cost Effectiveness

1. The ratio of hospital costs of angioplasty to bypass surgery were 53% for patients with disabling claudication and 75% for those with critical ischemia [38].

2. A cost-effectiveness analysis demonstrated that, on average, performing PTA as initial procedure in technically feasible cases and reserving bypass surgery for those patients in whom PTA fails, would save lives, limbs, and dollars [39].

References

1. Schwarten DE, Tadavarthy SM, Castañeda-Zúñiga WR. Aortic, Iliac, and Peripheral Arterial Angioplasty. In WR Castañeda-Zúñiga, SM Tadavarthy (eds.), *Intervent Radiol* (2nd ed). Baltimore: Williams & Wilkins, 1992. Pp. 378–421.

2. Becker GJ, Katzen BT, Dake MD. Noncoronary angioplasty. *Radiology* 170:921–940, 1989.

3. Kaufman SL, et al. Hemodynamic measurements in the evaluation and follow-up of transluminal angioplasty of the iliac and femoral arteries. *Radiology* 142:329–336, 1982.

4. Kandarpa K, et al. Hemodynamic evaluation of arterial stenoses by computer simulation. *Invest Radiol* 22:393–403, 1987.

5. McDermott JC, Crummy AB. Complications of Angioplasty. In S Kadir (ed.), *Current Practice of Interventional Radiology*. Philadelphia: BC Decker, 1991. Pp. 57–61.

6. Kadir S. Angioplasty of Superficial Femoral Artery Stenoses and Occlusions. In S Kadir (ed.). *Current Practice of Interventional Radiology*. Philadelphia: BC Decker, 1991. Pp. 311–319.

7. Rutherford RB, Becker GJ. Standards for evaluating and reporting the results of surgical and percutaneous therapy for peripheral arterial disease. *Radiology* 181:277–281, 1991.

8. Rutherford RB, Flanigan DP, Gupta SK, et al. Suggested stan-

dards for reports dealing with lower extremity ischaemia. Prepared by the Ad Hoc Committee on Reporting Standards, Society for Vascular Surgery/North American Chapter, International Society for Cardiovascular Surgery. *J Vasc Surg* 4:80–94, 1986.

9. Creasy TS, et al. Is percutaneous transluminal angioplasty better than exercise for claudication?—Preliminary results from a prospective randomized trial. *Eur J Vasc Surg* 4:135–140, 1990.

10. Wilson SE, et al. Percutaneous transluminal angioplasty versus operation for peripheral arteriosclerosis: Report of a prospective randomized trial in a selected group of patients. *J Vasc Surg* 9: 1–9, 1989.

11. Wolf GL, et al. Surgery or balloon angioplasty for peripheral vascular disease: A randomized clinical trial. *J Vasc Interv Radiol* 4:639–648, 1993.

12. Johnston KW, et al. 5-year results of a prospective study of percutaneous transluminal angioplasty. *Ann Surg* 206:403–413, 1987.

13. Rutherford RB, Durham J. Percutaneous Balloon Angioplasty for Arteriosclerosis Obliterans: Long-term Results. In JST Yao, WH Pearce (eds.), *Technologies in Vascular Surgery*. Philadelphia: WB Saunders, 1992.

14. van Andel GJ, et al. Percutaneous transluminal dilatation of the iliac artery: Long-term results. *Radiology* 156:321–323, 1985.

15. Samson RH, et al. Management of angioplasty complications, unsuccessful procedures and early and late failures. *Ann Surg* 199: 234–240, 1984.

16. Hunink MGM, et al. Patency results of percutaneous and surgical revascularization for femoropopliteal arterial disease. *Med Decis Making* 14:71–81, 1994.

17. Hunink MGM, et al. Risks and benefits of femoropopliteal percutaneous balloon angioplasty. *J Vasc Surg* 17:183–94, 1993.

18. Gallino A, et al. Percutaneous transluminal angioplasty of the arteries of the lower limbs: A 5-year follow-up. *Circulation* 70:619–623, 1984.

19. Henriksen LO, et al. Percutaneous transluminal angioplasty of infrarenal arteries in intermittent claudication. *Acta Chir Scand* 154:573–576, 1988.

20. Jørgensen B, et al. Percutaneous transluminal angioplasty of iliac and femoral arteries in severe lower-limb ischemia. *Acta Chir Scand* 154:647–652, 1988.

21. Johnston KW. Femoral and popliteal arteries: Reanalysis of results of balloon angioplasty. *Radiology* 183:767–771, 1992.

22. Capek P, McLean GK, Berkowitz HD. Femoropopliteal angioplasty: Factors influencing long-term success. *Circulation* 83 (Suppl I):I-70–I-80, 1991.

23. Krepel VM, et al. Percutaneous transluminal dilatation of the femoropopliteal artery: Initial and long-term results. *Radiology* 156:325–328, 1985.

24. Horvath W, Oertl M, Haidinger D. Percutaneous transluminal angioplasty of crural arteries. *Radiology* 177:565–569, 1990.

25. Whittemore AD, et al. Limitations of balloon angioplasty for vein graft stenosis. *J Vasc Surg* 14:340–345, 1991.

26. Szilagyi DE, et al. A thirty-year survey of the reconstructive surgical treatment of aortoiliac occlusive disease. *J Vasc Surg* 3:421–436, 1986.

27. Nevelsteen A, et al. Aortofemoral grafting: Factors influencing late results. *Surgery* 88:642–653, 1980.

28. Donaldson MC, Mannick JA, Whittemore AD. Femoral-distal bypass with in situ greater saphenous vein. Long-term results using the Mills valvulotome. *Ann Surg* 213:457–465, 1991.

29. Whittemore AD, et al. What is the proper role of polytetrafluoroethylene grafts in infraguinal reconstruction? *J Vasc Surg* 10:299–305, 1989.

30. Kent KC, et al. Femoropopliteal reconstruction for claudication. The risk to life and limb. *Arch Surg* 123:1196–1198, 1988.

31. Taylor LM, Edwards JM, Porter JM. Present status of reversed vein bypass: Five-year results of a modern series. *J Vasc Surg* 11:193–206, 1990.

32. Veith FJ, et al. Six-year prospective multicenter randomized comparison of autogenous saphenous vein and expanded polytetrafluoroethylene grafts in infrainguinal arterial reconstructions. *J Vasc Surg* 3:104–114, 1986.

33. Weibull H, et al. Complications after percutaneous transluminal angioplasty in the iliac, femoral, and popliteal arteries. *J Vasc Surg* 5:681–686, 1987.

34. Hasson JE, et al. Lower extremity percutaneous transluminal angioplasty: Multifactorial analysis of morbidity and mortality. *Surgery* 108:748–754, 1990.

35. Plecha FR, et al. The early results of vascular surgery in patients 75 years of age and older: An analysis of 3259 cases. *J Vasc Surg* 2:769–774, 1985.

36. Raby KE, et al. Detection and significance of intraoperative and postoperative myocardial ischemia in peripheral vascular surgery. *JAMA* 268:222–227, 1992.

37. Fellmeth BD, et al. Postangiographic femoral artery injuries: Nonsurgical repair with US guided compression. *Radiology* 178:671, 1991.

38. Hunink MGM, Cullen KA, Donaldson MC. Hospital costs of revascularization procedures for femoropopliteal arterial disease. *J Vasc Surg* 19:632–41, 1994.

39. Doubilet P, Abrams HL. The cost of underutilization: Percutaneous transluminal angioplasty for peripheral vascular disease. *N Engl J Med* 310:95–102, 1984.

Peripheral Directional Atherectomy

DuckSoo Kim

A properly conducted (Simpson) peripheral directional atherectomy is able to achieve "complete" recanalization without the need for subsequent balloon angioplasty. This modality also can serve as an adjunct to other techniques, which may provide less complete recanalization.

Advantages [1–6]

1. Removal of plaque, without the usual elastic recoil that accompanies balloon angioplasty, provides a reliable immediate outcome.
2. Lower dissection rate with a lower risk of acute or subacute occlusion.
3. Smooth luminal surface may lower risk of in situ thrombosis.
4. Reduced need of anticoagulation.
5. More effective for graft stenoses than angioplasty.
6. Lower risk of vessel perforation than angioplasty.
7. Availability of histologic specimen.

Disadvantages [1,2]

1. More expensive than balloon angioplasty.
2. More time-consuming than balloon angioplasty.
3. Larger arteriotomy—more complications, such as hematoma, bleeding, or pseudoaneurysm, at the puncture site.
4. Learning curve is usually longer than for balloon angioplasty.
5. Technical limitations
   a. Due to the stiffness and diameter of the distal catheter (rigid housing)
      (1) Only ipsilateral iliac and femoral approaches are possible.
      (2) Tortuous arteries are difficult to negotiate.
      (3) Arteries with acute take-off are difficult to cannulate, and caution must be exercised when performing atherectomy at the origin of such vessels.
      (4) Large or dilated arteries (> 10 mm) and very small (< 2 mm) distal vessels cannot be treated.
   b. Extremely calcified lesions are difficult to treat.

Indications

BASED ON CLINICAL PRESENTATION [1–6]

1. Leg claudication or rest pain.
2. Foot ulcer or gangrene.
3. Asymptomatic stenoses of bypass grafts with abnormal

duplex US evaluation of vein bypass grafts (prophylactic recanalization).

BASED ON ANGIOGRAPHIC MORPHOLOGY [1–8]

1. Eccentric, bulky, or ulcerated stenoses.
2. Short occlusions (usually < 5 cm).
3. Lesions unresponsive to balloon angioplasty.
4. Restenoses following balloon angioplasty.
5. Vein bypass graft stenoses.
6. Balloon angioplasty complicated by excessive dissection, or removal of intimal flap from dissection due to other reasons.
7. Completion of procedure in which another modality provides a pilot track (adjunct procedure).
8. Embologenic atheromas causing "blue toe syndrome."

Contraindications [1,2,6]

1. Long occlusions (> 5 cm).
2. Diffuse stenotic lesions.

Preprocedure Preparation

1. Same as for balloon angioplasty (see Chaps. 6 and 8).
2. **The Simpson directional atherectomy catheter** [1,2,9,10] (Advanced Cardiovascular Systems, Temecula, CA). Consists of a rigid hollow cylindrical housing with a "cutting window" and a rotating cutter that rides coaxially in the housing. This housing is attached to a torquable catheter, which contains the cutter drive-cable. A support balloon is mounted opposite the cutting window.
   a. During atherectomy, balloon inflation presses the cutting window against plaque. The cylindrical cutter shaves plaque that protrudes into the housing through the window and compresses it into the collection chamber at the distal end of the catheter (Fig. 7-1). Perforation during atherectomy is extremely unlikely because of this design, since the cutter blade remains within the housing and travels parallel to the vascular wall.
   b. The catheter has separate ports for balloon inflation and catheter flushing. Inflation of the support balloon to 2–3 atm secures the housing against the vessel wall without dilating the stenosis. The working diameter is determined by the sum of the housing diameter and the inflated support balloon diameter (Table 7-1).
   c. The catheter shaft-housing unit is available in sizes ranging between 6–11 Fr. The cutter housing (10 or 20 mm in length) has a longitudinally oriented aperture, the cutter window, over one-third of its circumference. The cup-shaped cutter blade is attached to a drive cable that traverses the length of the catheter and is attached proximally to the separate motor drive unit. Activation of the motor drive unit rotates the cutter blade at 2000 revolutions per minute. The advancement control lever changes the position of the cutter

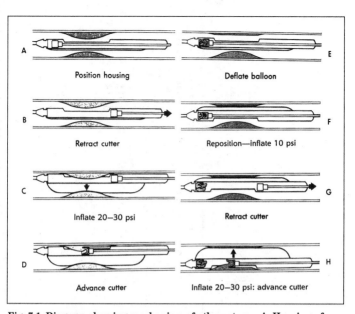

Fig. 7-1. Diagram showing mechanism of atherectomy. A. Housing of catheter in place across lesion. B. Cutter is retracted. C. Inflation of the balloon to 20–30 psi secures the housing against the vessel wall. D. Cutter is advanced with activation of the motor drive unit to cut atheroma. E. Excised tissue is collected in distal chamber and balloon is deflated. F. Housing is repositioned: balloon is inflated with low pressure (10 psi). G. Cutter is retracted. H. Cutter is advanced after inflation of the balloon up to 20–30 psi. (Modified from Devices for Vascular Intervention, Inc., Temecula, CA)

within the housing. The distal end of the housing is connected to a flexible collection chamber with a cone-shaped distal tip for storage of the resected material.

d. The original atherectomy catheter (Atherocath) had an 8 cm long, 0.018-in. fixed guidewire (spring-tip) attached to the distal end (nose-cone) of the collection chamber. Exchangeability of the fixed-guidewire and collection-chamber unit permits the replacement of damaged wires and facilitates removal of resected material. Although the fixed guidewire allows negotiation of severely stenotic segments quite easily, tortuous segments are difficult to negotiate and long lesions are difficult to traverse repeatedly during passes with the Atherocath. The later released over-the-wire atherectomy catheter (Atherotrack) addresses this problem. The 6–9 Fr. Atherotrack catheters contain a hollow channel, 0.014-in. or 0.018-in. in diameter, which allows passage of a guidewire (see Table 7-1). The larger Atherotrack catheters (10 and 11 Fr.) accept a 0.035-in. guidewire. The Atherotrack also has increased balloon size (see Table 7-1) relative to the Ath-

Table 7-1. Directional atherectomy catheter dimensions[1]

Shaft diameter (Fr.)	Housing diameter (mm)/(length [mm])	Inflated balloon diameter (mm)		Maximum working diameter (mm)		Diameter (in.) of movable guidewire (AT only)
		AC	AT	AC	AT	
6	2.0 (10)	*	1.5	*	3.5	0.014
7	2.3 (10)	*	1.7	*	4.0	0.014
7	2.3 (20)	2.5	3.0	4.8	5.3	0.018
8	2.7 (20)	3.0	4.0	5.7	6.7	0.018
9	3.0 (20)	3.0	4.0	6.0	7.0	0.018
10	3.3 (20)	4.0	6.0	7.3	9.3	0.035
11	3.7 (20)	4.0	6.0	7.7	9.7	0.035

AC = Atherocath; AT = Atherotrack.
*6 and 7 Fr. sizes for small vessels are only available with Atherotrack.

erocath which allows larger arteries to be treated with smaller catheters, requiring a smaller arteriotomy.

Procedure [1,2,9,10]

1. Preatherectomy angiography is performed with a reference ruler in place.
2. Confirm that the severity of the stenosis is angiographically or hemodynamically significant (by measurement of pressure gradient across the lesion, if possible).
3. Select a proper size of atherectomy catheter (see Table 7-1). This is critical because undersizing may result in an excessive residual stenosis. Working diameter should be equal to vessel diameter (corrected for magnification) on conventional cut-film angiogram.
4. Retrograde femoral approach is used for iliac lesions. Antegrade femoral approach is used for superficial femoral, popliteal, tibial, and peroneal arteries. Antegrade or retrograde approach with direct puncture of graft is used for bypass grafts. Sometimes, antegrade femoral approach is used for vein bypass grafts.
5. Following placement of an introducer sheath sized to accept the atherectomy catheter, the sidearm of the sheath is connected to a constant infusion of heparinized saline flush solution, and a bolus of heparin (5000–10,000 units) is administered intraarterially. Contrast media may be injected through the sheath sidearm during the procedure.
6. The atherectomy catheter is passed through the sheath and advanced to a point proximal to the obstructing lesion. Simple lesions may be crossed primarily with the fixed guidewire Atherocath, preferably under the guidance of digital road-mapping. The tip-guard provided with the set should be used to protect the fixed guidewire during passage through the hemostasis valve of the introducer sheath. When the over-the-wire system (Atherotrack) is used, the lesion should be crossed primarily with the guidewire. The Atherotrack can then be advanced over the guidewire and positioned at the level of the lesion. In cases of resistant lesions, initial passage of a straight catheter smaller than the atherectomy catheter shaft will allow subsequent passage of the device.
7. Once at the lesion, the cutting window is positioned tangential to the largest plaque volume and fluoroscopy is performed from the projection that best demonstrates the lesion.
8. The balloon is inflated to under 1 atm (approximately 10 psi) while the cutter blade is retracted proximally (see Fig. 7-1).
9. The balloon is then inflated to a maximum pressure of 2 atm (about 30 psi), the motor drive is turned on, and the cutter is advanced slowly along the course of the housing window, pushing the resected material into the collection chamber (see Fig. 7-1). The actual cutting may be detected by slowing of the motor and a tactile sensation.
10. The balloon is deflated and the cutter is retracted for another pass in the same position or following 30–45-degree

rotation (in a direction which keeps the collection chamber [nose-cone] from potentially unscrewing within the artery). These steps are continued until the collection chamber is full. This can be detected fluoroscopically as the point at which the cutter advancement is limited to the distal border of the housing aperture. Additional resection will overflow the chamber and risk distal embolization.

11. The catheter is removed and the collection chamber emptied.
12. Specimens are placed in formalin for subsequent histopathologic examination.
13. When the Atherotrack is used, the guidewire should be left across the lesion between passes, and the distal artery should be flushed intermittently with heparinized saline, as with balloon angioplasty.
14. The procedure is repeated until the desired angiographic endpoint (the least residual stenosis possible) is achieved.
15. The mean number of cutter passes required to adequately treat a focal stenosis is 6.7 [11]. The extended collection chamber can store up to 20 resected samples, enough for about 3 average focal stenoses.
16. Occluded segments should be initially treated by local thrombolytic therapy to uncover the underlying stenosis(es). Short (1–2 cm) occlusions may be crossed and treated primarily with the Atherotrack system.

Postprocedure Management [1,2,12]

1. Essentially the same as for balloon angioplasty.
2. The smooth, stable postatherectomy appearance of the luminal surface appears to justify reversal of heparinization and sheath removal at the end of the procedure [12], except for cases with long occlusions, for which anticoagulation should be continued for 48 hours.
3. Long-term antiplatelet medication should be administered just as following balloon angioplasty.

Results [1,2,6,9–19]

1. Initial technical success rate: 84–100%. The most common cause of failure is the use of an undersized device; this occurs most frequently in the common iliac artery. Most of these lesions can subsequently be successfully treated by balloon angioplasty [12,16].
2. Patency (results vary by lesion site, patient population, and operator experience): at 6 month, 45–99%; at 12 month, 69–92%; and at 24 month, 37–84%. The best results in the femoral-popliteal region are comparable to balloon angioplasty, albeit at considerably more cost per device. However, directional atherectomy may be more effective than angioplasty for vein bypass graft (anastomotic) stenoses. For cumulative long-term patency rates, see Table 7-2.
3. Higher restenosis rates are noted with improper debulking of plaque (> 10% residual stenosis). Restenosis rates are higher in diabetic than in nondiabetic patients.

Table 7-2. Peripheral directional atherectomy: cumulative patency [14]

	1 yr (%)	2 yr (%)	3 yr (%)	4 yr (%)	5 yr (%)
Iliac	90	90	75	—	—
Femoral-popliteal, tibial	88	80	65	52	52
Vein grafts	87	87	87	87	—

Table 7-3. Complications of peripheral directional atherectomy

Overall incidence of complications	3–21%
Death	0–1%
Acute occlusion of vessel	0–3%
Dissection	0–1%
Distal embolization	0–3%
Clinically significant emboli	0–1%
Vessel perforation	0%
Pseudoaneurysms at atherectomy site	0–1%
Pseudoaneurysms at puncture site	0–3%
Hematomas at puncture site	< 13%

4. In comparison with balloon angioplasty, lower major (e.g., dissection, abrupt occlusion) complication rates, but higher minor (e.g., groin hematomas) complication rates are reported.

Complications [1,2,6,9–16,17]

See Table 7-3.

References

1. Kim D, Orron DE. *Peripheral Vascular Imaging and Intervention.* St. Louis: Mosby–Year Book, 1992.
2. Kim D, et al. Peripheral directional atherectomy: 4-year experience. *Radiology* 183:773–778, 1992.
3. Barbano EF, et al. Correlation of clinical history with quantitative histology of lower extremity atheroma biopsies obtained with the Simpson atherectomy catheter. *Atherosclerosis* 78:183–196, 1989.
4. Dolmatch BL, et al. Blue toe syndrome: Treatment with percutaneous atherectomy. *Radiology* 172:799–804, 1989.
5. Maynar M, et al. Use of safety wire in atherectomy procedure for recanalization of complete arterial occlusions. *Semin Intervent Radiol* 5:256–259, 1988.
6. Graor RA, Whitlow PL. Transluminal atherectomy for occlusive peripheral vascular disease. *J Am Coll Cardiol* 15:1551–1558, 1990.
7. Maynar M, et al. Percutaneous atherectomy as an alternative treatment for postangioplasty obstructive intimal flaps. *Radiology* 170:1029–1031, 1989.

8. Breall JA, et al. Atherectomy of the subclavian artery for patients with symptomatic coronary-subclavian steal syndrome. *J Am Coll Cardiol* 21:1564–1567, 1993.

9. Simpson JB, et al. Transluminal atherectomy: A new approach to the treatment of atherosclerotic vascular disease. *Circulation* 72 (Suppl III):146, 1985.

10. Simpson JB, et al. Transluminal atherectomy for occlusive peripheral vascular disease. *Am J Cardiol* 61:96G–101G, 1988.

11. von Polnitz A, et al. Percutaneous peripheral atherectomy: angiographic and clinical follow-up of 60 patients. *J Am Coll Cardiol* 15:682–688, 1990.

12. Kim D, et al. Peripheral directional atherectomy: Five-year experience (abstract no. 1318). Presented at the Radiological Society of North America 79th Annual Meeting, Dec. 3, 1993; Chicago, IL.

13. Dorros G, et al. The acute outcome of atherectomy in peripheral arterial obstructive disease. *J Am Coll Cardiol* 13:102–108A, 1989.

14. Schwarten DE, et al. Simpson catheter for percutaneous transluminal removal of atheroma. *AJR* 150:799–801, 1988.

15. Hofling B, et al. Percutaneous removal of atheromatous plaques in peripheral arteries. *Lancet* 1:384–386, 1988.

16. McLean GK. Percutaneous peripheral atherectomy. *J Vasc Intervent Radiol* 4:465–480, 1993.

17. Katzen BT, et al. Long-term follow-up of directional atherectomy in the femoral and popliteal arteries. *J Vasc Intervent Radiol* 3:38–39, 1992. Abstract.

18. Maquin PR, et al. Peripheral atherectomy with the Simpson catheter: Midterm results. *Radiology* 181:294, 1991. Abstract.

19. Dorros G, et al. Percutaneous atherectomy for occlusive peripheral vascular disease: Stenoses and occlusions. *Cathet Cardiovasc Diagn* 18:1–6, 1989.

Renal Artery Balloon Angioplasty

Krishna Kandarpa
John E. Aruny

Percutaneous transluminal angioplasty of renal artery (PTRA) stenoses is indicated in the treatment of two major categories of renal disease that frequently coexist but may be present independently of each other: renovascular hypertension (for blood pressure control) and renal insufficiency (for salvage of renal function).

Renovascular Hypertension

Renovascular hypertension (RVH), which accounts for about 5% of all hypertensive patients [1,2], is usually due to atherosclerosis (75% of patients with RVH) or fibromuscular dysplasia in the renal artery. The diagnosis of RVH is often made retrospectively, based on improvement or cure of hypertension following either surgical revascularization or PTRA. The presence of a renal artery stenosis does not necessarily mean that it is the cause of hypertension. Patients with essential hypertension or other renal disease affecting the small vessels may develop main or large branch renal artery stenoses as part of a generalized atherosclerotic process. PTRA is not likely to achieve success in treating hypertension in the latter setting.

Indications [3–9]

Angiographically documented **renal artery stenosis** (RAS) or occlusion and a history of sustained **high BP** (140/95) in the setting of:
1. Failed medical therapy that is considered to have been optimized.
2. Multiple antihypertensive agents required to control BP (with an aim towards reducing, if not eliminating, the number of medications needed).
3. A positive radionuclide renogram with angiotensin-converting enzyme (captopril or enalaprilat [Vasotec]) challenge (see Chap. 27).
4. Renal vein renin secretion that lateralizes to one side with associated supression of renin secretion from the uninvolved side (see Renal Vein Renin Sampling).
5. A systolic pressure gradient of > 10 mm Hg measured across a segment of renal artery with a questionable stenosis. Areas of weblike stenosis that appear noncritical on angiography but have a significant systolic pressure gradient occur more often with fibromuscular dysplasia than with atherosclerosis.

Renal Insufficiency

Renal insufficiency may result from nephrosclerosis secondary to renal artery stenoses or occlusions. PTRA is indicated in order to either reverse the process or to prevent further decline of renal function secondary to impaired blood flow.

Indications [4–14]

Angiographically documented **RAS** or occlusion and **deteriorating renal function** or stable renal insufficiency while on ideal medical management with:

1. More than 50% renal artery diameter stenosis, or a measured systolic pressure gradient greater than 10 mm Hg across a stenosis that is difficult to grade visually. (Some investigators consider a systolic pressure gradient to be significant if it is equal to or greater than 15% of the aortic systolic pressure [8].)
2. Asymmetric loss of renal mass as demonstrated on serial imaging examinations. A long-axis kidney length of 8 cm is considered by some to be the lower limit at which function is likely to be retrieved [12,13].

Renovascular Hypertension, or Azotemia, or Both

Indications [4–16]

1. **Renal transplant arterial stenosis.** The location of these stenoses will occur at points of external compression from peritransplant fibrosis or more commonly at kink points that cause arterial injury when the transplant renal artery is anastomosed in an end-to-end fashion with the internal iliac artery. These lesions now appear to be less prevalent when the kinks are avoided by an end-to-side anastomosis of the transplant renal artery to the external iliac artery.
2. **Renal artery saphenous vein bypass graft stenosis.** These lesions occur most often at the points of anastomosis in a fashion similar to arterialized vein grafts in the arterial circulation. When angiography is indicated, the proximal and distal anastomosis must be thoroughly examined in multiple projections to clearly identify stenoses that may be difficult to demonstrate.
3. **Unexplained pulmonary edema.** These patients with renovascular hypertension and/or azotemia, and frequently severe coronary artery disease, have severe bilateral RAS rendering their kidney unable to excrete sodium and water [16].

Contraindications to renal angioplasty [4–16]

ABSOLUTE

1. Medically unstable patient.
2. Hemodynamically insignificant stenosis. Measurement of

the systolic pressure gradient across the stenosis is recommended when a lesion appears angiographically insignificant.

RELATIVE

1. Long-segment total occlusion.
2. Aortic atherosclerotic plaque extending into the renal artery (ostial lesion). Some workers [8] recommend an initial attempt at angioplasty, instead of directly going to surgery, because some (perhaps 25% of cases) of these apparently ostial lesions are actually renal artery-origin stenoses.
3. Severely diseased aorta—predisposing to increased risk of embolization of atheroma.
4. Contemplated surgical aortic replacement that may provide an opportunity for endarterectomy and/or reimplantation of the renal artery(ies).

Preprocedure Preparation

1. Discontinue long-acting antihypertensive medications prior to procedure; manage blood pressure with short-acting drugs as necessary (in consultation with referring physician).
2. Aspirin 325 mg PO qd (or dipyridamole 75 mg PO bid, optional), start 1 day prior to angioplasty (in consultation with referring physician).
3. Standard preangiography preparation (see Chap. 1).
4. Check prior studies (intravenous pyelogram, renal vein renin assays, radionuclide studies, angiograms). Alert your special chemistry laboratory if you wish to draw renal vein renins.
5. **Proteinuria, poorly controlled diabetes,** or serum Cr greater than 1.75 mg/dl: Nifedipine 20 mg PO 2 hours prior to procedure, and 25 g of mannitol in 1 liter of normal saline given IV at 500 ml/hour starting just before angioplasty [17].

Procedure (Fig. 8-1)

1. Standard Seldinger access to the right (preferred) common femoral artery. Place an arterial sheath (with a sidearm for flushing). Patients who have significant iliofemoral atherosclerosis have a higher chance of distal cholesterol embolization. In this case, use a long (20–30 cm) arterial sheath to minimize disruption of plaque during catheter exchanges and manipulations.
2. Document the grade and length of the stenosis with cut-film angiogram or intraarterial digital subtraction angiogram (DSA). When patients have bilateral significant stenoses, attempt angioplasty on the side with the larger kidney first (usually also technically easier since disease tends to be less severe); if this goes well, and if the patient can tolerate a prolonged procedure, attempt the other side.
3. Systolic pressure gradient across stenosis. This is usually not necessary; if an incidental stenosis of unclear significance is found in a hypertensive patient and renal vein

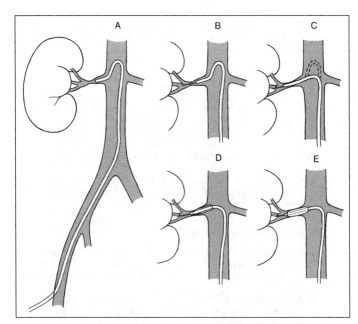

Fig. 8-1. Technique of renal angioplasty using shepherd's crook catheter.
After selection of an appropriate renal artery (A), a flexible-tip guidewire
is advanced through the lesion under fluoroscopic control (B). The
catheter is advanced across the stenosis by withdrawing the catheter at
the puncture site (C). The guidewire is then exchanged for a heavy-duty
tight J-wire (D), and an appropriate balloon catheter is inserted to dilate
lesion (E). (Redrawn from CJ Tegtmeyer, JB Selby. Percutaneous
Transluminal Angioplasty of the Renal Arteries. In WP Castañeda-Zúñiga
and TM Tadavarthy (eds.), *Interventional Radiology*, vol. 2 (2nd ed.).
Baltimore: Williams & Wilkins, 1992. P. 370.)

renins are not available or useful, then systolic pressure
gradients may be helpful.
4. Choice of balloon catheter system [17,18,19]
   a. Choose a **balloon diameter** equal to that of a nonstenotic segment of the vessel on a cut-film angiogram.
   (It has been recommended that the balloon be 1 mm
   greater than the nonstenotic segment [5] in vessels 4
   mm or greater in diameter. By making measurements
   on the cut-film, one automatically oversizes the required balloon dimension because of the intrinsic magnification on the film. Such oversizing may be too much
   for smaller vessels; a more accurate measurement
   should be made.)
   b. Older, **preshaped** 7 Fr. Simmons or Cobra catheters
   (purportedly to ease placement into renal arteries) with
   nontapered balloons are available. However, recent improvement in catheter design, such as **lower profile
   balloons** and 5 Fr. or **smaller shaft sizes,** have made
   these older, relatively poorly torquable balloon cathe-

ters less important to the armamentarium available for crossing even very tight stenoses.

c. **Guiding catheters** (7–9 Fr.) provide support and better seating within the ostium when using a **coaxial technique.** They have a blunt distal end, which minimizes arterial trauma, but are stiff and must be introduced through a larger arterial sheath. Additionally, the usable balloon size is limited to a maximum of 6 mm. However, the additional support provided can be helpful while negotiating very tight stenoses, which can be crossed with a wire but not the balloon. For example, with the guiding catheter seated in the renal ostium, a small vessel balloon (< 4 Fr. shaft) loaded with a high-torque floppy guidewire ($\leq$ 0.018 in.) can be negotiated across the stenosis, which can then be dilated in order to accommodate a bigger balloon. An open-ended guidewire (0.038-in. outer diameter) can be advanced over the 0.018-in. wire to provide support for the introduction of a 5 Fr. balloon catheter with the desired balloon diameter.

d. **Balloon-on-a-wire.** A balloon is mounted directly on a 0.035-in. wire. It can be passed coaxially through a standard catheter and then across a stenosis. This also is useful when angioplasty is performed in renal artery branch vessels. This system is not made to negotiate severe bends or tortuosity and performs best when the curves are relatively gentle.

5. Dilatation (see also Fig. 8-1; Chap. 6).

a. When ready to proceed with the angioplasty, administer 100–200 μg IA nitroglycerin through the diagnostic catheter, which should be engaged in the proximal renal artery. Oral nifedipine 10 mg given 1–2 hours or 10 mg sublingual nifedipine given 10–15 minutes before angioplasty may be useful in preventing **vasospasm.**

b. Using the "road-map" digital subtraction option on modern digital angiography/fluoroscopy machines facilitates cannulation and manipulation through a stenosis. Additionally, intraluminal position of the distal tip of the wire is also more easily confirmed.

c. Cross the lesion with a high-torque flexible-tip guidewire (0.035 in.) or a steerable tapered guidewire (0.018–0.035-in. TAD wire, Advanced Cardiovascular Systems, Temecula, CA). Alternatively, a torquable 0.014–0.018-in. wire can be used to cross the lesion and an open-ended wire can subsequently be passed over the smaller wire in order to provide support for advancing a catheter.

   If the wire advances with difficulty or the tip curves and is unable to be straightened, then stop all wire manipulations. Reassess the situation to determine if the wire has passed subintimally. If severe dissection or perforation has occurred, the procedure may have to be postponed for several days. If the renal artery has a caudal angulation and the stenosis is difficult to cross from below, consider using a better supporting catheter system (e.g., Simmons catheter, Cook,

Inc. Bloomington, IN; SOS-Omni catheter, Angiodynamics, Glens Falls, NY; or, on occasion, a renal guid-
ing-catheter system, Schneider USA, Inc., Minneapolis, MN) or a different approach to the lesion (e.g., low
axillary or high brachial artery, which should be needed
only on rare occasion).

d. Administer 5000 units IV heparin (70 units/kg) after
the wire has crossed the stenosis.

e. Advance the diagnostic catheter into the renal artery
across the stenosis. After the initial catheter has
crossed the stenosis, exchange one of the above wire
systems for a more rigid wire such as a 0.035-in. or
0.038-in. Rosen-exchange length wire.

f. Exchange the diagnostic catheter for the balloon catheter. Prevent motion of the distal wire tip by firmly
fixing it, otherwise spasm may be provoked in the distal
smaller vessels. Place balloon markers across lesion.

g. Inflate the balloon to specified pressure (4–10 atm for
high-pressure balloon) for 30–60 seconds × 3 (mechanical advantage of the balloon is about 2–6 times
greater).

h. Deflate the balloon immediately and completely to
avoid thrombus formation on balloon surface and possible vessel occlusion.

i. It is generally best to avoid recrossing the site of angioplasty after the vessel has been dilated. Therefore,
before retracting the balloon proximal to the stenosis,
if a "check" angiogram is to be performed or if a post-
PTA pressure gradient is to be measured, exchange the
above wire for a smaller diameter (0.025-in.) wire using
a proximal Y-connector.

j. Retract the balloon catheter over this wire.

k. Repeat angiogram (IA DSA is helpful) to check the
morphologic result. This angiogram is performed
through the balloon catheter (and is usually of suboptimal quality). If the result is thought to be acceptable,
remove the catheter and wire and insert a pigtail catheter to obtain a completion angiogram. Alternatively,
the wire can be left across the stenosis and a pigtail
catheter placed through a second puncture in the opposite femoral artery can be used to obtain the post-PTA
angiogram. A postangioplasty cleft is often seen, and
usually resolves in about 3 months [6].

l. If the angiographic result and post-PTA pressure gradient are acceptable, the procedure is terminated; otherwise, the balloon is reintroduced to the stenotic segment over the wire and the angioplasty is repeated
until satisfactory results are obtained.

m. Remember that if PTRA has failed or if the patient is to
undergo surgical revascularization without attempted
angioplasty, then the angiographer should demonstrate the vessels most likely to be used in the reconstruction. A good quality angiogram of the celiac axis
will demonstrate the splenic artery that can be used
to revascularize the left kidney [20], and the hepatic

and gastroduodenal arteries that have been used to reconstruct the right renal circulation [21,22].

n. While removing the balloon catheter from the artery, apply suction to the balloon and rotate the catheter in the direction in which the balloon wings tend to collapse; some manufacturers discourage application of suction to balloons made of polyethylene because this may actually worsen winging—consult package insert. The use of arterial sheath should prevent puncture-site trauma, but similar care must be exercised in retracting the balloon into the sheath.

Postprocedure Management

1. Monitor blood pressure for 24–48 hours [5].

    a. If initially high, then falling, and if blood pressure continues to drop below normal levels, administer normal saline by IV infusion.

    b. If increasing during or after procedure, consider captopril [5] (angiotensin-converting enzyme inhibitor) or short-acting medication (if BP > 100 mm Hg).

2. All patients are started on IV continuous drip heparin after the arterial sheath has been removed. Heparin is continued for 24 hours following the procedure.

3. Standard postangiography management also must be followed.

4. Continue aspirin 325 mg PO (and dipyridamole 75 mg PO bid, optional) for up to 6 months [4], in consultation with the referring clinician.

5. Follow BP response and renal function at frequent intervals initially. Most recurrences of hypertension tend to occur within 8 months [4].

Results

INITIAL

1. Initial **technical** success rate: 80–90% [4–8, 23].

2. Immediate **therapeutic** success rate

    a. Hypertension (favorable BP response as percentage of technical successes)

        (1) Fibromuscular dysplasia: 90–100% [4,5,7,8,15].

        (2) Atherosclerosis: 80% (success rates are much lower with true osteal lesions) [4,5,7,8].

        (3) Transplant renal artery: 70–100% [4,6].

    b. Azotemia (sustained decrease in Cr as percentage of technical success, which was noted in 82% of patients [14]) in setting of severe atherosclerosis: 58% [14].

3. Redilatation. In one study [4], about 13% of stenoses needed redilatation. Technical success was about 90%. The most important factor determining recurrence was a post-angioplasty residual diameter stenosis of 30% or greater.

LONG-TERM RESULTS (Table 8-1)

The criteria of the Cooperative Study of Renovascular Hypertension [24,25] as used to evaluate the results of PTRA are

Table 8-1. Long-term results for blood pressure response (as a percentage of patients with initial therapeutic success)

Study	Mean follow-up (months)	Fibromuscular dysplasia (%)			Atherosclerosis (%)			Comment
		C	I	F	C	I	F	
Sos et al. [5,14]	16	60	33	7	27	60	13	FD, n = 31; Ath., n = 20
Tegtmeyer et al. [4,15,19]	39	41	57	2	25	55	20	FD, n = 66; Ath., n = 65[a,b]
Miller et al. [8]	6	85	15	0	25	58	17	FD, n = 13; Ath., n = 12 Excluding ostial lesions
Cohn et al. [7]	16	—	—	—	17	30	53	Unilateral lesions
Kulhman et al. [9]	22	50	32	18	38	41	21	—
Average (%)	20	59	34	7	26	49	25	

C = cured; I = improved; F = failed by Cooperative Study of Renovascular Hypertension Criteria [25]; FD = fibromuscular dysplasia; Ath. = atherosclerosis.
[a]Tegtmeyer et al. [4] also have reported results in renal transplant recipients (up to 25% of them may develop renal artery stenoses [6]): cured, 0%; improved, 71%; failed, 29%.
[b]When the indication for angioplasty is renal failure, approximately 50% of patients show sustained improvement in renal function [4].
Note: Results of surgery are provided for comparison: overall—cured, 51%; improved, 15%; failed, 34% [17]. Later, Miller et al. [8] reported (at 6-month follow-up) surgical cures of 50% for atherosclerosis, 44% for ostial or mixed atherosclerotic lesions, and 100% for fibromuscular dysplasia.

Cured	Diastolic BP of 90 mm Hg or less without medication and decrease of at least 10 mm Hg in diastolic pressure
Improved	Diastolic BP between 90 and 110 mm Hg, with at least a 15% decrease
Failure	Diastolic BP greater than 90 mm Hg, or less than a 15% drop in a diastolic pressure of greater than 110 mm Hg

Complications

1. **Overall** incidence of complications: 13% [4,5,8,17,23].
2. Incidence of **major** complications (i.e., those requiring surgical intervention or having an altered hospital course): 3–11% [4,5,8,23] versus 20% for surgical bypass [8].
3. **Thirty-day mortality**: less than 1% [4,5,8,17,23]. Previously reported surgical mortality was 5.9% [10]; more recently, surgical mortality is reported as 0–5.4% [26,27].
4. **Angioplasty-site** complications
   a. Local thrombus: 1% [4,23].
   b. Angioplasty-related nonocclusive dissection: 2–4% [5,23]. When necessary, most of these patients have successful surgical bypass [5].
   c. Arterial rupture: 1–2% [4,23].
   d. Peripheral renal embolus: 2% [23].
   e. Guidewire-related dissection: 4% [23].
5. **Angioplasty-related** complications
   a. **Renal failure.** Acute renal failure or acute exacerbation of chronic renal failure: 1.5–6.0% [4,5,8,23]. Approximately 1% may go onto chronic dialysis [23].
   b. **Nephrectomy**: 1% [5] versus 15% for surgical bypass [8].
   c. Segmental **renal infarction** and **perinephric hematoma** without treatment or sequelae: 3% [8]. All patients were therapeutic successes.
6. Other complications
   a. Emboli to extremities: 1.5–2.0% [4,8].
   b. Cholesterol microemboli: 1% [14].
   c. Puncture-site trauma requiring surgery: 1–3% [5,17].
   d. Myocardial infarction: 1% [14].
7. **Management**
   a. If local thrombus occurs without significant dissection or vessel perforation, a trial of local intraarterial thrombolysis may be useful: 150,000 units of urokinase over 30 minutes, followed by 60,000 units/hour for up to 24 hours. Concomitant IV heparin also should be administered.
   b. If severe arterial rupture occurs, retroperitoneal hemorrhage may be prevented or slowed by retracting the balloon into the proximal renal artery and leaving it dilated until immediate surgery is performed (within 2 hours). Nonsurgical alternatives are available under special clinical circumstances [28].
   c. If the balloon ruptures and no arterial damage can be documented, quickly exchange the catheter for a new one and proceed with angioplasty.

d. Dissections. Angioplasty is always accompanied by a minor dissection that heals within months. Severe-looking nonocclusive angioplasty-related dissections may be managed conservatively [29]. A severe guide-wire-related dissection should call a halt to the procedure. A reattempt should be postponed by 1–2 weeks.

e. Chronic steroid therapy. Extra caution is urged when contemplating angioplasty in patients on chronic steroid therapy because they appear to be more prone to vessel rupture [30].

Renal Vein Renin Sampling

The usefulness of renal vein renin (RVR) activity to predict which patients will respond to revascularization remains controversial [31–37]. A recent review of 143 consecutive patients of whom 20 had renovascular hypertension (RVH) resulted in a sensitivity of 65%, a positive predictive value of 18.6%, and a negative predictive value of 89.3%. The authors concluded that the results were neither sensitive nor specific enough to exclude patients who do not have RVH [32]. Another study [33] of elderly patients (mean age of 60 years) found a very low specificity (21%) and negative predictive value (16%) of RVR analysis, limiting its use in this population. This same study also found that performing angioplasty without prior RVR analysis did not significantly affect clinical outcome.

However, RVR secretion that lateralizes to the affected side still carries a significant positive predictive value for curable hypertension and can influence decisions in the planning of revascularization.

Indications

1. To determine which patients with RVH may benefit from revascularization by either angioplasty or surgery.
2. To determine the physiologic significance of an angiographically proven renal artery stenosis that is difficult to grade.

Contraindications

1. Patients who are not candidates for revascularization will not benefit from selective RVR determination.
2. Lack of adequate access to the renal veins or inferior vena cava (IVC) (e.g., renal, caval, or bilateral iliofemoral vein occlusion, IVC filters placed both above and below the renal veins, or combinations thereof).

Preprocedure Preparation

1. Same as for renal angiography (see Chaps. 1 and 32).
2. Patients should ideally be off all antihypertensive medications for 2 weeks prior to sampling. (This is seldom achieved unless patients are hospitalized.) However, pa-

tients can usually be taken off of beta blockers and angiotensin-converting enzyme (ACE) inhibitors for several days prior to renin determination. The predictive value of RVR sampling is poor when plasma renin is stimulated by chronic administration of ACE inhibitors.

3. Captopril (1 mg/kg of body weight) administered 60–90 minutes before selective renal vein blood sampling appears to increase the diagnostic accuracy of renal vein catheterization by increasing the difference between the amount of plasma renin secreted by the two kidneys in cases of unilateral renal artery lesions [34]. Captopril stimulation [34] and sodium depletion [35], which may enhance the sensitivity of lateralization prior to renin sampling, may be useful.

Procedure

1. **Sterile technique.** Access with single-wall needle to avoid inadvertent puncture of the artery anterior to the vein and creation of an arteriovenous fistula.
2. **Selective catheterization**
   a. 6.5 Fr. Cobra 2 with a sidehole made in the distal tip approximately 2–3 mm from the end hole. If this catheter cannot be advanced into the renal vein to obtain adequate samples, then
   b. A 6 Fr. straight catheter may be directed into the renal vein with a tip-deflector wire.
3. The catheter must be advanced beyond the orifice of the left gonadal vein that empties most commonly into the proximal to middle-third of the left renal vein. The right renal vein can be sampled closer to the cava since the right gonadal vein enters directly into the IVC.
4. Catheterize the veins without the use of contrast, which affects the production of renin. Obtain an image with the catheter in each renal vein to document position. Search the IVC throughout its entire length to determine the location of the hepatic veins and the possibility of multiple renal veins or anatomic anomalies.
5. Obtain samples from the infrarenal IVC and the suprarenal IVC below the origin of the hepatic veins. Draw off at least 5 ml of blood into a syringe to be discarded before attaching the sample syringe.
6. Samples should be obtained as quickly and closely together as possible (within 20 minutes). Samples must be sent on ice to the laboratory for processing. Check with your own special chemistry laboratory as to how they wish to handle the samples.

Interpretation of Results

Results are commonly interpreted in one of two ways [3]:

1. **Simple ratio method.** The ratio of the RVR activity on the involved side divided by the activity in the other kidney. Many "thresholds" have been proposed but 1.5 : 1.0 is the ratio that most investigators regard as being positive (sensitivity 62%; specificity 60% [31]).

2. Incremental ratio method. Proposed by Vaughn [36] because of the poor performance of the simple ratio method:

$(V - A)/A$

where

V = right or left RVR activity
A = infrarenal IVC renin activity

A is the arterial renin activity, which is equal to the infrarenal IVC renin activity. An abnormally increased RVR content relative to arterial renin from the suspect kidney (step-up) can be used to reflect the degree of renal ischemia, if there is associated supression of renin secretion from the contralateral uninvolved kidney.

A ratio of greater than 0.48 that lateralizes to one side and has associated contralateral RVR activity supression is considered a positive result for the presence of renin secretion from an ischemic kidney and may have prognostic implications about the curability of the hypertension with surgical revascularization [32] and successful balloon angioplasty [31].

Pitfalls in RVR Sampling

1. Patient on chronic ACE inhibitors or beta blockers, and unable to safely be taken off medication for any period of time have RVRs with poor predictive values.
2. Failure to identify multiple renal veins or venous anatomic variants. Segmental renal artery stenoses may produce renin step-up in segmental veins and not be detected when main renal vein blood samples are obtained.
3. Samples obtained from the left renal vein proximal to the inflow from the left gonadal vein or samples inadvertently obtained from a low hepatic vein.
4. Failure to handle blood samples in an appropriate fashion, including delay in transporting samples to the laboratory for processing.

References

1. Berglund G, Anderson O, Wilhelmsen L. Prevalence of primary and secondary hypertension: Studies in a random population sample. *Br Med J* 2:554–556, 1976.
2. Lewin A, et al. Apparent prevalence of curable hypertension in the hypertension detection and follow-up program. *Arch Int Med* 145:424–427, 1985.
3. Pickering TG. Diagnosis and evaluation of renovascular hypertension: Indications for therapy. *Circulation* 83(Suppl I):I-147–I-154, 1991.
4. Tegtmeyer CJ, Kellum CD, Ayers A. Percutaneous transluminal angioplasty of renal arteries: Results and long-term follow-up. *Radiology* 153:77–84, 1984.
5. Sos TA, et al. Percutaneous transluminal renal angioplasty for renovascular hypertension due to atherosclerosis and fibromuscular dysplasia. *N Engl J Med* 309:274–279, 1983.

6. Gerlock AJ, et al. Renal transplant arterial stenosis: Percutaneous transluminal angioplasty. *AJR* 140:325–331, 1983.
7. Cohn DJ, et al. Transluminal angioplasty for atherosclerotic renal artery stenosis. *Semin Intervent Radiol* 1:279–287, 1984.
8. Miller GA, et al: Percutaneous transluminal angioplasty vs. surgery for renovascular hypertension. *AJR* 144:447–450, 1985.
9. Kuhlman U, et al. Long-term experience in percutaneous transluminal dilatation of renal artery stenosis. *Am J Med* 79:692–698, 1985.
10. Martin LG, Casarella WJ, Gaylord GM. Azotemia caused by renal artery stenosis: Treatment by percutaneous angioplasty. *AJR* 150:839–844, 1988.
11. Pickering TG, et al. Renal angioplasty in patients with azotemia and renovascular hypertension. *J Hypertension* 4:S667-S669, 1986.
12. Hallett JW, et al. Renovascular operations in patients with chronic renal insufficiency: Do the benefits justify the risks? *J Vasc Surg* 5:622–627, 1987.
13. Lawrie GM, Morris GC, DeBakey ME. Long-term results of treatment of the totally occluded renal artery in 40 patients with renovascular hypertension. *Surgery* 88:753–759, 1980.
14. Sos TA. Angioplasty for the treatment of azotemia and renovascular hypertension in atherosclerotic renal artery disease. *Circulation* 83(Suppl I):I-162–I-166, 1991.
15. Tegtmeyer CJ, et al. Results and complications of angioplasty in fibromuscular disease. *Circulation* 83(Suppl I):I-155–I-161, 1991.
16. Pickering TG, et al. Recurrent pulmonary edema in hypertension due to bilateral renal artery stenosis: Treatment by angioplasty or surgical revascularization. *Lancet* 9:551–552, 1988.
17. Martin LG. Angioplasty of Renal Artery Stenosis. In S Kadir (ed.), *Current Practice of Interventional Radiology* Philadelphia: B C Decker, 1991. Pp. 605–611.
18. Tegtmeyer CJ, Sos TA. Techniques of renal angioplasty. *Radiology* 161:577–586, 1986.
19. Tegtmeyer CJ, Selby JB. Percutaneous Transluminal Angioplasty of the Renal Arteries. In WR Castañeda-Zúñiga, SM Tadavarthy (eds.), *Interventional Radiology* (2nd ed.). Baltimore: Williams & Wilkins, 1992. Pp. 364–377.
20. Khauli RB, Novick AC, Ziegelbaum M. Splenorenal bypass in the treatment of renal artery stenosis: Experience with sixty-nine cases. *J Vasc Surg* 2:547–551, 1985.
21. Moncure AC, et al. Use of the splenic and hepatic arteries for renal revascularization. *J Vasc Surg* 3:196–203, 1986.
22. Moncure AC, et al. Use of the gastroduodenal artery in right renal artery revascularization. *J Vasc Surg* 8:154–159, 1988.
23. Gardiner GA Jr, et al. Complications of transluminal angioplasty. *Radiology* 159:201–208, 1986.
24. Simon N, et al. Clinical characteristics of renovascular hypertension. *JAMA* 220:1209–1218, 1972.
25. Maxwell JP, et al. Cooperative study of renovascular hypertension: Demographic analysis of the study. *JAMA* 220:1195, 1972.
26. Stanley JC. Renovascular hypertension: Surgical treatment. *Urol Radiol* 3:205–208, 1981.
27. Novick AC. Management of renovascular disease: A surgical perspective. *Circulation* 83(Suppl I):I-167–I-171, 1991.
28. Dixon GD, Anderson S, Crouch TT. Renal arterial rupture second-

ary to percutaneous transluminal angioplasty treated without surgical intervention. *Cardiovasc Intervent Radiol* 9:83–85, 1986.

29. Gardiner GA Jr, Meyerovitz MF, Harrington DP. Dissection complicating angioplasty. *AJR* 145:627–631, 1985.

30. Lois JF, et al. Vessel rupture by balloon catheters complicating chronic steroid therapy. *AJR* 144:1073–1074, 1985.

31. Pickering TG, et al. Predictive value and changes of renin secretion in hypertensive patients with unilateral renovascular disease undergoing successful renal angioplasty. *Am J Med* 76:398–404, 1984.

32. Roubidoux MA, et al. Renal vein renins: Inability to predict response to revascularization in patients with hypertension. *Radiology* 178:819–822, 1991.

33. Martin LG, Cork RD, Wells JO. Renal vein renin analysis: Limitations of its use in predicting benefit from percutaneous angioplasty. *Cardiovasc Intervent Radiol* 16:76–80, 1993.

34. Thibonnier M, et al. Improved diagnosis of unilateral renal artery lesions after captopril administration. *JAMA* 251:56–60, 1984.

35. Strong CG, et al. Renal venous renin activity: Enhancement of sensitivity of lateralization by sodium depletion. *Am J Cardiol* 27:602–611, 1971.

36. Vaughn ED, et al. Renovascular hypertension: Renin measurements to indicate hypersecretion and contralateral suppression, estimate renal plasma flow, and score for surgical curability. *Am J Med* 55:402–414, 1973.

37. Foster JH, et al. Renovascular occlusive disease: Results of operative treatment. *JAMA* 231:1043–1048, 1975.

Aortoiliac and Renal Artery Stenting

Mohsin Saeed

General Technical Principles of Arterial Stent Deployment

The general principles governing the placement of the Palmaz stent [1] for arterial occlusive disease are outlined. Specific technical and clinical considerations related to the use of these stents for each anatomic location are addressed under the relevant headings. At the present time, the FDA has approved only the Palmaz stent (Johnson & Johnson, Warren, NJ) for use in iliac arteries and the use of other stents remains investigational.

Preprocedure Preparation

Same as for percutaneous transluminal balloon angioplasty (see Chap. 6). Oral aspirin (325 mg) should ideally begin 24–48 hours before the procedure.

Procedure

1. Perform standard diagnostic angiography to evaluate the lesions.
2. Document pressure gradients across the lesion. A resting gradient of > 10 mm Hg, or a gradient > 20 mm Hg after 25 mg of IA tolazoline (Priscoline) is hemodynamically significant.
3. Cross the lesion with a wire and administer an IV heparin bolus of 3000–5000 units, followed by an infusion of 750–1000 units/hour. Target activated clotting time (ACT) should be about 2.5 times baseline.
4. Perform angioplasty with the appropriate balloon (Fig. 9-1a). This will test the lesion's compliance and make room for subsequent devices for stent deployment.
5. Repeat angiography following angioplasty. Do not stent if extravasation of contrast is noted, or if lesion is totally noncompliant. Stenting is also not indicated if there is no residual pressure gradient, or a minimal residual stenosis (< 30%).
6. Use fascial dilators at the femoral puncture site to facilitate the placement of a sheath of appropriate size and length across the lesion.
7. Crimp the Palmaz stent onto appropriate size balloon (see also Tables 21-2 and 21-3 for appropriate stent sizes). Crimping by hand is preferred. Test the stent for a snug fit prior to introducing it into the sheath. Preassembled balloon-mounted stents are now available.

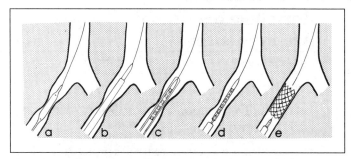

Fig. 9-1. Proper placement of stent. Dilation of stenosis with angioplasty
balloon (a); placement of introducer sheath (b); advancement of mounted
stent in sheath (c); withdrawal of sheath (d); withdrawal of balloon
after expansion of stent (e). (From Palmaz et al. Intraluminal stents in
atherosclerotic iliac artery stenosis: Preliminary report of a multicenter
study. *Radiology* 168:727–731, 1988.)

8. Carefully introduce the balloon-mounted stent across the
   hemostatic valve of the sheath. An appropriate introducer
   (metal sleeve) is used to protect the stent during this maneuver.
9. Keeping the sheath immobile, observe fluoroscopically as
   the stent is advanced through the sheath to the site of the
   lesion. Intermittent contrast injection through the side-
   arm of the sheath aids in positioning the stent. An external
   marker or digital road-mapping also may be useful.
10. After initial stent positioning, hold the stent immobile and
    retract the sheath to uncover approximately half the stent.
    This allows the stent to be safely moved in either direction
    for final adjustment in position (Fig. 9-1b, c).
11. Digital subtraction angiography may be performed
    through the sheath, if necessary.
12. After final stent positioning, retract sheath to completely
    uncover the stent. Confirm sheath position by contrast
    injection (Fig. 9-1d).
13. Using a mechanical inflating device, steadily inflate bal-
    loon under fluoroscopic monitoring until fully expanded
    (requires about 6 atm) and no waist is noted (Fig. 9-1e).
14. Deflate balloon completely, and aspirate with a 20-cc sy-
    ringe, if necessary. Carefully rotate balloon (in a direction
    that will refold the wings) to ensure it is free of stent.
    Retract balloon, keeping wire fixed, and remove through
    sheath.
15. Repeat angiogram, either through sheath or through cath-
    eter advanced over the wire above the stent. Evaluate wall
    contact and any residual stenosis.
16. If necessary, place larger balloon and expand the stent
    further.
17. If additional stent placement is necessary, the sheath must
    be first across the proposed site of stent deployment. If
    the sheath has to be advanced through a deployed stent,
    a sheath introducer must be used. If the stent has to be

crossed with a wire, a 3-mm J-wire must be used to avoid dissecting under the edge of the stent.

18. When stenting in series, approximately 1 mm of stent overlap is advisable. Avoid gaps as well as excessive overlap.

19. After deployment of stents to final desirable diameter, repeat arteriogram, measure pressure gradients across stented segment, and, if necessary, evaluate with intravascular US to detect any deficiency in appropriate wall contact or lack of full stent expansion in any region.

Postprocedure Management

1. Remove femoral sheath when the ACT is under 175. Obtain hemostasis by routine groin compression.

2. Overnight bed rest is advisable to avoid delayed hemorrhage from puncture site.

3. Continue daily aspirin (325 mg PO) indefinitely.

4. Obtain Doppler pulses and ankle brachial indices to document improvement and to establish a baseline for follow-up examination.

5. Encourage physical activity and discourage tobacco use following discharge from the hospital.

Special Clinical and Technical Considerations by Anatomic Location

Iliac Artery Stenting

INDICATIONS [2,3]

The patient selection criteria are similar to those for percutaneous transluminal (balloon) angioplasty (PTA). Stent placement is indicated for

1. Residual stenosis > 30% post-PTA.

2. Residual gradients exceeding 10 mm Hg post-PTA.

3. Dissection as a result of PTA [4].

4. Highly eccentric stenosis.

5. Recurrent stenosis following PTA.

6. Iliac artery occlusions (thrombolysis may or may not precede stent placement) [5,6].

CONTRAINDICATIONS

1. Coexisting aneurysmal disease of the abdominal aorta or iliac arteries necessitating surgical intervention.

2. Successful PTA.

3. Noncompliant vessels.

4. Contrast extravasation (perforation) noted following PTA.

5. Diffuse long-segment disease in small-caliber external iliac arteries.

6. Common femoral artery disease.

TECHNIQUE

The general technical principles of stenting apply. Specific considerations are:
1. Avoid stenting extremely tortuous vessels with rigid Palmaz stents.
2. Do not stent below the inguinal ligament.
3. For disease in the low external iliac location or common femoral artery location, consider endarterectomy.
4. When multiple stents are necessary, deploy them in the cephalocaudal direction.
5. When stenting long-segment iliac disease, it may be necessary to taper stent diameters from above downwards to avoid over-dilatation and abrupt step-off.
6. Generally, in addition to the usual criteria for stenting, stent placement is advisable for all iliac occlusions as well as for stenotic disease exceeding 5 cm in length.

Stenting of the Aortic Bifurcation [7,8]

Stenting of the aortic bifurcation reconstructs the aortic carina by dilating the terminal aorta and both iliac arteries and establishing favorable hemodynamics.

INDICATIONS

1. Lesions affecting the origin of both common iliac arteries.
2. Lesions in the terminal abdominal aorta impinging on iliac artery inlets.
3. Terminal abdominal aortic disease impinging on unilateral iliac origin necessitating high stent placement. This will frequently require a contralateral iliac stent even if no intrinsic disease of the contralateral vessel is present. Bilateral stenting in such a situation will prevent a unilateral stent from obstructing inflow to the contralateral vessel, and minimize turbulent flow.

TECHNIQUE

Again, the general principles of stent deployment apply. Special considerations include the following:
1. Obtain bilateral access from the common femoral arteries.
2. Perform kissing balloon angioplasty at the aortic bifurcation.
3. Position long vascular sheaths from each femoral access into the abdominal aorta.
4. Advance stents mounted on the appropriate size balloons into each vascular sheath and position within the vascular sheaths approximately 5 mm cephalad to the true aortic bifurcation.
5. Retract the sheaths and, after confirmation of stent position, deploy them by simultaneous inflation of balloons.
6. To avoid over-dilating a narrow terminal aorta, one may use a smaller balloon for initial deployment on one side and then switch balloon to achieve equal stent dilatation on each side.

Aortic Stenting [9]

Stents are not currently approved for use in the abdominal aorta. The large-caliber Palmaz iliac artery stents can safely be deployed up to an 18-mm diameter and are therefore applicable to aortic stenotic and occlusive disease.

INDICATIONS

The clinical criteria for patient selection are similar to those for aortic balloon angioplasty.
1. Residual stenosis < 30% following PTA.
2. Residual gradient exceeding 10 mm Hg following PTA.
3. Aortic dissections.
4. Graft anastomotic stenosis.
5. Highly eccentric stenosis.
6. Recurrent lesions following PTA.

CONTRAINDICATIONS

1. Diffuse aortic disease.
2. Extravasation of contrast following PTA.
3. Noncompliant lesions.
4. Diffuse iliac artery disease requiring bypass.
5. Aortic aneurysm requiring surgery.
6. Extreme aortic tortuosity.
7. Threatened occlusion of vital aortic branches.

TECHNIQUE

The basic steps of aortic stenting are similar to iliac artery stenting. However, the following are additional considerations:
1. Use smallest adequate balloon for initial stent deployment, then expand further with larger balloon if needed. This will obviate the need for overly large sheaths in the femoral artery.
2. To facilitate the above requirement, the preliminary PTA may have to be very conservative or be skipped altogether.
3. If multiple stents are to be deployed, they should all first be deployed with the smallest adequate balloon, and final stent expansion should be undertaken after all stents are in place. This again will obviate the need for large vascular sheaths in the femoral artery.
4. For relatively noncompliant lesions, it is not necessary to expand the stents to the full aortic diameter. The smallest hemodynamically adequate diameter should suffice.
5. When stenting across graft anastomotic sites or other annular lesions, care must be taken to achieve the best wall contact possible. This may necessitate the use of different size balloons along the length of the stent.
6. Intravascular ultrasound is advisable to ensure a satisfactory position of the stent, particularly if residual unexplained pressure gradients are encountered.

Results

1. Arterial stenting achieves ideal hemodynamic and angiographic results, virtually eliminating pressure gradients and stenoses.
2. Stents have greatly enhanced the management of long-segment stenoses, and have revolutionized the endovascular treatment of iliac occlusions.
3. Stents are ideally suited for the management of long arterial dissections.
4. Technical success rate is approximately 90–100%.
5. Cumulative 5-year angiographic patency of 94% and clinical success of 93% have been reported with iliac artery stents. This is far superior to the comparable PTA rates of 65% and 70%, respectively [3,10].
6. Stent failure is more likely in long-segment disease, particularly when affecting small-caliber external iliac arteries.
7. Acute thrombosis is exceedingly uncommon, and can usually be attributed to limitation of inflow or outflow.

Complications

Generally, complications from stent placement have been comparable to those encountered in routine PTA. The following complications have been reported; in the aggregate, they account for the total complications reported in most series, with rates between 5–10% [3].

1. Groin hematomas.
2. Pseudoaneurysms.
3. Embolization of atherosclerotic or thrombotic material.
4. Acute stent thrombosis.
5. Dissection.
6. Vessel perforation.
7. Congestive heart failure.

With proper technique and vigilant patient management, complications of vascular stenting can be minimized to make the procedure as safe as routine balloon angioplasty. Occasionally, however, larger vascular sheaths are deployed in stent placement. This necessitates extreme care in prevention of complications from groin punctures.

Renal Artery Stent Placement

Indications [11–19]

The usual criteria for selection of patients for renal artery angioplasty apply (see Chap. 8). Renal artery stenting may be considered for the following specific indications:

1. Stenosis recurring after previous percutaneous transluminal angioplasty of renal artery (PTRA).
2. Ostial renal artery stenosis.
3. Postoperative stenosis (renal artery bypass and transplant renal arteries).
4. Highly eccentric renal artery stenosis.
5. Acute failure of PTRA due to
   a. Vessel recoil with threatened closure.

    b. Complex dissections.
    c. Residual stenosis greater than 30%.
6. Renal artery size 4–8 mm.
7. Disease limited to main stem renal artery.

Contraindications [11–19]

RELATIVE

1. Branch vessel disease.
2. Lesion length exceeding 2 cm.

ABSOLUTE

1. Renal artery size less than 4 mm.
2. Diffuse intrarenal vascular disease.
3. Noncompliant lesion.
4. Kidney size less than 6 cm.
5. Unfavorable renal artery anatomy, not permitting sufficient distal vessel length to allow surgical bypass, if
   needed.
6. Vessel rupture during PTA.

Preprocedure Preparation

1. Modifications in antihypertensive medication regimen
   may be indicated as would be with angioplasty (PTRA).
2. Begin aspirin 325 mg PO daily 24 hours before procedure
   and continue indefinitely following procedure.
3. Begin dipyridamole (Persantine) 75 mg PO starting 24
   hours before procedure and continue for 3 months following procedure.
4. Foley catheter is recommended for bilateral renal artery
   stenting.
5. Sublingual nifedipine (10 mg) may be considered before
   the procedure to prevent spasm.
6. **Equipment suggestions**
   a. Stents. Palmaz endovascular stents with expansion
   range of 4–8 mm. Device length varies from 1–2 cm.
   The nonarticulated stents are preferable for renal artery use (Johnson & Johnson Interventional System,
   Warren, NJ).
   b. Guidewires. Suitable wires include the TAD-1 and
   TAD-2 (Advanced Cardiovascular Systems, Temecula,
   CA), the Platinum Plus 0.018-in. wire (Medi-tech Corp.,
   Watertown, MA), and standard Rosen wire (USCI, Billerica, MA).
   c. Balloon catheters. Any 5 Fr. system of appropriate
   balloon diameter is acceptable for renal angioplasty.
   Balloon length should not exceed 2 cm in general. However, for stent deployment, the Cordis 5 Fr. balloons
   have proved durable in our experience (Opta 5 balloons,
   Cordis Corp., Miami, FL).
   d. Angiographic catheters. Catheters for initial diagnostic angiography and selective renal artery catheterization are chosen by the same criteria as for renal angioplasty.

      e. Guiding catheters. Either an 8 Fr. "hockey stick" renal guiding catheter (Cordis Corp., Miami, FL), or a 6 Fr. long vascular sheath (Daig Corp., Minnetonka, MN) are acceptable.

Procedure

1. Place 6 Fr. vascular sheath in femoral artery.
2. Perform a selective diagnostic angiogram, document the stenosis, and cross it with a wire.
3. Give IV heparin bolus of 3000–5000 units, and infuse 700–1000 units/hour during the procedure to maintain an activated clotting time ACT greater than 200 seconds.
4. Selective intrarenal artery nitroglycerin in 100 μg boluses may be given to counter spasm.
5. Perform a balloon angioplasty using standard techniques. Maintain wire access across the dilated lesion at all times.
6. The rest of the procedure may be done using *either:* (a) an 8 Fr. "hockey stick" renal guiding catheter (0.082-in. or 0.084-in. internal diameter), *or* (b) a long 6 Fr. vascular sheath (40–60 cm)—skip to **b.** below.
   a. If **using an 8 Fr. renal guiding catheter,** proceed as follows. Currently no renal guiding catheters are available with a hemostatic hub, therefore a Y-adapter is needed for hemostasis.
      (1) Dilate the femoral artery track (using fascial dilators) to 8 Fr. size and place an 8 Fr. Terumo sheath (Medi-tech Corp., Watertown, MA). Insert the renal guiding catheter over the wire, using a Y-adapter at the hub. With the guiding catheter tip adjacent to the renal artery, obtain a digital subtraction angiogram (DSA) to document the post-angioplasty result.
      (2) Remove renal guiding catheter, leaving 8 Fr. sheath and guidewire in place.
      (3) With the Y-adapter still attached to the 8 Fr. guiding catheter, preload the appropriate angioplasty balloon catheter through guiding catheter until the balloon shows at the distal end. Crimp the stent onto the balloon and retract balloon carefully into guiding catheter until only the tip of the balloon shows. Tighten hemostatic valve around the balloon catheter shaft.
      (4) Advance the guiding catheter and stented balloon together over a wire through the femoral sheath until guiding catheter is across the renal artery lesion.
      (5) Loosen the hemostatic valve on the Y-connector to allow partial retraction of guiding catheter so that approximately 50% of the stent length is uncovered, keeping balloon catheter immobile.
      (6) Perform a DSA through the guiding catheter. Adjust stent position as necessary.
      (7) Retract guiding catheter to fully uncover the stent.
      (8) After confirming accurate stent position, deploy

the stent by inflating the balloon to between 6 and 8 atm.

(9) Remove balloon catheter and repeat DSA through the guiding catheter.

(10) One may expand the stent to larger diameter if necessary, using a larger balloon. Maximum stent diameter should not exceed the renal artery diameter by more than 10%.

(11) Remove wire and guiding catheter, leaving femoral artery sheath in place.

b. If **using the long 6 Fr. arterial sheath** (instead of the 8 Fr. renal guiding catheter), the first five steps are identical to those in **a.** above. Proceed from thereon as follows:

(1) Replace the original 6 Fr. femoral sheath with long 6 Fr. sheath (Daig Corp., Minnetonka, MN) and advance it adjacent to renal artery orifice, keeping wire in place. Obtain DSA through sheath.

(2) Advance long vascular sheath across the renal artery lesion using the sheath introducer. Remove the introducer.

(3) Hand-crimp stent onto appropriate size angioplasty balloon.

(4) With the stent mounted on the balloon, advance the balloon into the sheath under fluoroscopic guidance so that stent is positioned at the level of the lesion.

(5) Retract the sheath so that approximately 50% of the stent length is uncovered, keeping balloon catheter immobile.

(6) Perform a DSA through the sheath. Adjust stent position as necessary.

(7) Retract the sheath to fully uncover the stent.

(8) After confirming accurate stent position, deploy the stent by inflating the balloon to between 6 and 8 atm.

(9) Remove balloon catheter and repeat DSA through the sheath.

(10) If necessary, expand the stent to larger diameter using a larger balloon. Maximum stent diameter should not exceed the renal artery diameter by more than 10%.

(11) Remove wire, leaving femoral artery sheath in place.

Note: Stents mounted on angioplasty balloons are also available, and the above procedure can be easily modified to allow use of these premounted stents with minor variations in technique.

Postprocedure Management

1. Remove the femoral sheath when ACT is under 170 seconds and obtain puncture site hemostasis.

2. Restart IV heparin 2–4 hours after hemostasis.

3. Continue aspirin 325 mg PO daily for 6 months and dipyridamole (Persantine) 75 mg 3 times a day for 3 months.
4. Start warfarin sodium (Coumadin) on evening of procedure with 10 mg PO initial dose. Adjust subsequent doses to achieve target PT of 16–18 seconds. Continue for 4 weeks.
5. Continue IV heparin until PT is in therapeutic range; this is usually achieved by the third day following the procedure.
6. Adjust antihypertensive medications as necessary.

Results [11–14]

1. Initial technical success approaches 100%.
2. Mean residual stenosis is less than 5%.
3. Improved BP is noted in approximately 75% of patients.
4. Renal function may improve in properly selected patients. Present data are limited.
5. A greater than 15% residual stenosis after initial stent implantation may be a predictor of restenosis.
6. Restenosis at 6 months has been reported in 10–40% of patients undergoing angiographic follow-up. These data are from patients with highly unfavorable lesions, with significant variations in patient characteristics. It appears that prior failed interventions may unfavorably affect the patency rates after stent deployment.
7. Dilatation of restenotic lesions is technically easy. However, the data on long-term outcome is limited.

Complications and Caveats [11–14]

1. In general, the complications associated with balloon angioplasty of renal artery stenoses also may apply to renal artery stenting.
2. Risk of renal failure may be enhanced by the greater contrast volume requirements. For high-risk patients, especially those receiving simultaneous bilateral renal stents, contrast volume can be severely curbed by using dilute contrast and DSA. Using an 0.018-in. wire (Platinum Plus Wire, Medi-tech Corp., Watertown, MA) and obtaining selective angiograms through a 5 Fr. catheter with a Y-adapter also may help.
3. Risk of renal artery side branch occlusion may exist if a stent is placed across a side branch.
4. Systemic hemorrhage, such as from the gastrointestinal tract, may occur due to extensive anticoagulation. Therefore, patients must be carefully screened before starting anticoagulation.
5. Careful attention must be paid to exact stent positioning with frequent intermittent DSA to avoid mal-deployment of the stent, especially for ostial lesions.
6. The articulated stent, if used, should be positioned so that the lesion does not overlap the articulation where no stenting effect is present. For this reason, nonarticulated stents of smaller length may be preferable.

7. Adequate predilatation of the renal artery lesion is a most important step as it will facilitate subsequent advancement of the guiding catheter as well as final corrections of stent position before deployment.

References

1. Palmaz JC. Balloon-expandable intravascular stent. *AJR* 150: 1263–1269, 1988.
2. Palmaz JC, et al. Placement of balloon-expandable intraluminal stents in iliac arteries: First 171 procedures. *Radiology* 174:969–975, 1990.
3. Palmaz JC, et al. Stenting of the iliac arteries with the Palmaz stent: Experience from a multicenter trial. *Cardiovasc Intervent Radiol* 15:291–297, 1992.
4. Becker GJ, et al. Angioplasty-induced dissections in human iliac arteries: Management with Palmaz balloon-expandable intraluminal stents. *Radiology* 176:31–38, 1990.
5. Colapinto RF, Harries-Jones EP, Johnston KW. Percutaneous transluminal angioplasty of complete iliac artery occlusions. *Arch Surg* 116:277–281, 1981.
6. Rees CT, et al. Angioplasty and stenting of completely occluded iliac arteries. *Radiology* 172:953–959, 1989.
7. Tegtmeyer CJ, et al. Percutaneous transluminal angioplasty in the region of the aortic bifurcation: The two balloon techniques with results and long-term follow-up study. *Radiology* 157:661–665, 1985.
8. Palmaz JC, et al. Aortic bifurcation stenosis: Treatment with intravascular stents. *J Vasc Intervent Radiol* 2:319–323, 1991.
9. Dietrich EB, et al. Preliminary observations on the use of the Palmaz stent in the distal abdominal aorta. *Am Heart J* 125:490–500, 1993.
10. Richter GM, et al. Randomized trial: Iliac stent placement versus PTA (Abstract). Presented at the Society of Cardiovascular and Interventional Radiology 18th Annual Scientific Meeting, February 1993; New Orleans, LA.
11. Saeed M, Knowles HJ, Schatz RA. Stent placement in renal artery stenoses. (Abstract). American Roentgen Ray Society Annual Meeting, May 1992; Orlando, FL.
12. Thomson KR, et al. Palmaz articulated stents for proximal renal artery stenoses. SCVIR Meeting Abstracts, *J Vasc Intervent Radiol* 4:47, 1993.
13. Richter GM, Roeren T, Brado M, Noeldge G. Renal artery stents: Long-term results of a European trial. Society of Cardiovascular and Interventional Radiology Meeting Abstracts, *J Vasc Intervent Radiol* 4:47, 1993.
14. Rees CR, et al. Palmaz stent in atherosclerotic stenoses involving the ostia of the renal arteries: Preliminary report of a multi-center study. *Radiology* 181:507–514, 1991.
15. Palmaz JC, et al. Normal and stenotic renal arteries: Experimental balloon-expandable intraluminal stenting. *Radiology* 164:705–708, 1987.
16. Joffre F, et al. The usefulness of an endovascular prosthesis for treatment of renal artery stenosis. *Diagn Intervent Radiol* 1:15–21, 1989.

17. Tegtmeyer CJ, et al. Percutaneous transluminal dilatation of the renal arteries: Techniques and results. *Radiology* 135:589–599, 1980.
18. Martin LG, et al. Percutaneous angioplasty in clinical management of renovascular hypertension. *Radiology* 155:629–633, 1985.
19. Martin EC, et al. Renal angioplasty for hypertension: Predictive factors for long-term success. *AJR* 137:921–924, 1981.

Dialysis Access Shunt and Fistula Recanalization

John E. Aruny

Thrombolysis of the Dialysis Access

Indications

1. Thrombosed synthetic (polytetrafluoroethylene [PTFE]) dialysis access.
2. Failed Brescia-Cimino (native vessel) fistula.

Contraindications

ABSOLUTE

See also Chap. 5.
1. Active internal bleeding.
2. Recent ($\leq$ 1 year) cerebrovascular accident.
3. Intracranial or intraspinal neoplasm, or recent ($\leq$ 2 months) intracranial or intraspinal surgery.
4. Open-heart surgery within the past 3 weeks.

RELATIVE [1]

See also Chap. 5.
1. Fistula that has thrombosed within 3 weeks of construction.
2. Suspected graft infection.
3. Dangerously elevated serum potassium ($>$ 5 mEq/L) that does not respond to appropriate medical therapy and may require emergency catheter dialysis.
4. Severe allergy to iodinated contrast material.
5. Any contraindication to lytic therapy such as:
   a. Severe impairment of hepatic function.
   b. Recent major trauma or CPR.
   c. History of emboli from cardiac source.
   d. Subacute bacterial endocarditis.
   e. Coagulopathy.
   f. Diabetic hemorrhagic retinopathy.
   g. Lactating females.
   h. Pregnancy or unexplained amenorrhea for 3 or more days beyond expected menses.

Note: Recent surgical thrombectomy should not be considered a contraindication to thrombolysis. We have performed thrombolysis with high-dose, pulse-spray administration of urokinase (UK) as early as 24 hours following failed surgical thrombectomy [2].

Preprocedure Preparation

1. Obtain informed consent.
2. Speak with the vascular surgeon or review the operative note regarding placement of the fistula to know its course,

internal diameter (ID), and if its ID tapers to a smaller diameter at the arterial anastomosis.

3. Draw blood for serum electrolytes. Dangerously elevated serum potassium may require emergency dialysis via percutaneous catheter or may be treated with potassium-lowering regimens of glucose and insulin with coadministration of sodium polystyrene sulfonate (Kayexalate).

4. All patients to undergo thrombolysis with UK receive the following premedication to prevent or lessen the intensity of the rigors associated with high-dose, rapid-infusion UK:
   a. Diphenhydramine (Benadryl) 50 mg IV.
   b. Aspirin 650 mg PO.
   c. Cimetidine (Tagamet) 300 mg IV.

5. Preparation of UK for infusion [2]
   a. Each vial of UK containing 250,000 units is reconstituted with 10 ml of nonbacteriostatic sterile water (25,000 units/ml) (7500 units/0.3 ml). To each vial is added 1250 units of heparin.
   b. If subsequent vials are reconstituted for pulse spray, they are done so to the same dilution but without heparin.
   c. Urokinase for infusion is prepared by reconstituting 3 vials of 250,000 units with 5 ml of nonbacteriostatic sterile water in each. The content of these vials (15 ml) are added to a bag of 235 ml of normal saline or D5W (3000 units/ml).

Procedure

CROSSED-CATHETER TECHNIQUE

1. Accessing the graft. Establish the two points where you wish to enter the graft. This will depend on the length of the graft.
   a. Length of the graft
      (1) Most grafts that have not been previously revised are between 30 and 40 cm in length. Entering the graft within 5–10 cm of the apex of the loop is usually technically easy and provides enough crossover to pulse-spray the entire graft with UK without moving the catheters.
      (2) Revised grafts have longer venous limbs. Grafts of 50–60 cm may be encountered. In this case, place both punctures on the venous limb of the graft, angled toward each other and separated by at least 8–10 cm. This will allow technically easier access to the venous anastomosis if it is high in the axillary region or even to the internal jugular vein. Where to place the access sites is a skill developed largely by experience.
   b. Configuration of the graft. Access a straight graft in its center with the catheters separated by at least 5–8 cm.
      (1) Accessing any graft is usually quite simple since it has a large diameter (6–8 mm) and is only a few mm below the skin surface. Use a small-vessel

access set (Microvascular Access Set, Cook, Inc., Bloomington, IN) that comes with all of the components already together.

   (2) The needle used to puncture a looped graft on the venous limb is angled 45 degrees toward the apex of the graft and away from the venous anastomosis. The puncture on the arterial limb of the graft is angled 45 degrees toward the apex of the graft and away from the arterial anastomosis.

2. Preparing the access site

   a. Use a syringe with a 25-gauge needle to raise a wheal with a small amount of 1% lidocaine at the proposed entry site. Grasp the graft between the thumb and third finger of the hand holding the needle and advance the 22-gauge needle until you feel the definite "pop" of the needle passing through the graft wall. The patient should feel little discomfort. If the patient complains of pain then the needle has gone through both walls of the graft and should be withdrawn slightly.

   b. Intraluminal position is confirmed by the easy passage of the 0.018-in. platinum-tip guidewire. The clot is usually less than 48 hours old and is soft so that the tip of the guidewire meets with little resistance when it is advanced. Advance the wire, under fluoroscopy, until it curves within the apex of the graft loop.

   c. It is preferable to place the guidewire/catheter system first across the venous anastomosis before crossing the arterial anastomosis.

3. Place the 4 Fr. dilator with the 3 Fr. inner stylet over the guidewire until the hub is at the skin. Remove the inner stylet and the 0.018-in. platinum-tip guidewire.

4. The 4 Fr. dilator will accept a 0.035-in. guidewire; a hydrophilic, coated, and angled wire is preferred. The wire is gently negotiated through the anticipated location of the venous anastomosis and well into the native vein. Keep in mind that there is almost always a tight mechanical stenosis at the venous anastomosis and care must be taken to keep the course of the guidewire intraluminal.

5. Remove the 4 Fr. dilator and place 5 Fr. vascular dilator over the guidewire.

6. Remove the 5 Fr. vascular dilator and advance a 5 Fr. pulse-spray catheter to a point past the venous anastomosis well into the native vein. Remove the guidewire and flush the catheter. Inject a small amount of contrast to confirm that the tip is within a patent vein.

7. Perform a venogram of the central venous system through the pulse-spray catheter to determine if there is a central vein stenosis.

8. Withdraw a sample of blood and perform a baseline activated clotting time (ACT).

9. Withdraw the pulse-spray catheter under fluoroscopic guidance, periodically hand-injecting a small volume of contrast, until the tip of the catheter is just beyond the limits of the thrombus. This may be just at the venous anastomosis or within the native vein (Fig. 10-1).

10. Perform a second graft puncture into the venous limb

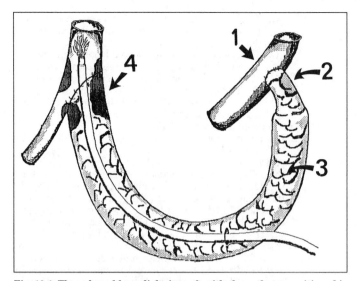

Fig. 10-1. Thrombosed loop dialysis graft with the catheter positioned in a patent vein just distal to the venous anastomosis. 1. Arterial anastomosis. 2. Platelet-rich thrombous often found near the arterial anastomosis. 3. Thrombus within the graft. 4. Intimal hyperplasia at the venous anastomosis.

    angled toward the arterial anastomosis. In a similar fashion place the guidewire across the anticipated location of the arterial anastomosis. This is done carefully so as not to dislodge any thrombus into the distal arterial circulation.

11. Position the second pulse-spray catheter with its tip at a point such that a gentle injection of contrast will faintly opacify the native artery distal to the graft anastomosis (Fig. 10-2).

12. Assemble the pulse-spray delivery system on the catheters.

13. Administer 2500 units of heparin IV or through the catheter with its tip at the venous anastomosis.

14. Begin pulse-spray pharmacomechanical thrombolysis with 0.3 ml of UK pulsed through each catheter every 30 seconds (Fig. 10-3).

15. Withdraw or advance the catheters as necessary to accomplish a uniform distribution of the 500,000 units of UK throughout the thrombus.

16. The end point of thrombolysis is the demonstration of antegrade flow of contrast, regardless of how slow, through the graft. If antegrade flow is not achieved, an additional 250,000 units of UK, divided between the two catheters are pulse-sprayed into the thrombus.

17. If minimal antegrade flow is not achieved after a total of 1 million units of UK has been administered, begin a constant drip infusion of 240,000 units/hour (80 ml/hr of the infusion mixture) through the catheter with its tip just

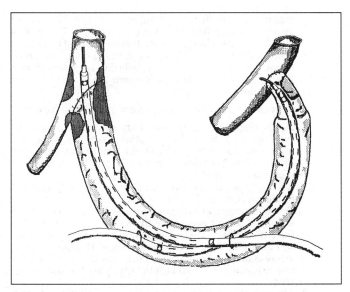

Fig. 10-2. The arterial pulse-spray catheter has been placed, completing the crossed-catheter system.

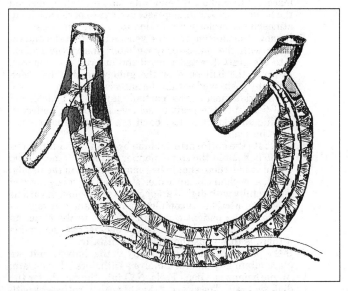

Fig. 10-3. Pulse-spray pharmacomechanical thrombolysis being performed through crossed, slit-hole catheters. Note that the entire thrombus burden is being treated. The catheters may have to be moved to treat the entire graft if it is longer than the segment of the catheter with the slits.

within the graft at the arterial anastomosis. The patient
may be removed from the angiography suite. The graft is
monitored with a Doppler probe for the return of blood flow.

18. When a Doppler signal is detected, the patient is returned
to the angiography table. Antegrade flow is confirmed with
a contrast injection. The graft is now ready for treatment
with balloon angioplasty.

BALLOON ANGIOPLASTY FOR MAINTENANCE OF ACCESS PATENCY

1. Use an angioplasty balloon with the same diameter as the
synthetic graft being dilated. Most are either 6 mm or 8
mm; some taper to 4 mm at the arterial anastomosis.
This information must be obtained from the surgeon who
inplanted the graft.

2. Advance the balloon over a guidewire directly into the
fistula without using an introducer sheath.

3. Treat the venous anastomosis first. There is almost always
a stenosis at this point or in the native vein just distal to
the actual anastomosis. Our experience shows that most
will dilate completely at between 8 and 10 atm; however,
an occasional stenosis will require a balloon that can sustain pressures of 17–20 atm to fully dilate the lesion (Fig.
10-4).

4. After dilating the venous anastomosis, withdraw the balloon and serially hand-inflate and deflate along the entire
length of the venous limb to detect intragraft stenoses and
macerate thrombus. If hand-inflation fails to fully distend
the balloon, use the angioplasty syringe to perform a high-
atmosphere, prolonged inflation to resolve the waist.

5. Remove the balloon from the venous anastomosis and replace with the pulse-spray catheter. Insert the balloon
into the graft directed toward the arterial anastomosis.
Advance the balloon over the guidewire that has been
carefully positioned within the native artery. Once beyond
the arterial anastomosis, partially inflate the balloon and
pull back into the graft to achieve a "Fogarty" effect of
pulling any clot that may be at the arterial anastomosis
into the graft.

6. Evaluate the entire arterial limb by serial hand-inflations
of the balloon in the same manner as on the venous side.

7. By this time, there should be rapid flow within the fistula.
If not, a mechanical cause (i.e., stenosis) must be searched
for carefully with digital angiograms performed in various
oblique projections. A completion angiogram is always obtained. If the patient complains of pain in the hand, an
angiogram of these distal vessels is necessary to determine
if there is thrombus that has gone distally.

8. If the patient needs to go directly to the dialysis unit, we
place minimally modified dialysis catheters (Hemo-Cath;
AngioDynamics; Glens Falls, NY) into the fistula for the
dialysis staff. These are 7 Fr. high-flow catheters with
internal stiffeners that can be passed over the same 0.035-
in. guidewire and through the same puncture sites used
during the salvage procedure (Fig. 10-5). The catheters are
placed in a crossed configuration, flushed with heparinized

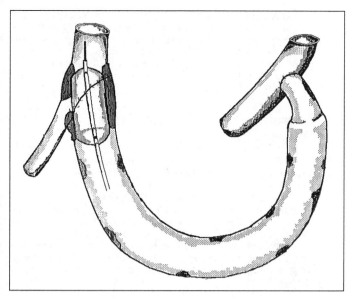

Fig. 10-4. Balloon angioplasty of the fibrointimal hyperplastic stenosis at the venous anastomosis.

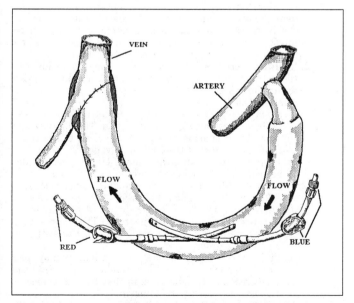

Fig. 10-5. Crossed dialysis catheters have been placed into the graft with the tips of the catheters at least 3 cm apart to prevent recirculation within the graft.

saline, and clamped. The clamps and luer-lock fittings are color coded for easy recognition by the dialysis staff.

The placement of these catheters in the angiography suite at the time of salvage has greatly facilitated the transition of the patient to the dialysis center. This is particularly true when the patient's arm is edematous and the graft is difficult to palpate.

Brescia-Cimino (Native Vessel) Dialysis Fistula

These fistulas have a unique anatomy and present different problems in achieving effective salvage. Distal to the arterial-venous (A-V) anastomosis the vein arborizes into multiple run-off vessels. A variable number of these channels will contain thrombus of varying age, thus complicating the process of thrombolysis. There may be multiple sites of venous stenosis each of which needs to be dilated with the angioplasty balloon to achieve optimum patency of the fistula. The results are not as reliable as with the synthetic group of fistulas and many surgeons and interventional radiologists would not attempt salvage.

Procedure

1. **Access** with an 18- or 19-gauge Teflon sheath angiocath used for IV access. The entry point is positioned antegrade near the construction of the A-V anastomosis. If there is clot at the anastomosis itself, a second catheter can be introduced retrograde pointed toward the anastomosis and the dose of UK is split between the two catheters.
2. **Frequent contrast injections** are needed to identify the network of anastomosing veins that are patent prior to thrombolysis.
3. Thrombolysis
   a. Do not use pulse-spray technique unless a thrombosed main venous trunk can be identified. This diagnosis is made by comparing previous venograms to the venogram performed at the time of salvage.
   b. Perform with constant infusion of UK prepared as described in **1**. The following protocol is followed:
      (1) 240,000 units/hour (80 ml/hr) for 2 hours then
      (2) 120,000 units/hour (40 ml/hr) for 2 hours then
      (3) 80,000 units/hour (27 ml/hr) until the patient is restudied, usually the next day. The end point for thrombolysis is less clear than in the synthetic fistula group.
   c. Probing the venous network with a guidewire may open small channels through the thrombus and speed lysis by increasing the surface area that the UK comes in contact with during the infusion.
4. After completing thrombolysis perform a fistulogram to determine if any new channels have been opened. Identify stenoses and dilate with a balloon of appropriate size as determined by the native vessel caliber.

Postprocedure Management

1. Measure ACT; remove catheters when 170 seconds or less. Observe the patient for 45 minutes after complete hemostasis is achieved.
2. Almost all patients are discharged home or directly to the hemodialysis unit for unrestricted hemodialysis. Patients are admitted only if they are not capable of obtaining assistance in case of a delayed complication.
3. We schedule patients to return in 30 days for a repeat fistulagram and possibly maintenance angioplasty.

Results

1. **Procedure times** cover a wide range and depend on the operator's experience. Times from 2–3 hours have been reported [2,3].
2. For **synthetic grafts** the immediate technical success in achieving patency following thrombolysis and angioplasty is greater than 90%. Surgical series describe successful salvage as a fistula that remains persistently patent for 1 month. The 30-day primary patency rate for thrombolysis and angioplasty is approximately 70%, and the 1-year primary patency rate is approximately 30%. Secondary patency rates of approximately 50% can be expected with repeated interventions to maintain fistula patency [3].
   Other studies have reported a primary patency of 40% at 6 months and 20% at 1 year that was similar to both surgically treated and percutaneously treated patients who received thrombolysis and angioplasty [4].
3. For **angioplasty** of Brescia-Cimino fistulas, the 1-month primary patency reported by Gmelin, et al. was 70% overall and higher with stenoses (89%) than with complete occlusions (46%) [5].
   Secondary patency among these patients was 93% at 6 months, 91% at 1 year, and 57% at 2 years for patients with stenoses. For patients with occlusions the secondary patencies for the same time period were 80%, 50%, and 14%, respectively. These were in fistulas that would otherwise have been abandoned.
4. **Doses of UK** range from 250,000 to 1 million units depending on the length of the fistula and thus the volume of thrombus to be treated.

Complications

1. **Bleeding**
   a. From sites distal to the site of local thrombolysis.
2. Local bleeding during the procedure—from puncture sites in the graft or at site of previous surgical graft entry for thrombectomy. These sites are treated with local manual pressure during the procedure. The best treatment is to restore rapid blood flow within the graft as soon as possible.
3. **Difficulty achieving hemostasis** at the puncture site. Placing a piece of Gelfoam over the puncture site during compression may speed hemostasis.

4. Rupture of the fistula. This has rot been a problem in our group of patients. Depending on the severity, it could be treated with prolonged balloon inflation at the rupture site, isolation of the graft with balloons occluding the arterial and venous ends, or inflation of a BP cuff above the arterial anastomosis.

5. Distal embolization of thrombus toward the hand from the region of the arterial anastomosis has been reported in approximately 0.8% of a large series [3].

6. Systemic complications related to the volume status of the patient such as angina and pulmonary vascular congestion are rare.

References

1. Kumpe DA, Cohen MAH. Angioplasty/thrombolytic treatment of failing and failed hemodialysis access sites: Comparison with surgical treatment. *Prog Cardiovasc Dis* 34:263–278, 1992.
2. Berger MF, Aruny JE, Skibo LK. Recurrent thrombosis of PTFE dialysis fistulas after recent surgical thrombectomy: Salvage by means of thrombolysis and angioplasty. *J Vasc Interv Radiol* 5: 725–730, 1994.
3. Valji K, et al. Pharmacomechanical thrombolysis and angioplasty in the management of clotted hemodialysis grafts: Early and late clinical results. *Radiology* 178:243–247, 1991.
4. Summers S, Drazan K, Gomes A. Urokinase therapy for thrombosed hemodialysis access grafts. *Surg Gynecol Obstet* 176:534–538, 1993.
5. Gmelin E, Winterhoff R, Riast E. Insufficient hemodialysis access fistulas: Late results of treatment with percutaneous balloon angioplasty. *Radiology* 171:657–660, 1989.

Acute Mesenteric Ischemia

Krishna Kandarpa

Clinical Signs and Symptoms

Patients who present with acute mesenteric ischemia (AMI) are generally elderly and commonly have cardiac problems (valvular or atherosclerotic) causing hypotension or embolic events. A history of a recent myocardial infarction, prior arterial embolization, hypovolemia, or concurrent digitalis therapy may be elicited. On examination, the classic finding is abdominal pain out of proportion to physical signs. Peritoneal signs, usually associated with bowel infarction, may be seen in up to 25% of patients [1]. A silent abdomen is occasionally noted [1–3]. A metabolic acidosis may be noted in 50% of patients [4]. Nonspecific findings include occult gastrointestinal bleeding, leukocytosis, and elevated serum phosphate. An elevation of serum amylase suggests bowel necrosis [5,6]. When mesenteric ischemia is suspected, angiography is the test of choice and should be performed emergently [5–9].

Note: Arteriography should precede contrast studies of the gastrointestinal track since residual barium within the lumen may obscure angiographic findings.

Indications (for Angiography) [5–9]

1. Diagnosis and determination of the cause for mesenteric ischemia
   a. Superior mesenteric artery (SMA) embolus (50%).
   b. In situ SMA thrombosis in the setting of underlying atherosclerosis (20%).
   c. Nonocclusive (vasospastic) ischemia (20%).
   d. Superior mesenteric venous thrombosis (10%).
2. Management of nonocclusive mesenteric ischemia (NOMI) with papaverine infusion. Perioperative papaverine infusion in the surgical management of occlusive emboli or thrombi.
3. Potential treatment of emboli with thrombolysis (IA or systemic) [10] and stenoses with percutaneous transluminal angioplasty (PTA). PTA has more commonly been used in the setting of chronic intestinal angina [11]. Potential treatment of SMV thrombosis with IA thrombolysis. The experience with these new forms of therapy is limited. They are currently indicated in a few highly selected circumstances.

Relative Contraindications

Patient's severely compromised medical status (e.g., multisystem failure) or prior severe reaction to iodinated contrast media.

Preprocedure Preparation (Resuscitation and Evaluation)

1. Stop oral intake.
2. Start large-bore IV access.
3. Initiate supportive therapy (e.g., correct hypotension, congestive heart failure).
4. Initiate physiologic monitoring (BP, ECG, arterial oxygenation).
5. Standard preangiography workup and preparation. Assess ability of patient to tolerate potential use of papaverine infusion.
6. Analgesia/sedation, preferably IV, prior to angiogram.
7. Check plain films of abdomen to aid diagnosis of bowel ischemia (wall thickening and thumb printing) or infarction (intramural or portal venous gas). Only about one-third of these studies will be positive [1,2,8,12]. A negative examination does not rule out AMI.

Procedure

1. **Imaging.** Obtain a biplane abdominal aortogram; the lateral projection provides the best view to rule out proximal embolic/occlusive disease of the mesenteric and celiac arteries while the AP projection splays open the distal branches optimally [4,7–9,13–15]. An IA digital subtraction aortogram in the lateral view can quickly rule out proximal lesions. Angiography has a true negative rate of 30–50% for detecting AMI [13].

   a. If a proximal SMA embolus is found (the majority of emboli lodge at the origin [20%] or proximal branches [70%]), the patient will need surgical embolectomy—for which mortality is 82% [1–6,16].

   b. If significant stenoses ($\geq$ 50% by diameter) involving at least two of the mesenteric arteries are found (usually in patients with chronic intestinal angina), consider transluminal angioplasty or vascular reconstruction [6,16]. In patients with chronic occlusions, collateral vessels may be noted.

   c. Spontaneous dissection of the SMA, although rare, can occur—surgical "intimectomy" may be needed [17].

2. If step **1** above does not provide a diagnosis, perform a **selective SMA angiogram** (with a catheter that can retain stable position, e.g., Simons 1, to ensure a better study and avoid a later exchange, if papaverine is to be infused) looking for vasospastic changes (NOMI), distal branch occlusion by emboli (about 10% of SMA emboli), or SMV thrombosis [9,13–15].

   a. **Nonocclusive mesenteric ischemia** (NOMI) [4,7–9,13–15]. The arterial lumen will have segmental sausage-like narrowings or diffuse nonspecific vasoconstriction (often seen with hypotension or pressor therapy). Focal narrowing at the origins of branches may be seen. Contrast may reflux from the SMA into the aorta because of the high resistance in the peripheral bed. Bowel wall staining and venous opacification may be delayed. To lazoline (Priscoline) challenge (optional) [4,13]: IA bolus of 25–50 mg tolazoline (over 1–2 minutes) serves as a rapid test for the effectiveness of vasodilator therapy; quickly repeat the SMA angiogram to assess response. (This same pharmacologic maneuver is used for improving the visualization of the superior mesenteric vein [SMV]; see **c** below.)

b. **Distal branch embolization.** Multiple peripheral filling defects with characteristic convex menisci [4,7,13].

c. **Superior mesenteric venous thrombosis.** Poor visualization of the SMV, prolonged opacification of venules or larger regional tributory veins may be noted. An SMA angiogram with IA tolazoline injection (see **a** above) and attention to late filming will usually demonstrate a fixed intraluminal filling defect, the only definitive sign of SMV thrombosis [4,7,13]. CT and Doppler US are alternative imaging modalities. However, flow-sensitive (e.g., gradient refocused pulse sequences) MRI is ideally suited for demonstrating the SMV and portal veins.

3. **Papaverine infusion**
   a. **Indications.** Intraarterial papaverine infusion is indicated for the management of AMI regardless of the etiology. It is clearly indicated in the setting of nonocclusive ischemia (with or without peritoneal signs) and serves a beneficial vasodilatory and antispasmodic function perioperatively (pre-, intra-, inter-, and post-) when surgery is necessary. When there is a chronic occlusion with good collateral formation, or when a minor occlusion or embolus is present without peritoneal signs, the decision to use papaverine should be individualized [4–6].

   b. **Contraindications**
   Complete atrioventricular heart block is an absolute contraindication [4,13]. Relative contraindications are:
   (1) Severe cardiac disease (especially with severe hypotension).
   (2) Concomitant infusion of alkaline substances (e.g., Ringer's lactate, heparin, urokinase) [4,9,13].
   (3) Narrow-angle glaucoma.

   c. **Infusion technique**
   (1) Check that large IV access and physiologic monitors are functioning properly.
   (2) Make sure that the infusion catheter has a stable position in the SMA. It may need to be secured at the groin.
   (3) Start IA infusion of papaverine at 30–60 mg/hour via constant infusion pump (at a concentration of 1 mg/ml NS, or adjust per fluid status of patient). Plan on an initial treatment for 12–24 hours. **Note:** Papaverine in Ringer's lactate will result in precipitation [4,9,13].

(4) Nifedipine 10–20 mg PO q6h may have an additive vasodilatory effect (optional) [13].

Postprocedure Management

Papaverine infusion may serve as the primary treatment for nonocclusive AMI when no peritoneal signs are present. However, close monitoring during therapy is essential. If peritoneal signs are persistent or worsening, the patient should have exploratory surgery. Most patients with occlusive causes for AMI (e.g., emboli and thrombi) and those with bowel infarction will need surgery. In either case, papaverine infusion may be started preoperatively. Clinical and angiographic assessment (as necessary) at 12–24 hours should determine further management [4–7,9].

1. If peritoneal signs are absent or resolve quickly (> 30 minutes after institution of papaverine), conservative nonsurgical management of nonocclusive AMI is indicated. Admit patient to ICU, and monitor vital signs and central venous pressure. Successful reperfusion of the bowel may cause abdominal pain and diarrhea during infusion [13].
2. If peritoneal signs are persistent or worsening, the patient should have exploratory surgery [5,6,16].
3. In all cases, maintain a patent IV access in the event of vascular dilatation and hypotension due to systemic effects of papaverine.
4. Assess patient and repeat angiogram at 12–24 hours or as indicated.
   a. If vasoconstriction is relieved, stop the infusion and remove the catheter (see **5** below).
   b. If there is no improvement, continue IA papaverine infusion for another 12–24 hours, with frequent assessment of the patient's status [9]. At the end of the second 24 hours, clinical and angiographic reevaluation of the patient should again determine the course of action. Occasionally, the infusion may be prolonged over several days [6].
5. Termination of papaverine infusion: When the patient's clinical status has improved and no peritoneal signs are present, replace papaverine with normal saline for 30 minutes before a repeat arteriogram. If the patient's condition remains stable and the arteriogram no longer demonstrates vasoconstriction, the catheter may be removed.

Results

1. With aggressive workup and intervention, including early supportive therapy and angiography with vasodilator infusion, mortality is down to 46% [4–6,9]. Prior to such intervention, in the mid-1970s, mortality was 70–90% [4–6,9].
2. In the presence of a low-flow state (i.e., NOMI) [1–6,9]
   a. Without peritoneal signs, outcome is generally good.
   b. With peritoneal signs and extensive bowel infarction (greater than 50% of small bowel), mortality is 60%.

Complications [4,9,13]

1. Vascular collapse due to vasodilation in hypovolemic patient.

2. Cardiac arrythmias.

References

1. Andersson R, et al. Acute intestinal ischemia: A 14-year retrospective investigation. *Acta Chir Scand* 150:217–221, 1984.

2. Khan AH, Rubinstein PC. Ischemic bowel disease: Diagnosis and prognosis. *Geriatrics* 39:63–72, 1984.

3. Boley SJ, Brandt LJ, Veith FJ. Ischemic disorders of the intestines. *Curr Probl Surg* 15:1–85, 1978.

4. Nemcek AA, Vogelzang RL. Interventional Management of Acute Mesenteric Ischemia. In DE Strandness, A van Breda (eds.), *Vascular Diseases: Surgical and Interventional Therapy.* New York: Churchill Livingstone, 1994. Pp. 785–793.

5. Durham JR, Flinn WR. Surgical Management of Acute Mesenteric Ischemia. In DE Strandness, A van Breda (eds.), *Vascular Diseases: Surgical and Interventional Therapy.* New York: Churchill Livingstone, 1994. Pp. 775–783.

6. Kayela RN, Sammartano RJ, Boley SJ. Aggressive approach to acute mesenteric ischemia. *Surg Clin North Am* 72:157–201, 1992.

7. Bakal CW, Sprayregen S, Wolf EL. Radiology of intestinal ischemia: Angiographic diagnosis and management. *Surg Clin North Am* 72:125–141, 1992.

8. Wolf EL, Sprayregen S, Bakal CW. Radiology of intestinal ischemia: Plain film, contrast and other imaging studies. *Surg Clin North Am* 72:107–124, 1992.

9. Athanasoulis CA. Bowel Ischemia, Management with Intraarterial Papaverine Infusion and Transluminal Angioplasty. In CA Athanasoulis et al. (eds.), *Interventional Radiology.* Philadelphia: Saunders, 1982. Chap. 24.

10. Schoenbaum SW, et al. Superior mesenteric artery embolism: Treatment with intraarterial urokinase. *J Vasc Interv Radiol* 3:485–490, 1992.

11. Sniderman KW. Transluminal angioplasty in the management of chronic intestinal ischemia. In DE Strandness, A van Breda (eds.), *Vascular Diseases: Surgical and Interventional Therapy.* New York: Churchill Livingstone, 1994. Pp. 803–809.

12. Levine MS. Plain film diagnosis of the acute abdomen. *Emerg Med Clin North Am* 3:541–562, 1985.

13. Morse SS, Clark RA. Management of Nonocclusive and Occlusive Mesenteric Ischemia. In S Kadir (ed.), *Current Practice of Interventional Radiology.* Philadelphia: B C Decker, 1991. Pp. 394–400.

14. Clark RA, Gallant TE. Acute mesenteric ischemia: Angiographic spectrum. *AJR* 142:555–562, 1984.

15. Morano JU, Harrison RB. Mesenteric ischemia: Angiographic diagnosis and intervention. *Clin Imag* 15:91–94, 1991.

16. van Lanschot JJ, van Urk H. Vascular reconstruction in intestinal angina. *Neth J Surg* 36:151–155, 1984.

17. Krupski WC, Effeney DJ, Ehrenfeld WK. Spontaneous dissection of the superior mesenteric artery. *J Vasc Surg* 2:731–734, 1985.

Acute Gastrointestinal Bleeding

Krishna Kandarpa

Indications [1–4]

1. Bleeding not responsive to conservative medical management, as manifested by clinical evidence of active life-threatening bleeding, continued blood requirements (> 500 ml in 8 hours) [2], etc. The large majority (75%) of patients with acute gastrointestinal bleeding will stabilize with supportive therapy and will not need angiographic intervention.
2. Endoscopy not available, contraindicated, failed, or inconclusive (15–20% of endoscopic procedures).

Relative Contraindications [1–4]

1. On rare occasion, the rate of bleeding is too brisk and severe for transcatheter intervention (which can be time-consuming); immediate surgical exploration may be preferable. Good clinical judgment is crucial in these cases.
2. Residual barium from recent gastrointestinal examination may obscure subtle contrast extravasation.

Preprocedure Preparation

1. Patient is stabilized and supportive therapy started (e.g., large-bore IV, nasogastric tube, gastric ice-water lavage, transfusion, correction of coagulopathy [5]).
2. Rule out overlooked obscure bleeding sources such as hemorrhoids, rectal fissures, etc.
3. Obtain report (preferably directly from the operator) of endoscopic examination and attempted treatment (e.g., cauterization, direct epinephrine injection). Review history for prior gastrointestinal surgery [6].
4. If endoscopy failed to reveal a lesion, obtain a radionuclide study (labeled Tc 99m RBC or Tc 99m SC); these studies are sensitive to bleeding rates of 0.1 ml/minute and, if positive, can guide arteriographic diagnosis and therapy [7,8]. When the rate of bleeding is around 500 ml/24 hours, the sensitivity of this test is 90% and specificity is 95% (see Chap. 27). Some authors will forgo the radionuclide study and go directly to angiography if the patient is bleeding acutely [2]. Radionuclide studies are especially helpful when the bleeding is intermittent, low-grade, or at sites that are generally inaccessible for endoscopy [2]. Newer cine scintigraphic techniques appear to increase sensitivity and accuracy of localization [9].
5. Standard preangiography workup, preparation, and monitoring (see Chap. 1). Discuss treatment plan with referring physician and patient, and obtain informed consent.
6. If a lower gastrointestinal (LGI) bleed is suspected, a Foley catheter will help keep the bladder empty. Thus, potential

contrast extravasation into a loop of bowel projected over the pelvis is not obscured by contrast-opacified urine. A Foley catheter is also useful for monitoring urine output during vasopressin therapy.

7. Caution is urged with sedatives/analgesics that may lower BP excessively, because they may cause the bleeding to temporarily cease before the angiogram is performed [10].

Procedure

1. Place a 5 or 6 Fr. **arterial sheath** within the femoral artery; this will facilitate catheter exchange, if necessary, and serve to maintain arterial access for repeat angiography, if it is needed at a later time.

2. **Document bleeding** with a selective arteriogram of the appropriate artery supplying the location of the bleed suggested by endoscopy or radionuclide scan. Otherwise use the following sequence: inferior mesenteric artery, superior mesenteric artery, celiac arteries. A biplane aortogram is unnecessary, with rare exceptions (e.g. aortoenteric fistula).

   a. Arteriography has an overall yield of 60% for localizing acute lower gastrointestinal bleeds; with active bleeding, the yield is 95% [1–4,10,11]. Arteriography accurately identifies 90% of acute upper gastrointestinal (UGI) bleeds [12]. Angiography can detect the source of chronic GI bleeding from an obscure origin in almost half the patients studied; it should be used early in the workup of such patients [13,l4].

   b. Bleeding rate required for visibility on arteriogram [1–10]:

      (1) UGI bleed, about 0.5 ml/minute.

      (2) Lower gastrointestinal (LGI) bleed, about 1 ml/minute.

3. **Localization of the bleeding site.** A bleeding site must be identified arteriographically (contrast extravasation into the intestinal lumen), with few exceptions, prior to transcatheter intervention.

   a. Transcatheter treatment can be performed for endoscopically documented bleeding from the gastroduodenal or left gastric artery territory (e.g., from ulcers and tumors), even though arteriography fails to demonstrate a bleed [15]. The prophylactic embolization of the left gastric artery, without prior localization of the specific site, has been advocated in the setting of massive UGI hemorrhage when the risk of multiorgan failure also exists [15], since 85% of UGI bleeds are supplied by this artery [11] and nearly 90% of these patients are expected to survive if the bleeding is controlled [16].

   b. In contradistinction, since bleeding from Mallory-Weiss tears is self-limited and the tears heal rapidly, failure to document a bleed angiographically means the bleeding has stopped [17] and transcatheter therapy is generally not indicated, even if prior endoscopy revealed bleeding [2].

4. Transcatheter treatment alternatives [18–26] are intraarterial vasopressin infusion or embolization (Table 12-1).

a. **Vasopressin** causes constriction of very small arteries, arterioles, and capillaries. This treatment is most successful when there is diffuse mucosal hemorrhage (e.g., gastritis) or bleeding from small vessels (e.g., LGI diverticular bleeds) [18]. Profuse bleeding from larger vessels (e.g., those eroded by peptic ulcers) is less likely to be controlled by IA vasopressin infusion, and embolotherapy is preferable [2,19,24,25].

b. **Embolotherapy** is especially useful in UGI bleeds because it stops bleeding immediately and the risk of bowel ischemia or infarction is minimal because of the extensive supply of collateral vessels [19,20,24,25]. Vasopressin may be used for UGI bleeds primarily, if the bleeding is from small vessels, or secondarily, if embolotherapy is not technically possible [24,25]. Conversely, if vasopressin fails to control a LGI hemorrhage, embolotherapy can be used in selected patients with careful attention to procedural detail (e.g., superselective Gelfoam embolization) [21–23].

c. **Intraarterial infusion of vasopressin** as initial treatment:
   (1) Indications
      (a) Diffuse mucosal bleeding at any site: gastritis [20], inflammatory processes (granulomatous) [10].
      (b) Lower gastrointestinal hemorrhage: small bowel (distal to ligament of Treitz) and colon. Vasopressin controls LGI diverticular bleeding in about 90% of cases, bleeding recurs in about 20% when infusion is discontinued [18].
   (2) Contraindications (see Chap. 40)
      (a) Severe atherosclerosis: coronary artery disease, congestive cardiomyopathy, peripheral vascular disease.
      (b) Severe hypertension or renal failure.
      (c) Prior GI surgery is a relative contraindication—a detail arterial road map is crucial [6,26].

d. **Transcatheter embolization** as initial treatment: brisk bleeding not responsive to conservative measures or vasopressin infusion. **Wait** 30 minutes after vasopressin infusion before embolization is attempted [2].
   (1) Indications
      (a) UGI bleeds. Mallory-Weiss tear, bleeding from large vessels eroded by gastric or duodenal ulcers, ulcerated tumors, and aneurysms.
      (b) Failure of vasopressin infusion in LGI bleeds. Superselective embolization with Gelfoam pledgets and peripherally placed microcoils can stop the bleeding primarily or stabilize the patient medically for elective surgery in selected cases with small bowel and colonic bleeding [21–23].

Table 12-1. Results of gastrointestinal hemorrhage: Intraarterial catheter-based therapy [2,3,4,17–25]

Site	Control rate			Overall control by transcatheter methods (%)
	Vasopressin alone (%)	Vasopressin and embolization (%)	Rebleed (%)	
Upper gastrointestinal				
Esophageal				
Mallory-Weiss tears	100	100	—	100
Esophageal varices	< 60[a]	—	—	
Gastroduodenal				
Gastric (discrete or multiple sites)	70–80	80–96	16–18[b]	96
Pyloroduodenal ulcer	35–60[c]	65–70	—	80
Lower gastrointestinal[d]				
Small-bowel ulcers, Meckel's diverticulum, diffuse hemorrhage	70	—	—	70
Cecal angiodysplasia, diverticulosis	80–90	—	30	90

[a]Intravenous vasopressin is just as effective and less invasive. There may be associated arterial bleeding sites in up to 20% of patients.
[b]Need embolization.
[c]Poor control reflects extensive collateral supply in this region and decreased contractility of inflamed mural tissue (latter also true of abscesses and tumors).
[d]Embolic therapy in the lower gastrointestinal system is generally not recommended because of poor collateralization and potential for bowel necrosis.

(c) Arteriovenous malformations of the colon [10].

(2) Contraindications [19]

(a) Inflow stenosis at the origin of the main mesenteric artery (e.g., celiac artery with reversal of flow in the pancreatic-duodenal arcade).

(b) Immediately after IA vasopressin infusion: wait 20–30 minutes for vasoconstriction to resolve. This will minimize false-positive result after embolization.

(c) Prior GI surgery (relative)—a detailed arterial road map is crucial [6,26].

Vasopressin Infusion Technique

1. Place the catheter selectively (e.g., proximal superior mesenteric artery) into the bleeding artery for intraarterial infusion (see Chap. 40 for preparation of vasopressin) [2].

2. Infuse vasopressin at 0.2 units/minute for 20–30 minutes.

3. Repeat the arteriogram.

4. If bleeding has stopped, secure the catheter to the groin, admit patient to ICU, and follow Postprocedure Management, **1.a,** below.

5. If bleeding continues with the initial rate of infusion, double the infusion rate to 0.4 units/minute, and infuse for another 20–30 minutes.

6. Repeat the arteriogram.

7. If bleeding has stopped, secure the catheter to the groin, admit patient to ICU, and follow Postprocedure Management, **1.b,** below.

8. If bleeding is not controlled after infusion of 0.4 units/minute for 20–30 minutes, increasing the dose rate is not beneficial, and alternative methods (embolization [see Chap. 13] or surgery) should be considered depending on the location of the bleeding site and the clinical condition of the patient.

Technique of Embolization [19]

1. A digital subtraction angiographic road map is very helpful for selecting the target vessel.

2. Superselective catheterization is generally recommended (at least during initial Gelfoam embolization). However, in certain circumstances, subselective (e.g., gastroduodenal artery [GDA] and left gastric artery [LGA]) embolization is acceptable. Superselective catheterization is preferred and should be diligently pursued for LGI embolization since collaterals are more sparse in this region. Small bowel embolization should be at the level of a mesenteric branch proximal to the terminal arcade in order to reduce the chance of bowel ischemia [21–23].

3. Gelfoam (Upjohn, Kalamazoo, MI) is a temporary embolic material. Resorption occurs in about 14 days. This is a first-line embolic material which is cut into 1–2 mm pledgets, soaked in diluted contrast, and slowly delivered as peripherally as possible via small-caliber coaxial catheters

(T3, Cook, Inc., Bloomington, IN; Tracker-18, Target Therapeutics, San Jose, CA) using a tuberculine syringe. Permanent occlusion can be obtained by placing microcoils (Hilal Coils, Cook, Inc.; or Flower Coils, Target Therapeutics, Freemont, CA), again as peripherally as possible. Permanent proximal occlusion, when not contraindicated, also can be obtained by placing larger Gianturco stainless steel coils (Cook, Inc.), for example, in the GDA or LGA. Care should be taken to closely match the lumen diameter of the catheter and wire diameter of the coil, so that the coils do not get impacted within the catheter.
4. Sterile technique is absolutely essential. Some authors advocate soaking Gelfoam pledgets in antibiotics (e.g., cefamandole) [2,12,19,20].

Postprocedure Management

SPECIFIC TO VASOPRESSIN INFUSION

1. Once bleeding is controlled, continue intraarterial vasopressin therapy as follows [2]:
   a. If initial rate of infusion is 0.2 units/minute, continue for up to 12–24 hours; then, if bleeding has stopped completely, curtail as follows:
      (1) Vasopressin at 0.1 units/minute for up to 12–24 hours, then heparinized D5W at 20 ml/hour for 4–6 hours.
      (2) Remove the catheter, if there is no further bleeding.
   b. If initial rate of infusion is at 0.4 units/minute, continue for 6–12 hours, then, if bleeding has stopped, curtail as follows:
      (1) Taper vasopressin by 0.1 units/minute every 6–12 hours.
      (2) Infuse heparinized D5W at 20 ml/hour for 4–6 hours.
      (3) Remove the catheter, if there is no further bleeding.
2. Patient must remain in ICU during vasopressin infusion.
3. The antidiuretic hormone side effect of vasopressin may manifest itself within 6–8 hours after the initiation of infusion, causing decreased urine output and electrolyte imbalance. Monitor fluid input and output, and electrolytes (sodium). Treat water retention with furosemide; replenish electrolytes as needed.

ALL PATIENTS

1. Watch for signs of rebleeding and other potential complications. The patient may pass melanotic stools long after the bleeding has been stopped by transcatheter treatment [10]. Stability of vital signs and Hct is more important.
2. Transient fever is not uncommon following Gelfoam embolization. Persistent fever should be worked up and treated.
3. Check puncture site for hematoma or thrombosis. Standard postangiography care.

Results (see Table 12-1) [3,4,17–24]

CAUSES FOR FAILURE OF VASOPRESSIN INFUSION

1. Large or abnormal vessels (e.g., cecal angiodysplasia) may not respond to vasopressin infusion [10].
2. A poorly placed or unsecured catheter could result in the infusion of the wrong vessel, and suboptimal treatment of the bleeding site.
3. Failure to recognize collateral supply to region of bleed.
4. Improper dose or regimen.

CAUSES FOR FAILURE OF EMBOLIZATION

1. Failure to recognize collateral supply to region of bleed.
2. Incomplete occlusion; failure to recognize spasm resulting in decreased blood flow and transient cessation of bleeding [2].
3. Failure to recognize and correct coagulopathy, especially in setting of extensive transfusion [2,5].

Complications

VASOPRESSIN INFUSION

Serious complications requiring discontinuation of infusion include [1–5,17–25]:
1. Cardiovascular (myocardial infarction, severe arrhythmia, or hypertension): 4%.
2. Bowel ischemia/infarction: 0.8%. It is not unusual for the patient to complain of abdominal cramps during the initial 30 minutes of infusion. Superselective infusion into the bleeding branch is associated with intestinal infarction [2].
3. Peripheral vascular ischemia manifested by mottling and pain: 0.5%.
4. Antidiuretic hormone side effect of vasopressin: 1%. Cerebral edema is rare.
5. Catheter-related thrombosis, false aneurysm, sepsis: 2%.

EMBOLIZATION [2,10,19,20]

1. Reflux of embolic material proximal to origin of intended branch.
2. Ischemia/infarction of embolized region (this risk is greater with LGI embolization, which should be used judiciously).
3. Rupture of aneurysms.

References

1. Baum S. Angiography and the GI bleeder. *Radiology* 143:569–572, 1982.
2. Kadir S. Principles of Management of Gastrointestinal Bleeding. In S Kadir (ed.), Current Practice of Interventional Radiology. Philadelpia: B C Decker, 1991. Pp. 408–414.
3. Rahn NH, et al. Diagnostic and interventional angiography in acute gastrointestinal hemorrhage. *Radiology* 143:361–366, 1982.

4. Clark RA, Colley DP, Eggers FM. Acute arterial gastrointestinal hemorrhage: Efficacy of transcatheter control. *AJR* 136:1185–1189, 1981.

5. Encarnacion CE, et al. Gastrointestinal bleeding: Treatment with gastrointestinal artery embolization. *Radiology* 183:505–508, 1992.

6. Encarnacion CE. Treatment of Postoperative Bleeding. In S Kadir (ed.), *Current Practice of Interventional Radiology.* Philadelpia: B C Decker, 1991. Pp. 436–439.

7. Wingelberg GC, et al. Radionuclide localization of lower gastrointestinal hemorrhage. *Radiology* 139:465–469, 1981.

8. McKusick KA, et al. ^{99m}Tc red blood cells for detection of GI bleeding: Experience with 80 patients. *AJR* 137:1113–1118, 1981.

9. Maurer AH, et al. Gastrointestinal bleeding: Improved localization with cine scintigraphy. *Radiology* 185:187–192, 1992.

10. Cardella JF, et al. Vasoactive Drugs and Embolotherapy in the Management of Gastrointestinal Bleeding. In WR Castañeda-Zuñiga, SM Tadavarthy (eds.), *Interventional Radiology.* (2nd ed.). Baltimore: Williams & Wilkins, 1992. Pp. 201–225.

11. Kelemouridis V, Athanasoulis CA, Waltman AC. Gastric bleeding sites: an angiographic study. *Radiology* 149:643–648, 1983.

12. Bennett JD, Kadir S. Treatment of Colorectal Bleeding. In S Kadir (ed.), *Current Practice of Interventional Radiology.* Philadelpia: B C Decker, 1991. Pp. 428–436.

13. Rollins ES, et al. Angiography is useful in detecting the source of chronic gastrointestinal bleeding of obscure origin. *AJR* 156: 385–388, 1991.

14. Lau WY, et al. Repeat selective visceral angiography in patients with gastrointestinal bleeding of obscure origin. *Br J Surg* 76:226–229, 1989.

15. Lang EV, et al. Massive upper gastrointestinal hemorrhage with normal findings on arteriography: Value of prophylactic embolization of the left gastric artery. *AJR* 158:547–549, 1992.

16. Lang EV, et al. Massive arterial hemorrhage from the stomach and lower esophagus: Impact of embolotherapy on survival. *Radiology* 177:249–252, 1990.

17. Keller FS, Routh WD. Treatment of Mallory-Weiss Tears. In S Kadir (ed.), *Current Practice of Interventional Radiology.* Philadelpia: B C Decker, 1991. Pp. 411–414.

18. Athanasoulis CA, et al. Mesenteric arterial infusions of vasopressin for hemorrhage from colonic diverticulosis. *Am J Surg* 129: 212–216, 1975.

19. Kadir S. Treatment of Pyloroduodenal Bleeding. In S Kadir (ed.), *Current Practice of Interventional Radiology* Philadelpia: B C Decker, 1991. Pp. 418–424.

20. Hilleren DJ. Treatment of Gastric Bleeding. In S Kadir (ed.), *Current Practice of Interventional Radiology.* Philadelpia: B C Decker, 1991. Pp. 414–418.

21. Cho KJ, Doenz F. Treatment of Small Intestinal Bleeding. In S Kadir (ed.), *Current Practice of Interventional Radiology.* Philadelpia: B C Decker, 1991. Pp. 424–428.

22. Guy GE, et al. Acute lower gastrointestinal hemorrhage: Treatment by superselective embolization with polyvinyl alcohol particles. *AJR* 159:521–526, 1992.

23. Okazaki M, et al. Emergent embolotherapy of small intestine hemorrhage. *Gastrointest Radiol* 17:223–228, 1992.

24. Ecstein MR, et al. Gastric bleeding: Therapy with intra-arterial vasopressin and transcatheter embolization. *Radiology* 152:643–646, 1984.
25. Gomes AS, Lois JF, McCoy RD. Angiographic treatment of gastro-intestinal hemorrhage: Comparison of vasopressin infusion and embolization. *AJR* 146:1031–1037, 1986.
26. Oglevie Sb, Smith DC, Mera SS. Bleeding marginal ulcers: Angiographic evaluation. *Radiology* 174:943–944, 1992.

Transcatheter Arterial Embolization

Clement J. Grassi
John E. Aruny

Indications

1. Uncontrolled bleeding
   a. Where medical therapy is unsuccessful or inappropriate.
   b. Where surgical intervention would carry an unacceptably high morbidity or mortality, such as
      (1) Bronchial artery hemorrhage [1–5].
      (2) Obstetric hemorrhage not responsive to packing and suture ligation [6,7].
      (3) Trauma [8] — iatrogenic and noniatrogenic — specifically involving
         (a) Liver [9–13].
         (b) Spleen [12,14].
         (c) Kidney [15–18].
      (4) Gastrointestinal bleeding [19–22].
      (5) Bleeding from dysplastic or neoplastic lesions involving
         (a) Urinary bladder [23].
         (b) Cervix [24].
         (c) Prostate [25].
         (d) Pelvis [26,27].
2. Treatment of vascular malformations including
   a. Arteriovenous malformations [28].
   b. Pulmonary arteriovenous (AV) malformations (which more closely resemble AV fistulas) [29].
3. Preoperative devascularization procedures to minimize blood loss
   a. Metastatic bone lesions [30,31].
   b. Renal cell carcinoma (controversial) [32].
   c. Obstetric [6,33].
   d. Spleen [34].
4. As a primary mode of therapy in various conditions
   a. Chemoembolization of liver tumors
      (1) Metastatic endocrine tumors [35,36].
      (2) Primary hepatocellular carcinoma [37,38].
   b. Therapeutic embolization of bone tumors for relief of pain and primary ablation [39,40].
   c. Treatment of hypersplenism [41,42].
   d. Testicular vein embolization; testicular varicoceles (see Chap. 17).

Contraindications

1. Inability to position the most distal tip of the catheter in a secure position to ensure low risk of nontarget organ embolization.

2. Use of an embolic agent that is too small and will pass through the target site of embolization into the nontarget distal circulation (e.g., Gelfoam powder is contraindicated in the embolization of AV fistulas with large channel(s) of communication). The embolic agent will pass through the fistula into the lungs.

Preprocedure Preparation

1. Routine preangiography preparation.
2. Analgesia/sedation with standard doses of narcotics and benzodiazepines for most adults. However, for complicated AV malformations and for all procedures performed on children, we recommend general anesthesia.
3. Antibiotic prophylaxis. Cefotetan (cefotan) 1 g IV q12h. First dose prior to the procedure and one dose 12 hours after the procedure. Then discontinue if the patient does not appear infected.
4. Review the imaging workup.

Embolic Material* and Its Use

1. **Particulate material**
   a. **Polyvinyl alcohol foam** (Ivalon, Contour) is an inert substance that is FDA approved and in general use. Particle sizes range from 100–1000 μ. It can be injected through diagnostic catheters or through coaxial 3 Fr. microcatheters.
      (1) **Purpose.** The material blocks the smallest vessel that it impacts against. There is an inflammatory response with fibroblast invasion and coexisting thrombus formation as well as a dense fibrous connective tissue formation [43]. Recanalization of the thrombus can occur over time. Once difficult to prepare, the commercial preparations now available are homogeneous as to size and suspend with adequate ease to allow uncomplicated use.
      (2) **Procedure**
         (a) Suspend the vial of particles with 30–40 ml of contrast agent and 1–2 ml of sterile saline to help avoid "clumping" of particles that may be a function of contrast dilution volume.
         (b) Use a 3-way stopcock to construct a system with two syringes to allow mixing of the embolic suspension from one syringe to the other to homogeneously suspend the mixture. 1-ml syringes are used with a 3 Fr. microcatheter and 3- or 5-ml syringes can be used with a 4 or 5 Fr. catheter.
         (c) Visually inspect the suspension to be sure that the suspension is well mixed and free-floating.

*The materials listed are those currently available in the United States.

(d) Inject the mixture under direct fluoroscopic vision for control of flow.

b. Gelfoam sheets and Gelfoam powder (Upjohn, Kalamazoo, MI). The powder has a particle size between 40–60 μ. The site of embolization is at the capillary level where the agent aggregates and occludes vessels of 100–200 μ diameter.

(1) Purpose. This agent is used when organ or tumor infarction is the desired result [44]. Because of the small particle size, it should always be used with caution and may most safely be introduced with balloon occlusion to prevent reflux of the embolic material into a nontarget vessel [45]. Gelfoam powder causes thrombosis that averages 3–4 months [46].

(2) Procedure

(a) Gelfoam sheets come in various sizes. Cut pledgets or "torpedoes" into suitable sizes with a scissor or scalpel.

(b) Soak pledgets with contrast medium. The Gelfoam will become less visually opaque and soft or jellylike.

(c) Connect a clear plastic tube to the end of the catheter, and introduce the Gelfoam pledget into the tube from a syringe. Observing the pledget in the tube confirms that it has been evacuated from the syringe.

(d) Flush the pledget by hand through the catheter to the site of embolization with a syringe of dilute contrast material. Regulate injection speed so that the particle will not reflux out of the vessel to be embolized.

(e) The end point of embolization is a significant reduction of the blood flow in the target vessel. Do not attempt to pack the vessel with Gelfoam because injection into a stagnant column of blood will cause the pledgets to reflux out of the target vessel.

(f) Gelfoam causes a panarteritis that promotes thrombosis. The occlusion lasts from a few days to a few weeks.

c. Avitene (Medchem Products) is microfibrillar collagen. Commonly used with other agents such as polyvinyl alcohol foam or with liquid agents such as Sotradecol (Elkins-Sinn, Cherry Hill, NJ). Causes immediate vascular occlusion but is rapidly degraded; reperfusion of the embolized territory usually occurs in a relatively short time [47].

d. Angiostat (Regional-Therapeutics) is another form of microfibrillar collagen. This bovine preparation is cross-linked using glutaraldehyde, which permits a more stable mass of embolic material.

2. Coil emboli. Many types and sizes are available. The coils are chosen for a specific application based on vessel diameter, blood flow rate, and the size of the catheter that was used to select the target vessel to be embolized. Coils are made of either stainless steel or platinum and may come with Dacron fibers to increase their thrombogenicity.

   a. Stainless steel coils come in 0.038-, 0.035-, and 0.025-in. diameters (minicoils). Stainless steel coils are relatively inexpensive but cause serious artifacts on MRI and are subject to magnetic torque.

   b. Platinum coils are available in 0.010- and 0.018-in. diameters (minicoils) and are formed into various configurations and unrestrained diameters. They are more expensive than stainless steel but cause less severe artifact on MRI and are not subject to magnet torque while in the scanner.

   c. Technique. Coils are introduced into a catheter with either a guidewire (0.038–0.025-in.) or a specialized coil pusher (0.010-in. and 0.018-in.) The coil is pushed along the catheter and deployed under direct fluoroscopic observation. Gentle forward and backward manipulation of the catheter is often necessary as the coil is being deployed to permit it to assume its intended shape. Coils can perforate the catheter, especially the microcoils, and any resistance to the advancement of the coil within the catheter should be carefully investigated.

3. Liquid embolic material

   a. Dehydrated ethanol (Abbott Laboratories, North Chicago, IL) is used when tissue necrosis, vessel thrombosis, and arterial wall sclerosis is the desired outcome. It is not radiopaque and must be carefully controlled. It is most effective in slow flow vascular lesions: venous malformations, esophageal varices, or where the flow can be slowed by using an occlusion balloon to permit time for adequate contact of the alcohol with the vessel wall. Careful angiographic delineation of the vascular territory to be embolized is required. Ethanol that contacts nontarget tissues will cause tissue necrosis or chronic painful neuritis.

   Note: Injection of ethanol causes extreme pain and we recommend general anesthesia when its use is contemplated.

   b. Sotradecol (Elkins-Sinn, Cherry Hill, NJ) sodium tetradecyl sulfate is a sclerosant. Usual application is for varicosities and venous malformations. Less pain is associated with its use than with ethanol, and larger volumes may be used [48].

Catheters

1. Diagnostic catheters. 4 and 5 Fr. catheters will accept coils appropriately sized to the internal diameter of the catheter (0.035 and 0.038-in.)

2. Coaxial systems. Utilized when subselection of a higher order vessel is necessary. They can be inserted through 5 Fr. or larger diagnostic catheters or through specially constructed guiding catheters.

   a. Cragg wire (Medi-Tech, Watertown, MA). Inner diameter is 0.027-in. and it accepts 0.025-in. coils as well as polyvinyl alcohol particles.

b. Tracker system (Target Therapeutics, Fremont, CA). Allows selection of high-order vessels with 0.016-in. and 0.014-in. guidewires. This system is ideal to deliver 0.018-in. platinum coils for superselective embolization. Larger internal lumen sizes have been introduced to permit the introduction of 0.025-in. coils as well as larger particle embolic material.

The Tracker-18 Unibody can be passed through a 6 Fr. guiding catheter. A Tuohy-Borst adapter allows for injection of contrast around the Tracker for monitoring the progress of the embolization.

3. Double-lumen balloon occlusion catheters. Available from several manufacturers in sizes of 5–8 Fr. Inflating the balloon slows blood flow distally and allows greater control of the embolic material. It also prevents reflux of the material into nontarget vessels.

Procedure (general guidelines)

1. Perform baseline diagnostic arteriogram of the region to be embolized.

2. Precise catheter placement (sub- or superselective) is essential and may by aided by digital subtraction angiographic "road map."

3. Maintain strict aseptic technique. Change gowns and gloves before embolization is performed. Keep working area sterile and free of blood.

4. Take extreme care not to contaminate diagnostic equipment (catheters, guidewires, or syringes) with embolic material. A separate sterile "interventional" table is useful because it allows separation of embolic material from the diagnostic catheters.

5. Embolization

a. Solids. Begin by occluding more peripheral branches with smaller embolic particles. Coils can be used if one desires to occlude the artery proximally and permanently. Coils also prevent the reflux of Gelfoam pledgets out of the target territory.

b. Liquids. Balloon occlusion catheter is necessary to avoid reflux and to control the flow of the agent.

6. Repeat arteriogram after embolization to estimate the degree of occlusion.

Postprocedure Management

1. Treatment of the postembolization syndrome. Virtually all patients experience, in varying degrees, symptoms of pain, nausea, vomiting, and fever (especially with Gelfoam). These symptoms tend to be self-limited. Therapy is supportive, including IV fluids, analgesia, and nasogastric (NG) tube if necessary. Symptoms usually resolve in 1–5 days.

2. Alert house staff and clinical staff to potential complications and expected course. The interventional radiologist should see the patient several times in the postembolization period and should offer support and suggestions for management.
3. Follow-up imaging may be necessary to document morphologic changes in the target region, organ, or tumor.

Results

1. Gastrointestinal bleeding (see Chap. 12); varicocele embolization (see Chap. 17).
2. Trauma. Large embolization experience at an inner-city trauma center with various types of injuries using various embolic agents had successful embolization of 82.2% of injuries [8].
3. Preoperative renal tumor embolization. Complete alcohol embolization significantly reduced the volume of blood transfused during nephrectomy for large hypervascular renal cell carcinomas [32].
4. Obstetric. Acute bleeding controlled in 8 of 9 patients [6].
5. Splenic embolization for hypersplenism. With carefully controlled infarction of 50–70%, 41 patients were successfully treated with no mortality. Complications were seen in 10 patients. An increase in platelet and WBC count was noted in the first postembolization day [49].
6. Pulmonary hemorrhage. Immediate control of bleeding in 75–90% of patients [2]. Twenty percent rebleed within 6 months.

Complications

1. **Pain** (moderate to severe) is experienced by many patients with infarction of a high percentage of organ volume. In addition to ischemia, this is likely related to organ capsule distention with edema. Paradoxically, repeat embolization may reduce pain.
2. **Infarction/ischemia of nontarget tissue**
   a. Thorax
      (1) Spinal cord injury/infarction during bronchial artery embolization, possibly from inadvertent embolization; one reported case causing paraplegia.
      (2) Loss of embolic material into systemic circulation.
   b. Liver
      (1) Hepatic infarction, with deaths reported after Gelfoam embolization [50]. Most deaths were in those with recent hemorrhagic shock from bleeding.
      (2) Parenchymal or intraperitoneal hemorrhage.
      (3) Portal vein thrombosis during transhepatic embolization of varices in 5 of 60 patients studied [51].
   c. Gallbladder. Infarction can occur during hepatic artery embolization for cancer.
   d. Stomach, duodenum. Unpredictable; gastric infarction is more likely in elderly patients with severe atherosclerosis or prior gastric surgery but overall is rare.

    e. Small bowel, large bowel. Therapeutic primary embolization is controversial because of the risk of bowel infarction. This risk must be weighed against the patient's condition. Generally, embolization is considered only after failure of vasopressin when surgery is contraindicated. Subselective catheter placement technique is mandatory, and even with such precautions, one series from five hospitals reports 3 of 23 cases (13%) required later surgery for acute bowel infarction [52].

    f. Urinary bladder. Infarction is uncommon, especially considering the frequency of pelvic embolizations for trauma [53].

    g. Peripheral nerve. Likely mechanism of injury is occlusion of the vasa nervosum; possible when Gelfoam powder or alcohol are used.

3. Postembolization abscess formation

    a. Spleen. Can effectively be prevented with antibiotic prophylaxis and scrupulous aseptic technique [49].

    b. Liver. Rare.

    c. Renal. Rare, reported in a patient with ongoing urinary tract infection [54].

4. Postembolization renal compromise. Renal failure and transient hypertension (lasting 24 hours) are well-recognized complications. Acute tubular necrosis may be secondary to large volumes of contrast.

5. Mechanical problems (e.g. coil migration, vessel dissection, subintimal material).

References

1. Rabkin JE, et al. Transcatheter embolization in the management of pulmonary hemorrhage. *Radiology* 163:361–365, 1987.
2. Stoll JF, Bettmann MA. Bronchial artery embolization to control hemoptysis: A review. *Cardiovasc Intervent Radiol* 11:263–269, 1988.
3. Uflacker R, et al. Bronchial artery embolization in the management of hemoptysis: Technical aspects and long term results. *Radiology* 157:637–644, 1985.
4. Hickey NM, et al. Percutaneous embolotherapy in threatening hemoptysis. *Cardiovasc Intervent Radiol* 11:270–273, 1988.
5. Tonkin ILD, et al. Bronchial artery and embolotheray for hemoptysis in patients with cystic fibrosis. *Cardiovasc Intervent Radiol* 14:241–246, 1991.
6. Mitty HA, et al. Obstetric hemorrhage: Prophylactic and emergency arterial catheterization and embolotherapy. *Radiology* 188:183–187, 1993.
7. Greenwood LH, et al. Obstetric and non-malignant gynecologic bleeding: Treatment with angiographic embolization. *Radiology* 164:155–159, 1987.
8. Panella T, et al. Percutaneous transcatheter embolization for arterial trauma. *J Vasc Surg* 2:54–64, 1985.
9. Rubin BE, Katzen BT. Selective hepatic artery embolization to control massive hepatic hemorrhage after trauma. *AJR* 129:253–256, 1977.

10. Sclafani SJA, Shaftan GW, McAuley J. Interventional radiology in the management of hepatic trauma. *J Trauma* 24:256–262, 1984.

11. Bass EM, Crosier JH. Percutaneous control of posttraumatic hepatic hemorrhage by Gelfoam embolization. *J Trauma* 17:61–63, 1977.

12. Sclafani SJA. Angiographic control of intraperitoneal hemorrhage caused by injuries to the liver and spleen. *Semin Intervent Radiol* 2:138–147, 1985.

13. Walter JF, Paaso BT, Cannon WB. Successful transcatheter embolic control of massive hematobilia secondary to liver biopsy. *AJR* 127:847–849, 1976.

14. Sclafani SJA. Angiographic hemostasis: Its role in the salvage of the injured spleen. *Radiology* 141:645–650, 1981.

15. Triller J, Krebs T, Ackermann D. Superselective embolization of traumatic renal pseudoaneurysm with a Tracker-18 catheter and microcoils. *Eur Radiol* 3–3:261, 1993.

16. Larsen DW, Pentecost MJ. Embolotherapy in renal trauma. *Semin Intervent Radiol* 9:13, 1992.

17. Eastham JA, et al. Angiographic embolization of renal stab wounds. *J Urol* 148:268–270, 1992.

18. Rosen RJ, Feldman L, Wilson AR. Embolization for postbiopsy renal arteriovenous fistula: Effective occlusion using homologous clot. *AJR* 131:1072–1073, 1978.

19. Eckstein MR, et al. Gastric bleeding: Intra-arterial vasopressin and transcatheter embolization. *Radiology* 152:643–646, 1984.

20. Waltman AC. Transcatheter embolization versus vasopressin infusion for the control of arteriocapillary gastrointestinal bleeding. *Cardiovasc Intervent Radiol* 3:289–297, 1980.

21. Encarnacion CE, et al. Gastrointestinal bleeding: Treatment with gastrointestinal arterial embolization. *Radiology* 183:505, 1992.

22. Guy GE, et al. Acute lower gastrointestinal hemorrhage: Treatment by superselective embolization with polyvinyl alcohol particles. *AJR* 159:521, 1992.

23. Lang EK, et al. Transcatheter embolization of hypogastric branch arteries in the management of intractable bladder hemorrhage. *J Urol* 121:30–36, 1979.

24. Athanasoulis CA, et al. Angiographic control of pelvic bleeding from treated carcinoma of the cervix. *Gynec Oncol* 4:144–150, 1976.

25. Mitchell ME, et al. Control of massive prostatic bleeding with angiographic techniques. *J Urol* 115:692–695, 1976.

26. Miller FJ Jr. et al. Selective arterial embolization for control of hemorrhage in pelvic malignancy: Femoral and brachial catheter approaches. *AJR* 126:1028–1032, 1976.

27. Pisco JM, Martins JM, Correia MG. Internal iliac artery: Embolization to control hemorrhage from pelvic neoplasms. *Radiology* 172:337–339, 1989.

28. Kaufman SL, et al. Transcatheter embolization in the management of congenital arteriovenous malformations. *Radiology* 137:21, 1980.

29. White RI Jr, et al. Pulmonary arteriovenous malformations: Technique and long-term outcome of embolotherapy. *Radiology* 169:663–669, 1988.

30. Rowe DM, et al. Osseous metastases from renal cell carcinoma:

Embolization and surgery for restoration of function. *Radiology* 150:673–676, 1984.

31. Dick HM, et al. Adjuvant arterial embolization in the treatment of benign primary bone tumors in children. *Clin Orthop* 139:133–144, 1979.

32. Bakal CW, et al. Value of preoperative renal artery embolization in reducing blood transfusion requirements during nephrectomy for renal cell carcinoma. *J Vasc Interv Radiol* 4:727–731, 1993.

33. Meyerovitz MF, et al. Preoperative uterine artery embolization in cervical pregnancy. *J Vasc Interv Radiol* 2:95, 1991.

34. Hickman MP, et al. Preoperative embolization of the spleen in children with hypersplenism. *J Vasc Interv Radiol* 3:647, 1992.

35. Therasse E, et al. Trancatheter chemoembolization of progressive carcinoid liver metastasis. *Radiology* 189:541, 1993.

36. Stokes KR, Stuart K, Clouse ME. Hepatic arterial chemoembolization for metastatic endocrine tumors. *J Vasc Interv Radiol* 4: 341, 1993.

37. Venook AP, et al. Chemoembolization for hepatocellular carcinoma. *J Clin Oncol* 8:1108–1114, 1990.

38. Vetter D, et al. Transcatheter oily chemoembolization in the management of advanced hepatocellular carcinoma in cirrhosis: Results of a western comparative study in 60 patients. *Hepatology* 13:427–433, 1991.

39. Chuang VP, et al. Arterial occlusion in the management of pain from metastatic renal carcinoma. *Radiology* 133:611–614, 1979.

40. Chiang V, et al. Arterial occlusion: Management of giant-cell tumor and aneurysmal bone cyst. *AJR* 136:1127–1130, 1981.

41. Kumpe DA, et al. Partial splenic embolization in children with hypersplenism. *Radiology* 155:357–362, 1985.

42. Grassi CJ, Boxt LB, Bettman MA. Partial splenic embolization for painful splenomegaly. *Cardiovasc Intervent Radiol* 10:291–294, 1987.

43. Quisling RG, et al. Histopathologic analysis of intra-arterial polyvinyl alcohol microemboli in rat cerebral cortex. *AJNR* 5:101–104, 1984.

44. Kunstlinger F, et al. Vascular occlusive agents *AJR* 136:151–156, 1981.

45. Greenfield AJ, Athanasoulis CA, Waltman AC. Transcatheter embolization: Prevention of embolic reflux using balloon catheters. *AJR* 131:165–168, 1978.

46. Barth KH, Strandberg JD, White RI Jr. Long-term follow-up of transcatheter embolization with autologous clot, oxcel, and Gelfoam in domestic swine. *Invest Radiol* 12:273–280, 1977.

47. Kaufman SL, Strandberg JD, Barth KH, White RI Jr. Transcatheter embolization with microfibrillar collagen in the swine. *Invest Radiol* 13:200–204, 1978.

48. Chow KJ, et al. Transcatheter embolization with sodium tetradecyl sulfate. Experimental and clinical results. *Radiology* 153:95–99, 1984.

49. Spigos DG, et al. Splenic embolization. *Cardiovasc Intervent Radiol* 3:282–288, 1980.

50. Trojanowski JQ, et al. Hepatic and splenic infarctions: Complication of therapeutic transcatheter embolization. *Am J Surg* 139: 272–277, 1980.

51. Widrich WC, Robbins AH, Nabseth DC. Transhepatic embolization of varices. *Cardiovasc Intervent Radiol* 3:298–307, 1980.
52. Rosenkrantz H, et al. Postembolic colonic infarction. *Radiology*
142:47–51, 1982.
53. Braf ZF, Koontz WW Jr. Gangrene of bladder. Complication of
hypogastric artery embolization. *Urology* 9:670–671, 1977.
54. Chuang VP, Wallace S. Current status of transcatheter management of neoplasm. *Cardiovasc Intervent Radiol* 3:256–267, 1980.

Percutaneous Intervention in Erectile Dysfunction

John E. Aruny

Penile Angiography

Indications

1. Evaluation of **ischemic erectile dysfunction** in men who are candidates for surgical revascularization or possible percutaneous angioplasty (see **1** under Preprocedure preparation).
2. Evaluation for possible therapeutic transcatheter embolization in patients with **high-flow priapism.**

Contraindications

A very small percentage of patients with erectile dysfunction are candidates for arteriographic evaluation. The contraindications for penile angiography are the same as for penile vascular surgery [1].

1. Long-standing diabetes mellitus.
2. Priapism in the past.
3. Peyronie's disease.
4. Age greater than 60.
5. Collagen vascular disease.

Ischemic Erectile Dysfunction

Preprocedure Preparation

1. **Preliminary evaluation criteria** will vary depending on the urologist's preferences. Patients should be screened with a group of tests which may include:
   a. **Psychometric asssessment** to exclude psychogenic causes of impotence.
   b. **Hormonal screening** to identify patients with depressed testosterone secretion as well as follicle-stimulating hormone and luteinizing hormone (FSH/LH) levels to distinguish between primary (gonadal) and secondary (hypothalamic) gonadal failure ($< 1\%$ of cases of erectile dysfunction).
   c. **PGE_1 test.** The injection of 20 µg of PGE_1 into the left corpus cavernosum, followed by visual sexual and masturbatory stimulation to evoke a rigid functional erection. When combined with history and physical (especially neurologic) examination, the PGE_1 test excludes neurologic causes for erectile dysfunction.
   d. **Screening tests** to assess penile arterial blood supply
      (1) Penile-brachial index (PBI; normal value ≥ 0.7) is the ratio of the systolic pressure within the

cavernosal arteries (determined with an inflatable cuff around the base of the penis and a Doppler probe) divided by the brachial systolic pressure.

(2) Nocturnal penile tumescence monitoring during sleep on three consecutive nights. Patients who have at least one 15 minute erectile episode on any of the three nights (characterized by greater than a 1.5 cm increase in penile circumference with more that 550 grams of axial rigidity) most likely have psychogenic erectile dysfunction, if hormonal and neurologic screening are normal.

(3) Color-assisted duplex ultrasound examination of the cavernosal arteries following the intracavernosal injection of 45 mg of papaverine. In our experience, peak systolic velocities of less than 35 cm/second (some investigators have used 30 cm/second) have been associated with significant arterial stenoses [2] in the internal iliac arterial system. Arteriography is useful for locating the exact site of the lesion(s). Patients with higher velocities, who are yet unable to attain an erection, should then be evaluated by pharmacocavernosometry to determine if incompetent draining veins are allowing rapid outflow (up to 50% of patients with erectile dysfunction in some series).

2. **Preparation for standard angiography.** Most studies can be done safely on outpatients. They are scheduled as the first case of the day in order to allow adequate time for postprocedure observation in the recovery unit. Patients are told to be prepared for possible stay overnight in case there is a problem or in the event that a balloon angioplasty is performed.

3. Place a Foley catheter to drain contrast, which may obscure the internal pudendal vessels, from the bladder. In addition, the catheter will provide support for the penis during manipulation for optimal imaging and to extend the vessels linearly to avoid kinking.

4. Begin administering anxiolytic drugs (e.g., diazepam, midazolam) early—preferably before entering the angiography suite. Fear and anxiety cause adrenergic stimulation which can cause spasm of the cavernosal arteries and be a cause of a false-positive examination.

5. Be prepared for possible balloon angioplasty of the iliac arteries and their larger branches.

Procedure

1. Retrograde common femoral artery access (preferably right) using sterile Seldinger technique. 5 Fr. catheters are preferred in order to minimize puncture-site caliber in outpatients. Arterial sheaths are used only if pericatheter leakage of blood is uncontrollable.

2. Barring specific indications for nonionic–low-osmolar contrast, conventional ionic contrast is used for the aortic and external iliac injections (see steps **3** and **4**). However, it is essential to use low-osmolar agents when selectively

injecting the internal pudendal artery in order to limit pain and minimize adrenergic vasospastic effects.

3. Obtain a single-plane frontal angiogram of the aortic bifurcation either with cut film or digital acquisition. This is performed with a 5 Fr. pigtail catheter placed just above the aortic bifurcation using standard methods. Evaluate the common iliac artery (CIA), external iliac artery (EIA), and internal iliac artery (IIA) circulaton, looking for stenoses and consequent shunting and collateral formation to the lower extremity, which may steal blood from the internal pudendal circulation. Patients with iliac steal syndrome have been treated successfully with balloon angioplasty [3–5].

4. If the iliac arteries do not contain significant stenoses, the catheter is exchanged for a 5 Fr. Berenstein catheter. Using a 0.035-in. angled Terumo wire, the catheter is advanced past the contralateral IIA into the EIA. A selective injection in the EIA is done to evaluate the inferior epigastric artery, which is the donor artery used for revascularization procedures.

5. The catheter is then withdrawn to the origin of the IIA. A 0.035-in. Wholey high-torque floppy guidewire (Advanced Cardiovascular Systems, Temecula, CA) is used to select the IIA and the catheter is then advanced. Position the penis by taping the Foley catheter to the contralateral thigh—make sure it is straight. The C-arm is then rotated into the ipsilateral 30-degree anterior oblique position. Using the "road map" feature of the digital angiography unit and a 5-ml contrast injection by hand, the anterior division of the IIA is identified.

6. Using the "road map" display, select the internal pudendal artery (IPA) with the Wholey wire and advance the Berenstein catheter to the origin. Test inject with approximately 3 ml of low-osmolar contrast to identify if the catheter has occluded the artery. If so, pull back the catheter to allow washout of contrast and inject at this location.

7. Pharmacoangiography. Inject 60 mg of papaverine into the corpus cavernosum with a 25-gauge needle approximately 5 minutes before the arterial injection. Attach a three-way stopcock to the Berenstein catheter with one port to the contrast injector and the other port for intraarterial injection of tolazoline (Priscoline). Dilute 25 mg of tolazoline with 10 ml of saline and inject over 30 seconds through the arterial catheter directly into the IPA immediately before contrast injection.

8. Filming program: 2 frames/second for 4 seconds, 1 frame/second for 4 seconds, and every other second for 10 seconds. Inject low-osmolar contrast at a rate of 2–4 ml/second for a total volume of 15–20 ml. Rate and volume will depend on the degree to which the catheter is selectively placed in the IPA and the flow that is observed on a hand-test injection.

9. The ipsilateral IIA is catheterized by forming a "Waltman's loop" with the Berenstein catheter. Advance the stiff end of the guidewire to the apex of the catheter (bend) at the aortic bifurcation, then advance the catheter-wire assem-

bly as a unit until the catheter tip is disengaged from the contralateral CIA. Having the catheter tip initially well into the contralateral iliac system facilitates the formation of generous loop within the aorta; if this is not done, a tight loop will kink the Berenstein catheter at the apex and prevent the passage of the guidewire or the injection of contrast. Remove the guidewire and point the catheter tip toward the ipsilateral CIA. Advance the Wholey wire to select this CIA in a anterograde manner and follow with the catheter.

10. Change the orientation of the penis by taping the Foley catheter to the opposite thigh, again making sure it is straight. Angle the C-arm 30 degrees in the ipsilateral anterior oblique projection and do a hand injection using the "road map" display to identify the anterior division of the IIA. Catheterize the IPA as described previously in step **6**. Contrast injection is again preceded by 25 mg tolazoline. However, it is not necessary to reinject intracavernosal papaverine.

11. Pull the catheter back into the ipsilateral EIA just above the puncture site and selectively inject at this location to opacify the ipsilateral inferior ipigastric artery.

Postprocedure Management

1. Standard postangiography and, if applicable, postangioplasty management.
2. Standard monitoring and evaluation criteria are used for potential same-day discharge (see Chap. 1, Outpatient Angiography).
3. Remove Foley catheter.
4. Evaluate the penis to confirm that it has returned to the flaccid state before the patient is discharged (see complications).

Results

1. The technical success rate for catheterizing of both IPAs from a single puncture site is over 95% in our experience. A technique of nonselective evaluation of the IPAs has been described [6]. However, this should not often be necessary, and there may be difficulties with vessel overlap and identification.
2. The importance of adequate sedation to limit anxiety, pain, and subsequent adrenergic stimulation with associated vasoconstriction cannot be overemphasized. Results should be interpreted with these factors taken into account when certain vascular territories are not demonstrated angiographically.
3. A thorough knowledge of the normal anatomy, including normal variants, is essential to the interpretation of results [7–9]. Anatomic variants are frequent—as in any small vascular territory. If the common penile artery or the origin of any of its branches is not seen during injection of the IPA, the catheter should be pulled back into the common anterior division of the IIA for a less selective

injection. The accessory IPA has been reported in 6–29% of internal iliac arteriograms [10,11]. It is often bilateral and can arise from the IIA, the obturator, or the ischial arteries, or from the proximal portion of the IPA [12].

4. The most common points of stenosis are where the IPAs penetrate the urogenital diaphragm, raising the question of external compression as an etiology of the stenosis. Also, this is the segment of the IPA most vulnerable to external straddle injuries and must be evaluated carefully in patients who relate a history of trauma. Angioplasty of small arterial branches has been noted to fail rapidly.

5. Diabetes produces two types of lesions:
   a. A nonspecific atheromatous obliterative lesion that occurs in the older patient.
   b. A generalized decrease in the caliber of the vessels, termed *hypoplastic arteries,* characteristic of the young diabetic [12].

Complications

1. Potential complications similar to those during angiography of small vessels (e.g., spasm, dissection).
2. Priapism following the injection of papaverine into the corpus cavernosum (more likely in younger patients). Therapy is direct irrigation of the corpus cavernosum with a solution of 1 mg of epinephrine diluted in 1 liter of saline.

High-Flow Priapism

Indications for Embolization

A large number of cases of high-flow priapism are due to perineal straddle injuries, resulting in arterial trauma and subsequent pseudoaneurysm formation [13]. Internal pudendal artery embolization should not be considered the first line of treatment for idiopathic priapism, as the following limited indications suggest.

1. Idiopathic priapism that does not respond to aspiration and irrigation of the corpus cavernosum with epinephrine and saline.
2. Idiopathic priapism that does not respond to a glandular-cavernosum shunt procedure.
3. Recurrent priapism shortly after successful detumescence by either indication **1.** or **2.** above.

Procedure

1. An arteriogram of the pelvis is performed to demonstrate increased flow to either the right or left IPAs. The side with increased flow is selected for embolization. If flow is equal, either side may be selected. Pseudoaneurysms are commonly seen in cases with prior local trauma.
2. Superselective catheterization of the culprit IPA is performed in a fashion similar to diagnostic angiography for

the evaluation of ischemic erectile dysfunction (see Ischemic Erectile Dysfunction).
3. Blood is aspirated and 10 ml is allowed to coagulate in a sterile basin. A volume of 3–6 ml of clot is injected into one IPA. Continued cavernosal irrigation is performed. If there is no response over 12–24 hours, the other IPA can be embolized in a similar fashion. Bilateral embolization should be limited to the most difficult cases.

Results

Several cases have been reported in which autologous clot has been used to embolize the IPA [14]. Autologous clot is at least partially reversible, and the intent is that potency can be maintained after the episode of priapism has subsided [15,16]. Results from large series are not presently available.

Complications

1. Penile gangrene can occur after bilateral embolization [17].
2. Inadvertent spillage of embolic material into the other branches of the hypogastric artery.
3. The standard complications of superselective catheter placement.

References

1. Sarlip ID. The role of vascular surgery in arteriogenic and combined arteriogenic and venogenic impotence. *Semin Urol* 8:129–137, 1990.
2. Benson C, Vickers MA, Aruny J. Evaluation of impotence. *Semin Ultrasound, CT, MR* 12:176–190, 1991.
3. Angelini P, Fighali S. Early experience with balloon angioplasty of internal iliac arteries for vasculogenic impotence. *Cathet Cardiovasc Diagn* 11:401, 1985.
4. Goldwasser B, et al. Impotence due to the pelvic steal syndrome: Treatment by iliac transluminal angioplasty. *J Urol* 133:860–861, 1985.
5. Van Unnik JG, Marsman JWP. Impotence due to the external iliac steal syndrome treated by percutaneous transluminal angioplasty. *J Urol* 131:544–545, 1984.
6. Schwartz AN, Freidenberg D, Harley J. Nonselective angiography after intracorporal papaverine injection: An alternative technique for evaluating penile arterial integrity. *Radiology* 167:249–253, 1988.
7. Bookstein JJ, Lang EV. Penile magnification pharmacoarteriography: Details of intrapenile arterial anatomy. *AJR* 148:883–888, 1987.
8. Bookstein JJ. Penile angiography: The last angiographic frontier. *AJR* 150:47–54, 1988.
9. Rosen MP, et al. Arteriogenic impotence: Findings in 195 impotent men examined with selective internal pudendal angiography. *Radiology* 174:1043–1048, 1990.
10. Rosen MP, et al. Radiologic assessment of impotence: Angiogra-

phy, sonography, cavernosography, and scintigraphy. *AJR* 157: 923–931, 1991.

11. Curet P, et al. Technical and anatomic factors in filling of distal portion of internal pudendal artery during arteriography. *Urology* 29:333–338, 1987.

12. Juhan CM, Padula G, Huget JH. Angiography in Male Impotence. In AH Bennett (ed.), *Management of Male Impotence*. Baltimore: Williams & Wilkins, 1982. P. 79.

13. Witt MA, et al. Traumatic laceration of intracavernosal arteries: The pathophysiology of non-ischemic, high-flow, arterial priapism. *J Urol* 143:129–132, 1990.

14. Walker TG, et al. "High flow" priapism: Treatment with super-selective transcatheter embolization. *Radiology* 174:1053–1054, 1990.

15. Belgrano E, et al. Percutaneous temporary embolization of the internal pudendal arteries in idiopathic priapism: Two additional cases. *J Urol* 131:756–758, 1983.

16. Wear JB, Crummy AB, Munson BO. A new approach to the treatment of priapism. *J Urol* 117:252–254, 1976.

17. Burt FB, Schirmer HK, Scott WW. A new concept in the management of priapism. *J Urol* 83:60, 1960.

Systemic and Portal Venous Procedures

Percutaneous Placement of Inferior Vena Cava Filters

Clement J. Grassi

Indications

ABSOLUTE

1. Contraindication to anticoagulant therapy in patients with known pulmonary emboli or significant deep venous thrombosis (DVT) [1–3].
2. Failure of anticoagulation. Patients with recurrent pulmonary emboli despite adequate anticoagulation [1–3].
3. Complications of anticoagulation. Patients with a complication of previously instituted anticoagulant therapy, such as:
   a. Intracranial or central nervous system (CNS) hemorrhage.
   b. Gastrointestinal or retroperitoneal hemorrhage.
   c. Heparin-induced thrombocytopenia [4].

RELATIVE

1. Large free-floating iliofemoral or inferior vena cava (IVC) thrombus [5].
2. Progression or extension of DVT despite adequate anticoagulant therapy [6].
3. Failure of an indwelling IVC filter (i.e., patients with recurrent pulmonary emboli where abnormality of an existing filter is discovered); if anticoagulation is contraindicated, a second filter should be added [7].
4. Patients undergoing pulmonary embolectomy surgery, especially those with severe bilateral pulmonary embolism [8].
5. Patients with chronic pulmonary hypertension and cor pulmonale with prior pulmonary embolism—individuals who may not survive further embolic episodes [8,9].
6. Situations where long-term anticoagulant therapy is problematic (e.g., patients with syncope, elderly patients with unsteady gait).

PROPHYLACTIC* PLACEMENT

1. Prophylactic placement in high-risk, immobilized patients (e.g., postoperative hip and knee [10], neurosurgical), or those with multiple pelvic trauma [11] can be considered on an individualized basis until temporary filters, which are better suited for this role, are available.
2. Preoperative prophylactic placement of permanent filters is controversial. It has been advocated for some patients

---

*The definition of the term *prophylaxis* varies in the literature according to the author. As used here, it refers to placement of a filter in a patient who is at increased risk for venous thromboembolic disease, but has no documented clot within the extremity deep veins or the pulmonary arteries.

(hip, knee, spine surgery) [9]. Temporary filters, when available, are the device of choice.

Contraindications (to percutaneous filter insertion)

ABSOLUTE

1. Severe blood coagulopathy, or coagulopathy unresponsive to therapy which may predispose the patient to bleeding from the puncture site (surgical venotomy and closure preferred).
2. Patients who cannot or will not comply with postprocedure rest orders, especially with a 24-Fr. system (surgical venotomy and closure preferred).

RELATIVE

1. Young patients with long life expectancy (traditionally, the use of permanent filters has been discouraged in such patients since there is limited information on the distant long-term sequelae). Temporary or retrievable filters may be indicated in the future.
2. Patients in early pregnancy. Fetal susceptibility to radiation exposure is highest.
3. Obstructive thrombus along all available routes of insertion, an uncommon occurrence.*

Preprocedure Preparation

1. **Prior imaging review.** Radionuclide perfusion-ventilation scan, pulmonary arteriogram, venous US, or venogram. A diligent effort should be made to objectively document the presence of thrombus. Objective medical indications, rather than the recent reduction in the size of introduction systems and simplification of insertion technology, should dictate the need for filter placement [7].
2. **Patients with suspected failure of prior indwelling filter.** Screen with an imaging study (e.g., CT with contrast, flow-sensitive MRI, color-flow US) to determine if the current filter and IVC are occluded. This information also will help to determine the site of access for the diagnostic cavogram and insertion of a second IVC filter, if needed. This approach saves steps, and unnecessary additional punctures.
3. **Obtain informed consent** from patient, guardian, or proxy (see Table 15-1).
4. **Laboratory check.** As guidelines: PT ($\leq$ 15 seconds), PTT close to control, platelets (> 100,000/μl or platelet transfusion on-hand), Hgb/Hct, WBC, BUN, Cr.
5. **Heparinized patient.** Stop heparin infusion approximately 4 hours prior to puncture; check PTT (at most

---

*Often, one route (e.g., right internal or external jugular vein) can be identified by ultrasound (US) or venography. Another option is to use the small Simon nitinol filter system (7 Fr., 9 Fr.), which can be placed via the antecubital vein access.

Table 15-1. Guidelines for timing of IVC filter placement as per Jones, Barnes, and Greenfield [3] after documented acute episode of PE or DVT*

Place within 24 hours
  Patients with acute pulmonary embolism in whom anticoagulation either is contraindicated or has failed. For patients with positive diagnostic pulmonary angiography, a filter should be placed immediately at the time of the procedure
  Patients with PE or high-risk DVT (e.g., free-floating iliofemoral thrombus) for whom anticoagulation is inadequate therapy by itself

Place within 48 hours
  Patients with DVT in whom anticoagulation is contraindicated or has failed

Elective
  Anticoagulation contraindicated in a patient at high risk for PE or DVT

PE = pulmonary embolism; DVT = deep venous thrombosis.
*Clinical judgment must be used according to the specific patient circumstances.

1.2 × control or activated clotting time of ≤ 200) (see General Principles in Chap. 1).

6. **Warfarinized patient.** As a guideline, PT ≤ 15 seconds is acceptable (see General Principles in Chap. 1). Reverse PT with fresh-frozen plasma, if necessary.

7. **Pre- and intraprocedural medication** at angiography suite. Midazolam (Versed) 1–2 mg IV, fentanyl 50 μg IV, or other sedative/analgesic of choice. Monitor vital signs and adjust maintenance doses accordingly.

8. **Lead radiopaque scale.** Can be useful as a guide to placement location and measurement of IVC diameter.

Procedure Steps for All Filters

1. Imaging of the IVC. Catheter access can be obtained by the femoral or jugular vein approach, preferably with a single-wall puncture technique [7] using an open-ended needle. If the access route is not obstructed by thrombus (determined by US or contrast test injection), a pigtail catheter or similar flush injection catheter can be used for the inferior vena cavogram (IVC-gram). Many angiographers position the pigtail catheter in the IVC above the iliac vein bifurcation; some angiographers place the pigtail catheter across the iliac vein bifurcation within the left iliac vein proper in order to exclude the possibility of an anomalous left IVC. Contrast injection of 18–20 ml/second, 36–40 ml total volume is used.

2. Check the IVC-gram for the following:
   a. Presence of significant thrombus.
   b. Location of the renal veins (commonly at the L1–L2 vertebral level); the optimal location of the filter's apex

is just at the level of the most inferior renal vein. At this point the venous flow rates are highest due to the confluence of the renal outflow and IVC return; such placement avoids venous stasis and facilitates dissolution of entrapped thrombus by the intrinsic lytic system.

    c. Infrarenal IVC diameter. The manufacturers' recommended maximum vena caval diameter for the Titanium Greenfield, Simon nitinol, Vena Tech, and stainless steel Greenfield filters is 28 mm (adjusted for film magnification). The Gianturco-Roehm bird's nest filter has a recommended maximum diameter of up to 40 mm; consequently, it is suitable for IVC diameters in the 29–40 mm range as well.

    d. Anatomic anomalies. E.g., double inferior vena cavae necessitate a filter in each IVC.

3. Use the spine as a reference for the renal vein level, or mark the location of the lowest renal vein with a radiopaque marker. A radiopaque ruler or scale may also be used; tape it onto the table under the patient prior to sterile preparation and draping.

4. Prepare the filter according to the manufacturer's directions. The reader is referred to the specific product directions. Users should be proficient with insertion and deployment of the filter (practice with models and review videotapes) and attain familiarity by first observing or assisting in procedures. In this way, difficulties can be avoided during actual filter placement.

5. Following filter insertion, a plain film of the abdomen is obtained for documenting its position. An IVC-gram obtained on completion of the procedure is useful for evaluation of filter patency.

6. Remove the introducer/sheath system from the patient. Compress the puncture site for 10–15 minutes.

**Procedural Suggestions and Technical Tips
for Specific Filters**

The reader is referred to each device's "Instructions for Use" from the manufacturer for complete descriptions of the steps for placement. The U.S. Food and Drug Administration (FDA) has approved the following five devices:

    1. Gianturco-Roehm bird's nest filter (BNF), (Cook, Inc.; Bloomington, IN).

    2. Simon nitinol filter (SNF), (Nitinol Medical Technologies, Woburn, MA, and Bard Inc., Billerica, MA).

    3. Stainless steel Greenfield filter (SSGF), (Medi-Tech/Boston Scientific, Watertown, MA).

    4. Titanium Greenfield filter (TGF), (Medi-Tech/Boston Scientific Corp., Watertown, MA).

    5. Vena Tech filter (VTF), (B. Braun Medical Division, Evanston, IL).

The following are additional technical suggestions which may or may not be applicable to all situations.

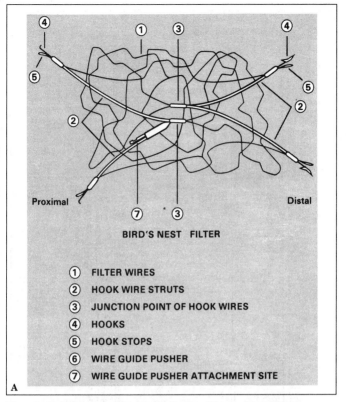

A

BIRD'S NEST FILTER

① FILTER WIRES
② HOOK WIRE STRUTS
③ JUNCTION POINT OF HOOK WIRES
④ HOOKS
⑤ HOOK STOPS
⑥ WIRE GUIDE PUSHER
⑦ WIRE GUIDE PUSHER ATTACHMENT SITE

Fig. 15-1. The Gianturco-Roehm bird's nest filter and introduction system. A. Bird's nest filter. B. Filter components. C. Cross-section of filter catheter with a preloaded filter. (Courtesy of Cook, Inc., Bloomington, IN.)

Free-form Filters (Figs. 15-1 and 15-2)

GIANTURCO-ROEHM BIRD'S NEST FILTER

1. When placing the BNF within the IVC, deploy the initial (superior) V-strut and fix with a slight to-and-fro motion; minimal manual force is required.
2. Avoid wire prolapse. Withdraw the filter/catheter back 4–6 cm (vs. 1–3 cm), but not inferior to the iliac vein bifurcation. This will provide room for the filter mesh formation within the vena cava, and helps to avoid wire prolapse superiorly.
3. Avoid potential entanglement of the tip of the filter metal pusher with the wire mesh. Following deployment of the final (inferior) V-strut within the vena cava, *slowly readvance the catheter/sheath assembly* to the base of the V-strut, and withdraw the central metal pusher within the catheter. This step ensures that the plastic catheter,

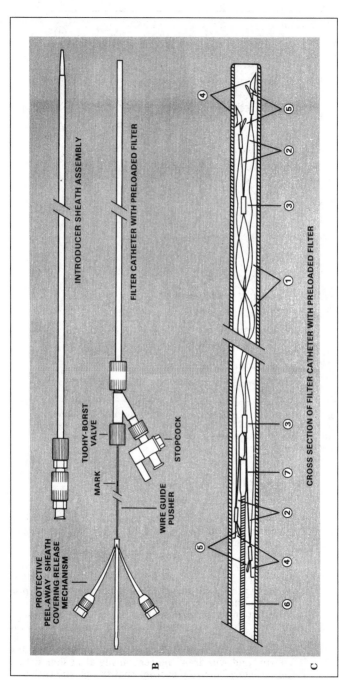

B

PROTECTIVE PEEL-AWAY SHEATH COVERING RELEASE MECHANISM

INTRODUCER SHEATH ASSEMBLY

FILTER CATHETER WITH PRELOADED FILTER

TUOHY-BORST VALVE

STOPCOCK

MARK

WIRE GUIDE PUSHER

C

CROSS SECTION OF FILTER CATHETER WITH PRELOADED FILTER

Fig. 15-1 (continued)

not the wire tip, passes by the mesh, preventing entanglement and potential scraping of the wall.

Fixed-form Filters

GREENFIELD TITANIUM FILTER/STAINLESS STEEL
GREENFIELD FILTER

1. Asymmetric leg opening. Occurs more frequently with the TGF than with the SSGF. The foot processes appear grouped or "crossed" on a frontal view of the IVC.
2. Suggestions to avoid asymmetric leg opening
   a. Flush the introducer frequently, preferably with continuous infusion of heparinized saline from a pressurized bag. If small amounts of thrombus form within the capsule around the filter legs, this may affect leg opening on release.
   b. An abrupt change in diaphragmatic position during deployment may perturb the TGF, allowing legs to contact one side of the IVC wall prematurely. Have the patient practice holding his or her breath at a comfortable level of inspiration. Prior to deploying the filter, instruct the patient to hold the breath as practiced. Having the patient perform a slight Valsalva maneuver during deployment will distend the IVC, increasing the room within the lumen and potentially avoiding asymmetric deployment.
3. If TGF filter legs appear "crossed" on the AP vena cavogram
   a. Obtain a plain film or fluoroscopy of the patient in a frontal projection with 30-degree craniocaudal angulation; in many cases the legs are not actually crossed, but superimposed or asymmetrically distributed [12].
   b. If leg hook crossing has occurred, be cautious before manipulating the filter with an angiographic catheter. Although improved leg position can be technically achieved, undesired caudal displacement of the filter has been reported in three cases [13]. Such unintended filter malposition often necessitates placement of a second filter.

SIMON NITINOL FILTER

1. "Caudal drop" of the SNF. Described originally as a technical problem with the SNF, in which the filter dropped inferiorly approximately 2–3 cm from the intended placement level [14,15]. Some operators have advocated correcting this inadvertent filter movement during unsheathing with a slight forward advancement of the pusher wire [15]. However, with experience, the angiographer will note that such "caudal drop" mainly occurs with larger diameter vena cavae. The forewarned operator can easily unsheath the filter dome, readjust the filter's infrarenal IVC position, and after readjustment, continue to unsheath the SNF feet for final deployment and fixation.
2. SNF 7 Fr. internal diameter/9 Fr. outer diameter size is the

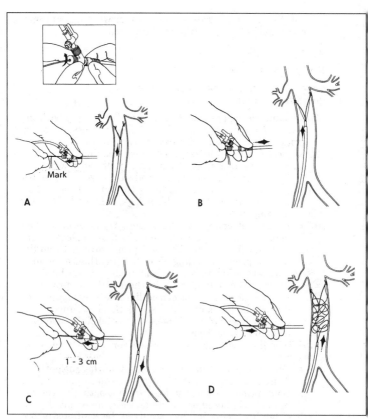

Fig. 15-2. A. After positioning of the 12 Fr. sheath/dilator appratus, the 12 Fr. dilator and guidewire are removed. The 11 Fr. introduction catheter is advanced fully and locked to the 12 Fr. sheath. Proximal struts are positioned below the renal orifices. The Tuohy-Borst valve securing the guidewire pusher is loosened. With the pusher wire fixed in a stationary position, the sheath catheter assembly is withdrawn to the suture tie or dark mark, as shown. This releases the proximal struts. B. Proximal struts are "set" with a 1–3 mm forward-backward motion. C. Introduction catheter/sheath assembly is withdrawn over the pusher wire 1–5 cm before filter discharge. D. Filter wires are discharged by slowly advancing the guidewire pusher into the stationary catheter/sheath assembly. The guidewire pusher is advanced until the proximal junction point of the distal struts is visualized in a distal end of the introduction catheter/ sheath. E. Entire wire guide pusher/catheter/sheath assembly is advanced until junction points overlap 1–3 cm. F. Distal struts are released by fully withdrawing catheter sheath assembly over stationary wire guide pusher. G. Distal prongs are set by a 1–3 mm forward–backward motion of the entire assembly. H. After carefully removing the protective peel-away sheath from the covering release mechanism, the filter is manually released. With one hand, the guidewire pusher is firmly grasped, and, with the other hand, the knob end is fully depressed to release the filter. Release should be confirmed fluoroscopically. (Courtesy of Cook, Inc., Bloomington, IN.)

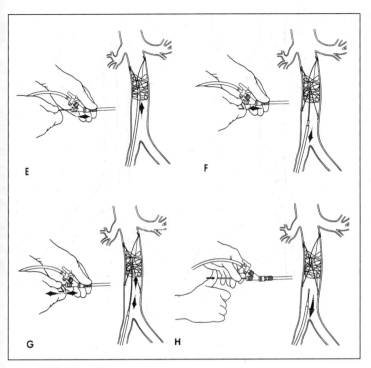

Fig. 15-2 (continued)

smallest introducer size available. Insertion by subclavian and antecubital vein access is possible.

VENA TECH FILTER (Fig. 15-3)

Incomplete opening and tilting. Modifications recently have been made in the side-rail length and leg chamber to avoid uneven contact with the IVC wall, potentially avoiding this problem.

Postprocedure Management

1. Bed rest for 6–8 hours is recommended.
2. If clinically needed (i.e., leg DVT) heparin may be restarted in 6–8 hours if there are no puncture-site bleeding or other complications.
3. Check pulses distal to the puncture site q15min for 1 hour, q30min for the next hour, and q1h for the next 2 hours.
4. Follow other pertinent postangiography orders (see Chap. 1).
5. Return the "product registration" material card by mail to the manufacturer. By federal requirements, all perma-

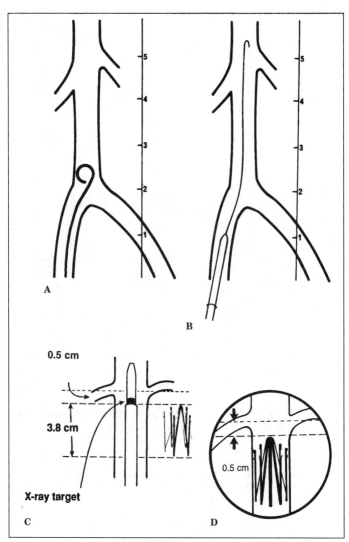

Fig. 15-3. Transfemoral placement of a Vena Tech IVC filter. A. An inferior vena cavogram is performed using a 5 Fr. pigtail catheter positioned above the iliac vein confluence. The right iliac vein and IVC are noted to be patent. The IVC diameter is measured (must be ≤ 28 mm), anatomic variants are ruled out, and renal veins are identified. B. The catheter is exchanged for a 0.038-in. J-guidewire, track dilatation is performed as needed, and the filter introducer is advanced. C. The filter capsule is introduced to below the renal veins, and, with the Vena Tech filter, the metallic marker (x-ray target) is positioned approximately 0.5 cm below the renal veins. In so doing, the 3.8-cm-long filter will be correctly positioned inferior to the renal veins. D. The filter is deployed and the introducer is removed; the groin is compressed for 10–15 minutes.

nently implanted medical devices must now be documented and registered.

Results

1. Vena caval filters can be placed percutaneously in the majority of patients in whom access is available, with technical success rates in the 95–100% range, depending on the specific device and the experience of the operator [16].
2. Although there are variations between devices and studies, the incidence of recurrent pulmonary embolism ranges between 3% and 6%, depending on length of follow-up [7,16]. The reader is referred to long-term clinical and radiographic follow-up data [16].

Complications

RELATED TO PERCUTANEOUS VENOUS ENTRY

1. Femoral vein thrombosis: 2–33% [17–21]. Early investigation of the incidence of procedure-related femoral vein thrombosis (puncture site) showed a 33% rate with in situ sonography [17]. Subsequent studies have shown rates of access-site thrombosis (AST), after placement of a 24 Fr. SSGF, of 14% [18] and 19% [19]. It was anticipated that with the new low-profile 12–14 Fr. filter, rates of AST would be lower. In 60 of 81 patients studied by US (either BNF, TGF, or VTF) 10% developed occlusive AST, 25% developed asymptomatic nonocclusive AST, and only 3% developed symptoms related to AST [20]. The BNF shows a 2% prevalence of femoral vein occlusion [21]. These studies [20,21] indicate that the risk of femoral vein thrombosis has not been eliminated, but it has been substantially lowered with the low-profile introduction systems.
2. Venous hemorrhage at puncture site: 5% or less [22].
3. Arteriovenous fistula, delayed: 1–3% [23].
4. Extraperitoneal hematoma: 2% [24].
5. Air embolism. Rare—associated with the right internal jugular vein approach and improper technique.

RELATED TO FILTER OR VENOUS THROMBOEMBOLISM*

1. Filter malposition. Varies with the device, 1–10% [2,7, 14,24–26].
2. Filter migration. Less than 1% in most series [14,25,26].
3. Recurrent pulmonary embolism: 5% or less; up to 3% can be fatal [27].
4. Vena caval occlusion/thrombosis: 3–9% [14,24–26,28].
5. Vena caval perforation: 1%; focal leg or strut penetration of the caval wall; although this may occur more frequently, it is usually asymptomatic.

*The following percentages are best used for approximate comparison. The reader should be aware that exact comparison of filter morbidity can be problematic since the quality of clinical data is quite variable [7], and is not always confirmed by imaging studies.

References

1. Goldhaber SZ, Grassi CJ. Management of Pulmonary Embolism. In DC Sabeston (ed.), *Textbook of Surgery* (8th ed.). Philadelphia: Saunders, 1990. Pp. 115–127.
2. Greenfield LJ. Current indications for and results of Greenfield filter placement. *J Vasc Surg* 1:502–504, 1984.
3. Jones TK, Barnes RW, Greenfield LJ. Greenfield vena caval filter: Rationale and current indications. *Ann Thorac Surg* 42:548–555, 1987.
4. Silver D, Kapsch DH, Tsoi EKM. Heparin-induced thrombocytopenia, thrombosis and hemorrhage. *Ann Surg* 198:301–305, 1983.
5. Norris C, Greenfield L, Hermanson J. Free-floating iliofemoral thrombosis: a risk of pulmonary embolism. *Arch Surg* 120:806–808, 1985.
6. Grassi CJ. Inferior Vena Caval Interruption. In SZ Goldhaber (ed.), *Prevention of Venous Thromboembolism.* New York: Marcel Dekker, 1993. Pp. 315–342.
7. Grassi CJ. Inferior vena caval filters: Analysis of five currently available devices. *AJR* 156:813–821, 1991.
8. Stewart JR, Greenfield LJ. Transvenous venal caval filtration and pulmonary embolectomy. *Surg Clin North Am* 62:411–430, 1982.
9. Golueke PJ, et al. Interruption of the vena cava by means of the Greenfield filter: Expanding the indications. *Surgery* 103:111–117, 1988.
10. Vaughn BK, et al. Use of the Greenfield filter to prevent fatal pulmonary embolism associated with total hip and knee arthroplasty. *J Bone Joint Surg* 71(A):1542–1547, 1989.
11. Webb LX, et al. Greenfield filter prophylaxis of pulmonary embolism in patients undergoing surgery for acetabular fracture. *J Orthop Trauma* 6:139–145, 1992.
12. Greenfield LJ, Cho KH (eds.). *Product Instructions: The Titanium Greenfield Vena Cava Filter and 12 French Introducer Systems.* Watertown, MA: Boston Scientific Corp., 1990. P. 50.
13. Sweeney TJ, Van Aman ME. Deployment problems with the Titanium Greenfield filter. *J Vasc Interv Radiol* 4:691–694, 1993.
14. Simon M, et al. Simon Nitinol inferior vena cava filter: Initial clinical experience. *Radiology* 172:99–103, 1989.
15. Kastan DJ, Forcier NJ, Kahn ML. Simon nitinol vena cava filter: Preliminary observations and suggested procedural modifications. *J Vasc Interv Radiol* 2:123–124, 1991.
16. Ferris EJ, et al. Percutaneous inferior vena cava filters: Follow-up of seven designs in 320 patients. *Radiology* 188:851–856, 1993.
17. Pais SO, et al. Percutaneous insertion of the Greenfield inferior vena cava filter: Experience with 96 patients. *J Vasc Surg* 8:460–464, 1988.
18. Dorfman GS, et al. Iatrogenic changes at the venotomy site after percutaneous placement of the Greenfield filter. *Radiology* 173:159–162, 1989.
19. Mewissen MW, et al. Thrombosis at venous insertion sites after inferior vena cava filter placement. *Radiology* 173:155–157, 1989.
20. Molgard CP, et al. Access-site thrombosis after placement of inferior vena filters with 12–14 F delivery sheaths. *Radiology* 185:257–261, 1992.
21. Hicks ME, et al. Prevalence of local venous thrombosis after trans-

femoral placement of a bird's nest vena caval filter. *J Vasc Interv Radiol* 1:63–68, 1990.

22. Grassi CJ, Rogoff P, Bettmann MA. Complications and pitfalls in transfemoral filter insertion. Presented at the 35th Annual Meeting of the Association of University Radiologists; Charleston, SC: March 1987. Abstract.

23. Grassi CJ, et al. Femoral arteriovenous fistula after placement of a Kimray-Greenfield filter. *AJR* 151:681–682, 1988.

24. Rose BS, et al. Percutaneous transfemoral placement of the Kimray-Greenfield vena cava filter. *Radiology* 165:373–376, 1987.

25. Ricco J, et al. Percutaneous transvenous caval interruption with the "LGM" filter: Early results of a multicenter trial. *Ann Vasc Surg* 3:242–247, 1988.

26. Roehm JOF, et al. The Bird's Nest inferior vena cava filter: Progress report. *Radiology* 168:745–749, 1988.

27. Geisinger MA, Zelch MG, Risino B. Recurrent pulmonary embolism after Greenfield filter placement. *Radiology* 165:383–384, 1987.

28. Grassi CJ, Matsumoto AH, Teitelbaum GP. Vena caval occlusion after Simon Nitinol filter placement: MRI demonstration in patients with malignancy. *J Vasc Interv Radiol* 3:535–539, 1992.

Transjugular Intrahepatic Portosystemic Shunt

John E. Aruny

Indications

ESTABLISHED BENEFIT

Patients with portal hypertension and variceal hemorrhage who have failed endoscopic variceal sclerotherapy [1] (i.e., sclerotherapy failed to control acute bleeding or there have been at least two episodes of rebleeding with repeated sclerotherapy, with each episode requiring blood transfusion)

POTENTIAL BENEFIT

1. Portal decompression prior to surgery [1–3].
2. Hepatorenal syndrome.
3. Intractable ascites.
4. Budd-Chiari syndrome [4].

Contraindications (Relative)

1. Portal vein thrombosis.
2. Significant pressure gradient between the hepatic veins and the right atrium that cannot be resolved with balloon angioplasty or surgery. These gradients may be caused by
   a. Inferior vena cava (IVC) narrowing secondary to hepatic parenchymal tumor (hepatoma or metastases)
   b. Hypernephroma growing into the IVC, or
   c. Lymphoma causing external compression of the IVC.

Preprocedure Preparation

1. Obtain informed consent. This procedure remains investigational as of this writing. A protocol for performing this procedure should be filed in advance with the Internal Review Board of your hospital.
2. Standard preparation for angiography, including ECG, oxygen saturation, and hemodynamic monitoring.
3. Replace blood loss adequately.
4. Place a Foley catheter in the bladder.
5. Prior to attempting a transhepatic puncture, it is helpful to opacify the portal venous system (PVS) with either hepatic wedge portography or arterial portography (via injection of the superior mesenteric and splenic arteries and delayed filming to capture the portal phase). This may be performed several days prior to shunt placement, if the patient is stable, or at the same session if the shunt is placed on an emergency basis. Color ultrasound (US) examination may be useful for determining portal vein patency and its relationship to the hepatic vein, but it is seldom useful for real-time guidance during transhepatic puncture of the portal vein.

6. Attempt to reverse coagulopathy (optional). Opinions vary regarding this since the risk of procedure-related bleeding appears to be low [1–3,5].
  a. The overwhelming majority of these patients will have coagulation disorders. The PT on initial presentation may be 20 seconds or higher. Two units of fresh-frozen plasma may be given prior to the procedure. A third and fourth unit may be given during the procedure. Often, a PT of approximately 15 seconds is the best that can be achieved, even with agressive therapy.
  b. Vitamin K, 25–50 mg IM, may be administered.
  c. Patients may be severely thrombocytopenic. Patients with counts of less than 50,000 μ/ml probably should receive platelet transfusion. Platelets are usually administered in an even number of units (2, 4, 6, etc.). They will be quickly sequestered in the enlarged spleen of these patients and therefore should be administered at the time of highest risk for bleeding. This is at the time of jugular vein and PV puncture as well as when the sheath is removed.
7. Preprocedure antibiotics are often already being administered by the referring service. If not, Cefotetan (Cefotan) 2 gm IV may be administered immediately prior to the procedure (optional, if the jugular sheath is removed immediately after the procedure).
8. A large percentage (70–80%) of patients will have ascites, which will be relieved by a successfully placed shunt within 3 weeks [1,5]. Paracentesis immediately prior to the procedure is not necessary, and it carries the added risk of peritonitis.
9. Assemble required components
  a. Micropuncture Coaxial Access set, Colapinto-Ring hepatic access set (Cook, Inc., Bloomington, IN).
  b. Palmaz Stents (Johnson & Johnson, Warren, NJ) or Wallstents (Schneider, Minneapolis, MN).
  c. 0.035-in. Amplatz Super Stiff and angled Glidewires (Medi-Tech, Watertown, MA).
  d. 5 Fr. Cobra-2 catheter.
  e. Appropriate balloon angioplasty catheters.

Procedure

1. The preferred access is via the right internal jugular vein by the anterior approach. The right external and left internal jugular veins also may be used. A directed US examination will quickly confirm the patency and location of the vein (behind the sternocleidomastoid muscle). Choose a point halfway between the insertion of this muscle on the clavicle and the angle of the mandible for puncture. Thoroughly sterilize the puncture site and ajacent skin. Use 1% lidocaine for local anesthesia at this point. Locate the pulsation of the right internal carotid artery and pull the artery medially with gentle traction to the skin. Enter the vein with a 5-cc syringe attached to a 22-gauge needle that is part of the Micropuncture Coaxial Access set. Direct the needle toward the ipsilateral nipple while performing gentle aspiration. Strong blood return with gentle aspiration indicates the position of the needle tip within the vein. Insert the guidewire and advance the coaxial dilator. Remove the inner portion of the dilator and insert a 0.035-in. guidewire past the right atrium into the IVC.

2. Advance a 5 Fr. Cobra end-hole catheter over the wire into the IVC and measure pressures from the IVC to the right atrium.

3. Enter the right (or largest middle) hepatic vein with the 5 Fr. Cobra catheter, advancing it over a 0.035-in. angled Glidewire (Medi-Tech, Watertown, MA). Measure hepatic wedge and right hepatic vein pressures. Obtain a hepatic venogram.

4. Exchange the Glidewire for a 0.035-in. Amplatz Super Stiff guidewire (Medi-Tech, Watertown, MA), placing its tip in the distal hepatic vein. Remove the 5 Fr. catheter and advance the 35 cm, 10 Fr. sheath supplied with the Colapinto-Ring hepatic access set into the selected hepatic vein.

5. Advance the Colapinto needle (16-gauge) over the wire (the stiff guidewire and the reverse bevel of the Colapinto needle protect the sheath from damage) until its tip protrudes out of the sheath.

6. Remove the guidewire and pull back the sheath inside the hepatic vein; the venous puncture site should be approximately 2 cm from the IVC-hepatic vein junction. Using the indicator (arrow) on the needle hub as a guide, turn the needle counter-clockwise (looking in the direction of the patient's head-to-feet) pointing it anteriorly toward a right portal vein branch.

7. Portal vein puncture can be difficult and time-consuming. Forcefully advance the needle through the hard cirrhotic parenchyma to enter the portal vein 1–3 cm peripheral to its bifurcation. Aspirate the needle as it is slowly withdrawn. When blood is aspirated, inject contrast to confirm the position of the needle tip within the lumen of the portal vein.

8. The choice of the guidewire that is advanced into the portal vein varies. A 0.035-in. floppy-tip guidewire is supplied with the introducer set. Alternatively, a 0.035-in. high-torque floppy-tip wire such as the Wholey guidewire (Advanced Cardiovascular Systems, Temecula, CA) may be used.

9. Advance a 5 Fr. catheter across the hepatic parenchyma into the portal vein. This may require considerable force (Fig. 16-1). If the catheter will not cross the hardened liver parenchyma, predilate the tract with a 4 mm angioplasty balloon and reintroduce the 5 Fr. catheter.

10. Measure portal pressure and calculate portal vein to right atrial pressure gradient. Perform a portal venogram, paying special attention to the splenic vein, dilated coronary vein(s), and varices.

11. Reintroduce the Super Stiff 0.035-in. guidewire and remove the 5 Fr. catheter. Then dilate the tract with a 10-mm diameter low-profile balloon catheter (Fig. 16-2).

12. Stent the tract formed in the parenchyma with either a

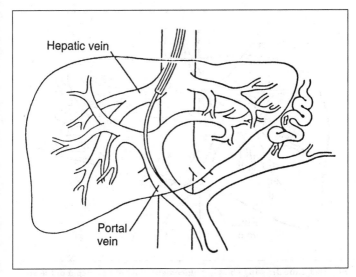

Fig. 16-1. Line drawing showing the 5 Fr. catheter passed over the guidewire from the right hepatic vein across the liver parenchyma into the right portal vein. (From G. Zemel et al. Technical advances in transjugular intrahepatic portosystemic shunts. *Radiographics* 12:615–622, 1992.)

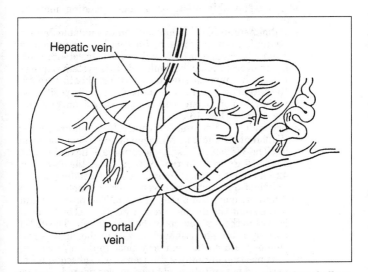

Fig. 16-2. Line drawing showing the low-profile 10-mm angioplasty balloon dilating the tract from the right hepatic vein to the portal vein in preparation for placement of the stent. The guidewire has been passed well into the splenic vein to maintain a secure position during passage of the angioplasty balloon. (From G. Zemel et al. Technical advances in transjugular intrahepatic portosystemic shunts. *Radiographics* 12:615–622, 1992.)

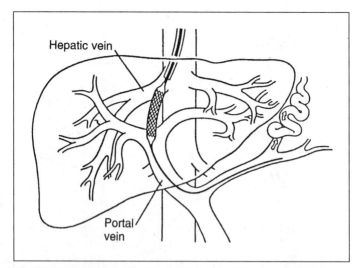

Fig. 16-3. Line drawing showing placement of a balloon-expandable stent across the shunt tract. (From G. Zemel et al. Technical advances in transjugular intrahepatic portosystemic shunts. *Radiographics* **12:615–622, 1992.)**

balloon-expandable stent or a self-expanding metallic stent:

    a. Palmaz stents. One 30-mm balloon-expandable Palmaz stent (Johnson & Johnson, Warren, NJ) mounted on a 10-mm balloon, or occasionally up to three stents (with 5-mm overlap), may be deployed. This system requires the preliminary passage of the 10 Fr. sheath through the parenchyma. The first stent is optimally positioned within the portal vein with no more than 5 mm protruding distally (Fig. 16-3).

    b. Schneider Wallstents. Alternatively, a self-expanding Wallstent (Schneider, Minneapolis, MN) may be used [6]. The Wallstent has the advantage of flexibility and a small 7 Fr. introduction system; either the 68-mm or 42-mm length or both may be used depending on the length of the tract to be covered. The diameter may be 8 mm or, more commonly, 10 mm. The proximal end of the stent should not extend into the IVC but should be within the first few cm of the hepatic vein. The distal portion of the stent should be within the right portal vein or main portal vein very close to the bifurcation. This position minimizes interference if subsequent hepatic transplantation should be considered. If two stents are used they must be telescoped within each other so that no portion of the parenchymal tract is left unstented.

13. Following shunt placement, repeat venogram and pressure gradient measurements across the shunt. A maximum portosystemic shunt gradient of 12 mm Hg is desired.

If the gradient is higher, or if varices continue to fill on the venogram, dilate the shunt with a 10-mm balloon, and repeat portal venogram and remeasure the gradient. The Wallstent may be expanded to 12 mm if necessary. However, there is shortening of the length of the stent if it is expanded to this diameter (see **4** under Complications). On occasion a second parallel shunt may be needed to reduce the gradient further.

14. If the patient is actively bleeding at the time of shunt placement, embolization of the coronary vein(s) and varices is indicated. Perform coil embolization via a catheter placed through the shunt. Coaxial technique may be needed to achieve adequate position of the catheter tip to safely deposit occlusion coils. Some choose to embolize varices that persistently opacify on the repeat venograms [2]; others do not, as long as the gradient is under 12 mm Hg [1].

Postprocedure Management

1. Patients need frequent monitoring of their vital signs, fluid input and output, bed rest for 24 hours, and Hct checks every 6 hours until stable.
2. We remove the 35 cm, 10 Fr. sheath and replace it with a 10 cm, 10 Fr. sheath. This allows for central vascular access. A triple-lumen catheter also can be placed through the central diaphragm of the sheath if needed. Remove this sheath when adequate peripheral venous access is achieved. Alternatively, some prefer to remove the jugular access immediately after the procedure in order to minimize the risk of infection.
3. Pay close attention to the clotting parameters that are corrected with the administration of fresh-frozen plasma and platelets.
4. Wean patients on IV vasopressin (Pitressin) infusion of this drug in the standard manner.
5. Use color duplex US to monitor the speed and direction of flow within the portal vein and the shunt. Perform the first study within 2 days of placing the shunt and then at 3, 6, 9, and 12 months. Normally, there is reversal of flow (hepatofugal) within the native portal veins toward the shunt. If the patient rebleeds, US is the examination of choice to determine if the shunt is patent. If velocities decrease from the initial values or color flow indicates reversal of the expected hepatofugal flow within the portal veins, perform a venogram to evaluate for hepatic vein or intrashunt stenoses. Acquired venous stenoses may have to be treated with additional stents.

Results

1. Immediate technical success (includes successful placement and gradient < 12 mm Hg): 96–100% [1–5].
2. Second parallel shunt required: 10% [2,3].
3. Thirty-day mortality, not necessarily related to the procedure: 13% (n = 100) [2,3].

4. Recurrent bleeding: 4–17% [1–3,5].
5. Primary shunt patency: 75% at 6 months, 50% at 1 year, and 32% at 2 years. Primary-assisted patency is 85% at 12 months after shunt creation [7].

Complications

1. New or worsening encephalopathy: 10–15% [1–5]. This can be treated successfully with a standard lactulose regimen.
2. Bleeding complications from the puncture site or from a misdirected portal vein puncture that perforates the hepatic capsule (< 1%).
3. Hepatic vein stenosis with subsequent shunt thrombosis.
4. If two self-expanding Wallstents are used, they may shorten enough to leave a segment of liver parenchyma unstented. Thrombosis of the shunt has been reported with 1 mm of parenchyma exposed just 10 days after placement [1].
5. Hemobilia: 1% [2,3].
6. Bacteremia: 3% [2,3].
7. Transient renal failure: 3% [2,3].

References

1. Zemel G, et al. Percutaneous transjugular portosystemic shunt. *JAMA* 26:390–393, 1991.
2. Ring EJ, et al. Percutaneous intrahepatic portosystemic shunts to control variceal bleeding prior to liver transplantation. *Ann Intern Med* 116:304–309, 1992.
3. Roberts JP, et al. Intrahepatic portocaval shunt for variceal hemorrhage prior to liver transplantation. *Transplantation* 52:160–162, 1991.
4. Peltzer MC, et al. Treatment of Budd-Chiari Syndrome with a transjugular intrahepatic portosystemic shunt. *J Vasc Interv Radiol* 4:263–267, 1993.
5. Zemel G, et al. Technical advances in transjugular intrahepatic portosystemic shunts. *Radiographics* 12:615–622, 1992.
6. LaBerge JM, et al. Creation of transjugular intrahepatic portosystemic shunt (TIPS) with the Wallstent endoprosthesis: Results in 100 patients. *Radiology* 187:413–420, 1993.
7. Haskal ZJ, et al. Transjugular intrahepatic portosystemic shunt stenosis and revision: Early and midterm results. *AJR* 163:439–444, 1994.

Testicular Vein Embolization for Varicoceles

John E. Aruny

Varicoceles occur from dilatation and tortuosity of the veins of the pampiniform plexus. Most are idiopathic, but some may be associated with incompetent or absent valves of the internal spermatic vein (Fig. 17-1). Diagnosis is made by clinical examination of the scrotum and can be confirmed with ultrasound. Approximately 10% of the male population is affected, usually on the left side. There is a rare association with left renal tumors that occlude the renal vein and obstruct inflow from the left spermatic vein.

The association of a varicocele with infertility is well documented [1,2]. Decrease in sperm motility and abnormal morphology with a minimal decrease in sperm count are the findings most suggestive of the effect of a varicocele [3].

Indications

1. Scrotal pain and edema.
2. Recurrent varicocele after surgical treatment and failure of semen analysis to improve 3 months after therapy.
3. Testicular atrophy in a pediatric patient with a large varicocele diagnosed on physical examination.

Contraindications

1. Severe abnormality of the coagulation system.
2. Demonstrated severe prior contrast reaction.

Preprocedure Preparation

1. Procedures are performed on an outpatient basis. Occasional overnight admission may be required to achieve hemostasis at the puncture site or to observe for other untoward reactions.
2. Standard preangiography workup and preparation.
3. Laboratory check: Hgb/Hct, platelet count, PT/PTT, BUN, Cr.
4. Place lead shielding to protect the testicles from radiation. The testicles and pampiniform plexus should never be fluoroscoped or seen on the film.

Procedure

1. A right common femoral vein puncture provides the best access for this procedure. Place an 8 Fr. arterial sheath and infuse the sideport with heparinized saline.
2. Catheters. Left varicocele, 7.3 Fr. Hopkins embolotherapy catheter (Cook, Inc., Bloomington, IN). A Simmons-1 (shepherd's crook) catheter is helpful for selecting the renal veins.

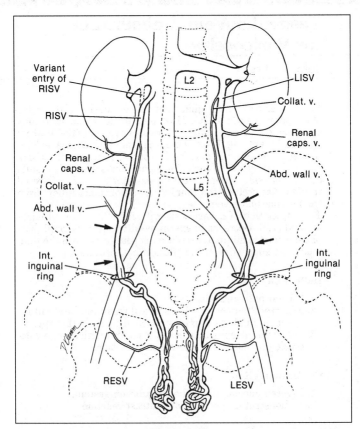

Fig. 17-1. Internal spermatic vein with insufficiency of valves on both left (LISV) and right (RISV), producing bilateral varicocele. Region between arrows on RISV and LISV is most common single-channel site for embolization with single balloon. Left (LESV) and right (RESV) external spermatic vein. (Reprinted from WR Castañeda-Zúñiga, SM Tadavarthy [eds.], *Interventional Radiology*, vol. 1 [2nd ed.]. Baltimore: Williams & Wilkins, 1992. P. 130.)

3. Position the catheter tip in the renal vein beyond the spermatic vein ostium. Perform a left renal venogram with the patient executing a Valsalva maneuver in order to demonstrate reflux down the spermatic vein. Collaterals that may originate from the renal hilum or paralumbar region may be noted.

4. Advance the catheter 2–3 cm into the spermatic vein and inject 15 cc of contrast with the patient executing a Valsalva maneuver. Contrast will flow in a retrograde fashion down the spermatic vein toward the testes. Measure the size of the vein and note the position of all parallel collateral channels.

5. Several methods of embolization have been proposed, each with its own advantages.

a. Metallic coils require relatively little experience to use effectively. However, many coils may be required (average, 6–12). Place a small coaxial catheter (e.g., 3 Fr. Teflon or Cragg convertible wire [Medi-Tech, Watertown, MA]) through the 7.3 Fr. outer catheter and deploy 0.025-in. wire coils appropriately sized to the diameter of the spermatic vein at the desired level of occlusion. Deposit the first coil near the superior pubic ramus, making sure that no draining collaterals are present beyond this point. Deploy additional coils as necessary above this level.

(1) Collateral veins. A repeat contrast injection after spermatic vein occlusion often will reveal new collaterals that have become visible with the higher pressure now present in the occluded spermatic vein. Each of these collaterals may cause failure of the procedure and, therefore, must be occluded either directly or at its opening into the spermatic vein. If the collaterals are large enough, they can be entered directly with the small catheter and a 0.018-in. or smaller guidewire. These veins can then be embolized with the appropriately sized coil placed as distally as possible. Place coils every 3–5 cm along the spermatic vein, working back toward the renal vein. Inject contrast after each coil placement to demonstrate parallel collateral vessels that have become newly visible. Place the last coil with care so as to occlude the most cephalad portion of the spermatic vein without protruding into the left renal vein. Poorly deployed coils may migrate into the central venous circulation, eventually lodging in the pulmonary circulation.

(2) All coils are placed with the patient performing a **Valsalva maneuver** to ensure that the maximum radius of the coil is achieved, thereby minimizing the risk of migration.

b. Detachable balloons require more skill and experience to place successfully without complications. Their advantage is that they can be positioned, inflated, and then deflated and moved to a more optimal position if necessary. A second balloon can be placed high in the spermatic vein with a 70% glucose solution "sandwiched" between the balloons to act as a sclerosing agent [3]. Only two balloons are required, thus reducing the procedure time significantly.

c. Spermatic vein occlusion with hot contrast material is reported to be successful in 94% of veins treated (n = 122); this is higher than the 63–96% reported with the other methods [4]. Introduce a 7 Fr. headhunter catheter with 6–8 distal sideholes (shaped with steam as necessary) via the right internal jugular vein. Place the tip in the middle of the spermatic vein for venography. During sclerotherapy the catheter is usually positioned at the level of the middle to upper part of the sacroiliac joint. From this location, inject body temperature contrast with firm compression of the vein against the superior pubic ramus; this confirms that no sclerosing agent will reflux into the pampiniform plexus. Inject 3–4 ml of 4% lidocaine into the vein to achieve a greater degree of local anesthesia. Empty the vein of blood by aspiration from the catheter for 5–10 seconds. Vigorously inject 8–12 ml of boiling, high-osmolar contrast material from a standard plastic syringe. Use fluoroscopic guidance during the injection to monitor that no material goes below the point of vein compression. Perform at least three injections. The main disadvantage of this method is that it is painful.

Postprocedure Management

1. Remove all catheters and the sheath; attain hemostasis at puncture site.
2. Monitor patient in the recovery room for **4 hours** prior to discharge (outpatient discharge evaluation criteria must be met).
3. Immediately evaluate any evidence suggestive of coil or balloon migration to the lung—with a chest radiograph if necessary.

Results

1. Technical success of embolization is almost 100%.
2. Pregnancy rates of 11–60% may be achieved [4–9].

Complications

1. Coils
   a. Misplacement of coil or migration into the central venous circulation.
   b. Venous perforation, usually self-limiting, may occur when venospasm is present, and one perseveres with catheter manipulation. The best option is to **stop** the procedure and wait about 5–10 minutes for the spasm to abate spontaneously. Rarely, direct infusion of small doses of nitroglycerin (100 μg) may be needed to break the spasm.
2. Balloons. Balloon migration into the lung, usually asymptomatic.
3. Hot contrast
   a. Phlebitis of the pampiniform plexus with testicular atrophy and aspermia.
   b. Thigh anesthesia, paresthesias.

References

1. Dubin L, Amelar RD. Varicocelectomy as therapy in male infertility: A study of 504 cases. *Fertil Steril* 217:217–220, 1975.

2. Formanek AG, et al. Embolization of the spermatic vein for treatment of infertility: A new approach. *Radiology* 139:315–321, 1981.
3. Halden W, White RI. Outpatient embolotherapy of Varicocele. *Urol Clin North Am* 14:137–144, 1987.
4. Hunter DW, et al. Spermatic vein occlusion with hot contrast material: Angiographic results. *J Vasc Interv Radiol* 2:507–515, 1991.
5. Marsman JWP. Clinical versus subclinical varicocele: Venographic findings and improvement of fertility after embolization. *Radiology* 155:635–638, 1985.
6. Schuman L, et al. Right-sided varicocele: Technique and clinical results of balloon embolotherapy from the femoral approach. *Radiology* 158:787–791, 1986.
7. Kunnen M, Comhaire F. Fertility after varicocele embolization with bucrylate. *Ann Radiol (Paris)* 29:169–171, 1986.
8. Riedl P, et al. Left spermatic vein sclerotherapy: A seven year retrospective analysis. *Ann Radiol (Paris)* 29:165–168, 1986.
9. Braedel HU, et al. Outpatient sclerotherapy of idiopathic left-sided varicocele in children and adults. *Br J Urol* 65:536–540, 1990.

Coronary Arterial and Cardiac Valve Procedures

Coronary Balloon Angioplasty

John A. Bittl

Indications

1. Stable angina pectoris
   a. Persistent symptoms despite medical therapy.
   b. Positive exercise test.
2. Unstable angina pectoris
   a. Direct angioplasty during the acute ischemic episode.
   b. Immediate angioplasty with thrombolytic therapy.
   c. Deferred angioplasty after prolonged heparin and aspirin for thrombus-containing lesions.
3. Acute myocardial infarction (MI)
   a. Direct angioplasty without antecedent thrombolytic therapy.
   b. Rescue angioplasty (thrombolytic therapy has failed).
   c. Cardiogenic shock.
   d. Postinfarction angina.
   e. Evidence of ischemia on postinfarction exercise testing.
4. Previous coronary artery bypass surgery
   a. Native vessel.
   b. Saphenous vein bypass graft.
   c. Internal mammary (thoracic) artery or gastroepiploic artery.

Determinants of Technical Feasibility

1. Lesion characteristics associated with increased likelihood of failure or with increased likelihood of complications [1,2].
   a. Total occlusion.
   b. Lesion containing thrombus.
   c. Degenerated vein graft with friable lesions.
   d. Angulated segment (especially in "shepherd's crook" of proximal right coronary artery).
   e. Bifurcation lesion.
   f. Lesion length greater than 20 mm.
   g. Calcification.
   h. Aorto-ostial location.
   i. Multivessel coronary artery disease (CAD).
2. Patient characteristics associated with increased likelihood of failure or complications [3,4].
   a. Advanced age (> 65 years).
   b. Depressed ejection fraction (< 30%).
   c. Unstable angina.
   d. Postinfarction angina.
   e. Hemodialysis.

Absolute Contraindications

1. Absence of angina or ischemia.
2. Unprotected left main CAD.

Preprocedure Preparation

1. Optimize medical therapy for angina.
2. Administer aspirin 325 mg PO qD (and dipyridamole 75 mg PO tid if stenting is considered).
3. Prepare for cardiac catheterization and angiography.
4. Use ear or finger oximetry continuously to determine whether supplemental oxygen is required to maintain arterial oxygen saturation greater than 90%.
5. For acute MI complicated by cardiogenic shock, support the systemic circulation with intraaortic balloon pumping and provide ventilatory support if indicated. For acute MI with ejection fraction less than 30%, strongly consider prophylactic intraaortic balloon pumping [5].
6. Confirm on-site capability for surgical backup.

Procedure

1. Insert sidearm sheath in the right femoral artery. Sizing of the sheath is based on the size and type of intracoronary devices that may need to be accommodated during the procedure.
   a. A 10 Fr. sheath is required if directional coronary atherectomy is considered.
   b. 9 Fr. sheath for flexible coil stents greater than 3.0 mm in diameter, for laser catheters 2.0 mm in diameter.
   c. 8 Fr. for smaller flexible coil or slotted tube stents, 1.7-mm laser catheters, or smaller rotational atherectomy devices.
   d. 7 Fr. for perfusion balloon catheters.
   e. 6 Fr. for nonperfusion balloon catheters.
2. Insert 5 Fr. right venous sheath to provide venous access, if needed, for ventricular pacing or rapid infusion of fluids to maintain intravascular volume.
3. Select coronary guide catheter.
   a. The short-tip Judkins left configuration is suitable for almost all lesions in the left anterior descending artery and most lesions in the circumflex coronary artery.
   b. The Amplatz left configuration is suitable for some circumflex and right coronary lesions, especially when totally or subtotally occluded or when proximal tortuosity exists.
   c. The right Judkins configuration is suitable for lesions in the right coronary artery that are easy to cross, especially in the absence of a prominent "shepherd's crook."
   d. The right Judkins or Amplatz configurations are suitable for saphenous vein grafts with an initial downward or horizontal take-off.
   e. The right or left bypass guides are alternative guide catheters for bypass grafts.
   f. The internal mammary guide is used for internal mammary lesions or, rarely, for bypass grafts that have a sharp upward take-off.
4. Connect an external Y-connector to the guiding catheter for introduction of guidewires and balloons through the

sealable port, and pressure monitoring, flushing, and contrast injection through the open port. The sealable port should be tightly closed except during catheter and wire movement.

5. Administer 10,000–12,500 units heparin IV. Measure activated clotting time (ACT) after 5 minutes. If the value is less than 300 seconds (Hemochron), administer supplemental heparin in a dose of 2500–5000 units and repeat ACT again. Place patient on a continuous infusion of heparin in a dosage of 800–1000 units/hour.

6. Document stenosis in at least two angiographic views and record the views on cine film, digital playback loop, or both. Optimize the projection, visualizing the stenosis and eliminating overlapping branches, for freeze-frame display on a slave-monitor.

7. Select balloon catheter to match reference diameter of vessel measured in adjacent normal segment to the nearest 0.5 mm. (For total occlusions, it may be necessary to use either a 1.5- or 2.0-mm balloon to predilate the lesion.)

8. Choose appropriate guidewire. Floppy guidewires are appropriate for most lesions except total occlusions, which may require stiff guidewires, catheter support, or both.

9. Cross lesion with guidewire and advance the tip as far distally as possible.

10. Advance the prepared balloon catheter to the target lesion. Ensure that the balloon is accurately centered in the lesion by aligning the central or tip radiopaque markers under fluoroscopic guidance.

11. Inflate the balloon slowly to 1 atm. Over the next 30–60 seconds, inflate the balloon slowly and gradually to 4 atm. If the patient tolerates the balloon inflation to this pressure without hemodynamic compromise or chest pain, maintain inflation for a total of 60–120 seconds. Deflate balloon and allow restoration of coronary flow for about 1–2 minutes before the inflation is repeated to a nominal pressure of about 8 atm or until the indentation or "waist" imposed on the balloon by the stenosis has been eliminated.

12. During full balloon inflation, monitor femoral arterial pressure closely and deflate the balloon promptly if BP falls abruptly.

13. After a successful dilatation, withdraw the balloon catheter into the guide catheter over the guidewire and perform angiography of the target lesion in two views. The entire vessel should be imaged in order to document whether guide-catheter–induced trauma has occurred proximally or evidence of embolization has appeared distally.

14. If vessel closure or dissection has occurred, repeat balloon dilatation and check the ACT. Balloon dilatation with a perfusion balloon for as long as 20 minutes (Stack perfusion balloon; Advanced Cardiovascular Systems, Temecula, CA) may be necessary to repair significant dissection. For focal dissections without significant contrast retention or reduction in thrombolysis in myocardial infarction (TIMI) flow grade, the subsequent in-hospital course may be benign [6]. For incomplete dilatation or flow-compro-

mising focal dissection, directional atherectomy may be used as a salvage approach. For more severe dissection, placement of a flexible coil stent after pretreatment with dipyridamole 75 mg PO tid and Dextran-40 at an infusion of 50 ml/hour may be required [7]. If bail-out strategies with perfusion balloon angioplasty, atherectomy, or stenting are unsuccessful, urgent bypass surgery should be strongly considered. Support of the coronary circulation with a perfusion and support of the systemic circulation with intraaortic balloon pumping are useful adjunctive measures in patients referred for emergency bypass surgery.

15. If evidence of intracoronary thrombus has appeared after balloon inflation, intracoronary urokinase (UK) should be considered. A bolus of 50,000 units followed by 2000 units/minute can be administered intracoronary through the guide catheter or via an infusion catheter for a total of 100,000–1,000,000 units [8].

16. If test injections demonstrate an angiographically satisfactory and stable appearance of the dilated site, perform a cine angiogram to document the final result, with wires and balloon catheters removed.

Postprocedure Management

1. Remove femoral sheaths and compress site for 30 minutes or more to stop bleeding if step **3** below does not apply.

2. Use ECG monitoring for 12–24 hours.

3. Keep pulmonary and femoral artery in place for ≤ 24 hours for patients with low cardiac output, class III congestive heart failure, or ejection fraction ≤0.35. Administer IV saline as needed to keep pulmonary artery wedge pressure between 14–20 mm Hg and BP greater than 100 mm Hg. Use intraaortic balloon pumping for patients at high risk for abrupt vessel closure [5].

4. Discharge the patient from hospital after 18–72 hours, when stable.

Results

1. Clinical success is defined by less than 50% stenosis at the treated site and the absence of major complications in hospital (death, MI, or need for bypass surgery); it ranges from 78%–92% and depends on clinical and angiographic variables [9,10].

Complications

1. Abrupt vessel closure occurs in up to 7% of patients treated with angioplasty and accounts for most of the morbidity of the procedure [4].

2. Death occurs in about 1% of patients, emergency bypass surgery in about 2% of patients, and MI in about 3% of patients [9,10].

3. Angiographic evidence of restenosis (> 50% diameter ste-

nosis) appears in approximately 50% of patients, and clinical restenosis occurs in about 30% of patients treated with balloon angioplasty within 6 months of the procedure [11–13]. In selected patients with discrete, de novo lesions in large coronary arteries greater than 3.0 mm in diameter, intracoronary stenting may reduce restenosis rates by approximately 30% [14,15].

References

1. Ellis SG, et al. Multivessel Angioplasty Prognosis Study Group. Coronary morphologic and clinical determinants of procedural outcome with angioplasty for multivessel coronary disease: Implications for patient selection. *Circulation* 82:1193–1202, 1990.

2. Ryan TJ, et al. Guidelines for percutaneous transluminal coronary angioplasty. A report of the American Heart Association/American College of Cardiology Task Force on Assessment of Diagnostic and Therapeutic Cardiovascular Procedures (Subcommittee on Percutaneous Transluminal Coronary Angioplasty). *Circulation* 88:2987–3007, 1993.

3. Ellis SG, et al. Predictors of success for coronary angioplasty performed for acute myocardial infarction. *J Am Coll Cardiol* 12:1407–1415, 1988.

4. Detre KM, et al. Incidence and consequences of periprocedural occlusion. The 1985–1986 National Heart, Lung, and Blood Institute Percutaneous Transluminal Coronary Angioplasty Registry. *Circulation* 82:739–750, 1990.

5. Ohman EM, et al. Use of aortic counterpulsation to improve coronary artery patency during acute myocardial infarction: Results of a randomized trial. *Circulation* 90:792–799, 1994.

6. Huber MS, et al. Use of a morphologic classification to predict clinical outcome after dissection from coronary angioplasty. *Am J Cardiol* 467–471, 1991.

7. Roubin GS, et al. Intracoronary stenting for acute and threatened closure complicating percutaneous transluminal coronary angioplasty. *Circulation* 85:916–927, 1992.

8. Schieman G, et al. Intracoronary urokinase for intracoronary thrombus accumulation complicating percutaneous transluminal coronary angioplasty for acute ischemic syndromes. *Circulation* 82:2052–2060, 1990.

9. Myler RK, et al. Lesion morphology and coronary angioplasty: Current experience and analysis. *J Am Coll Cardiol* 19:1641–1652, 1992.

10. Detre K, et al. Percutaneous transluminal coronary angioplasty in 1985–1986 and 1977–1981. The National Heart, Lung, and Blood Institute Registry. *N Engl J Med* 318:265–270, 1988.

11. Nobuyoshi M, et al. Restenosis after successful percutaneous transluminal coronary angioplasty: Serial angiographic follow-up of 229 patients. *J Am Coll Cardiol* 12:616–623, 1988.

12. Adelman AG, et al. A comparison of coronary atherectomy with coronary angioplasty for lesions of the proximal left anterior descending coronary artery. *N Engl J Med* 329:228–233, 1993.

13. Topol EJ, et al., on behalf of the CAVEAT Study Group. A comparison of balloon angioplasty with directional atherectomy in patients with coronary artery disease. *N Engl J Med* 329:221–227, 1993.

14. Serruys P, et al., for the BENESTENT Stud*j* Group. A comparison of balloon-expandable–stent implantation with balloon angioplasty in patients with coronary artery disease. *N Engl J Med* 331:489–495, 1994.
15. Fischman DL, et al., for the Stent Study Investigators. A randomized comparison of coronary-stent placement and balloon angioplasty in the treatment of coronary artery disease. *N Engl J Med* 331:496–501, 1994.

Balloon Valvuloplasty of Stenotic Cardiac Valves

John A. Bittl

Indications

1. Aortic stenosis, as a bridge to valve replacement
   a. Senile calcific.
   b. Rheumatic.
   c. Bicuspid.
2. Rheumatic mitral stenosis.
3. Pulmonic stenosis
   a. Typical dome deformity.
   b. Congenital dysplasia.

Contraindications

1. Aortic valvuloplasty should not be performed in patients who are candidates for valve surgery [1].
2. Patients with a low aortic valve gradient and depressed ejection fraction fail to show sustained clinical improvement [2].
3. Mitral or aortic valvuloplasty should not be performed in the presence of greater than 1^+ insufficiency of the mitral or aortic valve.
4. Transseptal catheterization should not be performed in the presence of left atrial thrombus or within 6 months of uninterrupted anticoagulation prescribed for systemic thromboembolism.
5. Mitral valvuloplasty should not be performed in surgical candidates with calcified, thickened, immobile leaflets and subvalvular involvement [3].
6. Pulmonary valvuloplasty should not be done in the setting of moderate pulmonary hypertension (systolic pressure > 50 mm Hg).
7. Although left-sided prosthetic valve stenosis has been treated successfully [4], only right-sided tissue prostheses should be dilated.

Preprocedure Preparation

1. Normalize PT, PTT, and Hct.
2. Optimize medical therapy for congestive heart failure.
3. Prepare for cardiac catheterization and angiography.

Procedure

AORTIC STENOSIS

1. Use the retrograde approach.
2. Insert 9 Fr. (for 15-, 18-, or 20-mm dilating balloons) or 14 Fr. (for 23- or 25-mm balloons) right femoral arterial sheath.

3. Insert 7 Fr. pulmonary artery line through 7 Fr. right venous sheath.

4. Insert 5 Fr. pacer through a second 5 Fr. right femoral venous sheath and advance to right ventricular apex. Set to demand mode at rate of 60 beats per minute (bpm) or 10 bpm below intrinsic heart rate.

5. Advance 7 Fr. pigtail catheter through right femoral sheath to descending aorta.

6. Administer 10,000 units IV heparin.

7. Using 0.035- or 0.038-in. straight guidewire, advance pigtail catheter into left ventricle. Remove guidewire.

8. Measure oxygen consumption, record simultaneous left ventricular and aortic pressures, and obtain blood samples from femoral artery and pulmonary artery to calculate cardiac output and aortic valve area.

9. Exchange pigtail for 260-cm (exchange length) 0.038-in. Amplatz extra-stiff guidewire (Cook, Inc., Bloomington, IN) or its equivalent with "left ventricular apex" configuration (Fig. 19-1).

10. Advance prepared 18–20-mm dilating balloon (sidearm-connected, 50-cc syringe with 1 : 4 mix of contrast medium and normal saline) over the extra-stiff guidewire to position the center of the balloon across the aortic valve.

11. Under fluoroscopy, the assistant should partially inflate balloon. The operator should advance or withdraw balloon catheter as necessary to keep the impression of the aortic valve centered on the balloon as the balloon is then rapidly inflated to its full extent.

12. Full balloon inflation usually causes a marked drop in cardiac output; systolic femoral arterial pressure falls to about 60 mm Hg within 8 seconds [5], necessitating prompt balloon deflation.

13. After a successful dilatation, exchange the dilating balloon catheter for a pigtail over the extra-stiff guidewire, remove wire, and record left ventricular versus femoral arterial pressure. Newer balloon catheters (Mansfield, Watertown, MA) have a pigtail configuration that allows the pressure gradient across the aortic valve to be assessed without catheter exchange.

14. For a doubling of the valve area, approximately a fourfold reduction in the gradient is needed. This can commonly be achieved by using a 20-mm or occasionally 23-mm balloon in women, and a 23-mm or rarely, 25-mm balloon in men. The risk of oversizing the balloon is the development of aortic insufficiency.

15. Optional—aortography can assess the severity of aortic insufficiency after the procedure.

16. Measure oxygen consumption, record simultaneous left ventricular and aortic pressures, and obtain blood samples from femoral artery and pulmonary artery to calculate cardiac output and aortic valve area after valvuloplasty.

17. Withdraw catheters and administer 75–100 mg protamine IV.

18. Remove 5 Fr. right femoral sheath and compress site for 30 minutes or more to stop bleeding.

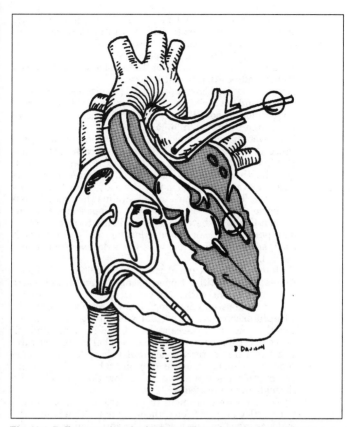

Fig. 19-1. Balloon aortic valvuloplasty. The pulmonary artery is cut away in order to reveal the placement of the 23-mm dilating balloon centered in the aortic valve orifice. The balloon catheter is stabilized by an 0.038-in. extra-stiff exchange wire with a modified apical curve. A 7 Fr. balloon-tipped catheter is placed across the interatrial septum and into the left ventricle for recording of left ventricular pressure (optional). A 5 Fr. bipolar pacer electrode is positioned in the right ventricular apex, and a 7 Fr. balloon-tipped catheter is passed to the pulmonary artery. Blood pressure is recorded from the left femoral artery.

MITRAL STENOSIS

1. Use the anterograde approach.
2. Place 6 Fr. sidearm sheath in right femoral artery.
3. Through 7 Fr. right femoral venous sheath, advance 7 Fr. balloon-tipped catheter to pulmonary artery.
4. Insert 5 Fr. pacer through a second 5 Fr. right femoral venous sheath and advance to right ventricular apex. Set to demand mode at rate of 60 bpm or 10 bpm below intrinsic heart rate.
5. Perform transseptal catheterization via the right femoral

vein with Brockenbrough needle, Brockenbrough catheter, and 8 Fr. Mullins sheath (United States Cardiac Instruments, Billerica, MA).

6. Administer 10,000 units heparin IV.

7. Advance 7 Fr. pigtail catheter through left femoral arterial sheath and position in left ventricle.

8. Measure oxygen consumption and simultaneous left ventricular and left atrial pressures, and obtain blood samples from femoral and pulmonary arteries to calculate mitral valve area before valvuloplasty.

9. If an over-the-wire balloon dilatation system is used, advance a 7 Fr. flow-directed balloon-tipped catheter through Mullins sheath to left ventricular apex. Advance the Mullins sheath over the balloon-tipped catheter across the mitral valve about 1–2 cm into the body of the left ventricle. Never leave the unprotected Mullins sheath in the left ventricle without protection by a J-tipped guidewire or balloon-tipped catheter so as to avoid inadvertent ventricular puncture. If an Inoue dilatation balloon system is used, advancing the guidewire to the left ventricle is not needed.

10. Exchange balloon-tipped catheter for 260-cm, 0.038-in. Amplatz extra-stiff J-tipped exchange-length guidewire or its equivalent with "left ventricular apex" configuration. Place a second 260-cm, 0.038-in. Amplatz extra-stiff J-tipped exchange-length guidewire through the Mullins sheath, which easily accepts both 0.038-in. wires, and advance to the left ventricular apex parallel to the first wire. The two wires enter the femoral vein through a single venotomy site; blood loss is minimized by gentle, continuous digital pressure above and below the venotomy site throughout the procedure (Fig. 19-2).

11. Option for wire placement in pediatric patients: Using a Cook deflector wire (Cook, Bloomington, IN), advance the balloon-tipped catheter across the aortic valve to the descending aorta and exchange this for the appropriate extra-stiff J-tipped exchange-length guidewire, and then proceed as above.

12. Dilate interatrial septum with 7-mm peripheral angioplasty balloon.

13. Sequentially advance two 18-mm balloon catheters (50-cc syringe containing 1 : 4 mixture of contrast medium and normal saline attached to sidearm) over the exchange wires to position the balloon across the mitral valve as viewed in the shallow right anterior oblique projection.

14. Inflate the balloons to 4 atm while the operator advances or withdraws the balloon catheter to maintain balloon position across the mitral valve. Blood pressure usually falls precipitously, requiring prompt deflation of the balloons. The operator then withdraws the completely deflated balloons into the left atrium, allowing an increase in cardiac output and BP, while the assistant advances the exchange wire to maintain position.

15. After a successful inflation, the left atrial pressure (recorded from a balloon-tipped catheter exchanged for one

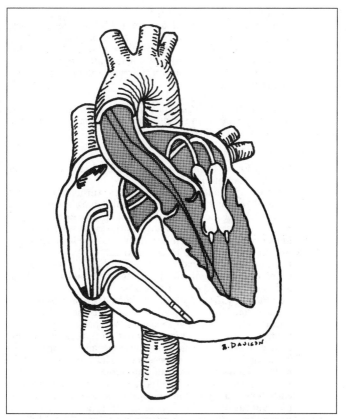

Fig. 19-2. Balloon mitral valvuloplasty. Two 15-mm dilating balloons are centered in the mitral valve orifice. Each balloon catheter is passed over a 0.038-in. extra-stiff exchange wire, which courses from the right femoral vein to IVC across the interatrial septum into the left ventricle with the distal J-tip positioned in the descending aorta. Other catheters needed during dilation include a femoral arterial monitor, a 5 Fr. right ventricular bipolar pacemaker, a 7 Fr. left ventricular pigtail catheter, and a 7 Fr. balloon-tipped catheter in the pulmonary artery (not shown).

balloon catheter) or pulmonary artery wedge pressure should be compared with pressure recorded from a 7 Fr. pigtail positioned in the left ventricle.

16. For a doubling of the valve area, approximately a fourfold reduction in the gradient is needed. If an inadequate reduction in the gradient is achieved, repeat dilatation with 18-mm and 20-mm balloons or two 20-mm balloons.

17. After successful dilatation of the mitral valve, remove the fully deflated dilating catheters across the interatrial septum.

18. Withdraw one guidewire to the left atrium and advance a balloon-tipped catheter to that position. Measure oxygen

consumption, simultaneous left ventricular and left atrial pressures, and obtain blood samples from femoral artery, pulmonary artery, and from the superior and inferior venae cavae to calculate mitral valve area and determine the presence of an atrial septal defect after valvuloplasty.

19. Perform left ventriculogram to assess the presence of mitral regurgitation.
20. Remove all catheters.
21. After the heparin effect has dissipated (with ACT < 180 seconds), remove the right femoral venous sheaths and compress until bleeding stops.

PULMONIC STENOSIS

1. Place 5 Fr. or 6 Fr. catheter in right femoral artery for arterial pressure monitoring.
2. Advance 7 Fr. balloon-tipped catheter through 9 Fr. right femoral venous sheath to either pulmonary artery.
3. Advance a second 7 Fr. balloon-tipped catheter through 9 Fr. left femoral venous sheath to the right ventricle.
4. Measure pulmonic valve gradient and cardiac output.
5. Administer 10,000 units IV heparin.
6. Position the second balloon-tipped catheter in the opposite pulmonary artery and exchange for two 260-cm, 0.038-in. J-tipped standard exchange wires.
7. Advance two 15-mm dilating balloon catheters (with 50 cc syringe containing 1 : 4 mixture of contrast medium and normal saline attached to the balloon ports) over the exchange wires to the pulmonic valve. Inflate both balloons slowly and maintain balloon position by advancing or withdrawing the catheters as necessary. Maintain full inflation of both balloons across the pulmonic valve for about 5 seconds. During rapid deflation, withdraw the balloon catheters rapidly to the inferior vena cava, allowing cardiac output and BP to increase, while the assistants advance the guidewires to maintain position (Fig. 19-3).
8. After successful inflation, replace the guidewires with balloon-tipped catheters, one positioned in the right ventricle and the other in the pulmonary artery.
9. Measure pulmonic valve gradient and cardiac output.
10. Optional—perform contrast injection in main pulmonary artery to assess presence of pulmonic insufficiency.
11. Withdraw all catheters unless further hemodynamic monitoring or pacing is indicated.
12. Reverse the heparin effect with 75–100 mg protamine IV.
13. Compress femoral sites for 20 minutes or until bleeding has stopped.
14. Discharge from the hospital after 48 hours or when the patient is stable.

Postprocedure Management

1. ECG monitoring for at least 24 hours for all patients.
2. For aortic and pulmonary stenosis, keep pulmonary (PA) and femoral artery lines in place for at least 24 hours for patients with low cardiac output, class III congestive heart

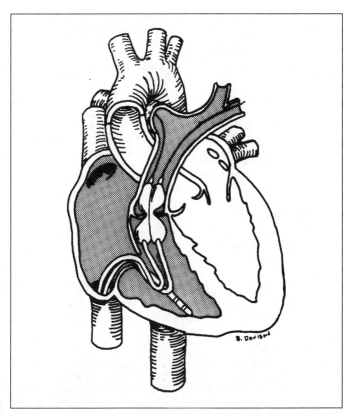

Fig. 19-3. Pulmonic balloon valvuloplasty. Two 15-mm balloons are centered in the pulmonary valve orifice over 0.038-in. exchange-length J-tip guidewires, which course from the right femoral vein to IVC through the right heart and into the left and right pulmonary arteries. A 5 Fr. bipolar pacemaker is positioned in the right ventricular apex and BP is recorded at the right femoral artery.

    failure (CHF), or ejection fraction <0.35. Administer IV saline as needed to keep PA wedge pressure between 14–20 mm Hg and BP greater than 100 mm Hg. (Not applicable to pulmonic stenosis.)

3. Discharge from hospital after 48–72 hours, when stable.

Results

1. Aortic valvuloplasty
    a. Valve area increases from 0.6 to 0.9 cm^2 acutely in most studies [1,5,6].
    b. Ejection fraction and other measures of left ventricular performance do not show sustained improvement [2,5].
    c. Event-free survival is probably not enhanced with aor-

tic valvuloplasty [1]. Hemodynamic evidence of restenosis occurs in about 80% of patients within 6
months [1,2,5,7,8].

2. Mitral valvuloplasty

  a. Valve area increases from about 0.9 to 1.8 cm² in most
  studies [9,10]. Almost 90% of patients with non-
  calcified, pliable leaflets will have a valve area greater
  than 1.5 cm² [3].

  b. Sustained functional improvement in seen after mitral
  valvuloplasty, especially in younger patients with non-
  calcified, pliable leaflets and no prior history of atrial
  fibrillation [11–13].

3. Pulmonic valvuloplasty

  Provides long-term relief of pulmonary valvular obstruction in the majority of patients [14].

Complications

1. Severe valvular insufficiency has been seen in 1–4% of
patients after mitral or aortic valvuloplasty [8,15].

2. Hemopericardium and cardiac tamponade has occurred in
1–2% of patients after mitral or aortic valvuloplasty [8,15].

3. Vascular repair may be needed in 5–10% of patients after
aortic valvuloplasty.

4. Stroke has been reported in 1–2% of patients.

5. Conduction defects have usually been transient.

References

1. Kuntz RE, et al. Predictors of event-free survival after balloon
   aortic valvuloplasty. *N Engl J Med* 325:17–23, 1991.
2. Davidson CJ, et al. Failure of balloon aortic valvuloplasty to result
   in sustained clinical improvement in patients with depressed left
   ventricular function. *Am J Cardiol* 65:72–77, 1990.
3. Palacios IF, et al. Follow-up of patients undergoing percutaneous
   mitral balloon valvotomy. Analysis of factors determining restenosis. *Circulation* 79:573–579, 1989.
4. Cox DA, et al. Improved quality of life after successful valvuloplasty of a stenosed mitral prosthesis. *Am Heart J* 118:839–
   841, 1989.
5. Bashore TM, Davidson CJ. Follow-up recatheterization after balloon aortic valvuloplasty. Mansfield Scientific Aortic Valvuloplasty Registry Investigators. *J Am Coll Cardiol* 17:1188–
   1195, 1991.
6. Bittl JA, et al. Peak left ventricular pressure during percutaneous
   aortic balloon valvuloplasty: Clinical and echocardiographic corre-
   lations. *J Am Coll Cardiol* 14:135–142, 1989.
7. Davidson CJ, et al. Determinants of one-year outcome from balloon
   aortic valvuloplasty. *Am J Cardiol* 68:75–80, 1991.
8. Safian RD, et al. Balloon aortic valvuloplasty in 170 consecutive
   patients. *N Engl J Med* 319:125–130, 1988.
9. Turi ZG, et al. Percutaneous balloon versus surgical closed commissurotomy for mitral stenosis. A prospective, randomized trial
   [see comments]. *Circulation* 83:1179–1185, 1991.

10. Reyes VP, et al. Percutaneous balloon valvuloplasty compared with open surgical commissurotomy for mitral stenosis [see comments]. *N Engl J Med* 331:961–967, 1994.
11. Pan M, et al. Factors determining late success after mitral balloon valvotomy. *Am J Cardiol* 71:1181–1185, 1993.
12. Cohen DJ, et al. Predictors of long-term outcome after percutaneous balloon mitral valvuloplasty. *N Engl J Med* 327:1329–1335, 1992.
13. Bittl JA. Mitral valve balloon dilatation: Long-term results. *J Card Surg* 9(Suppl):213–217, 1994.
14. McCrindle BW, Kan JS. Long-term results after balloon pulmonary valvuloplasty. *Circulation* 83:1915–1922, 1991.
15. Vahanian A, et al. Results of percutaneous mitral commissurotomy in 200 patients. *Am J Cardiol* 63:847–852, 1989.

Nonvascular Interventional Procedures

Percutaneous Nephrostomy and Antegrade Ureteral Stenting

Krishna Kandarpa
John E. Aruny

Percutaneous Nephrostomy

Indications [1–7]

1. External drainage of renal collecting system.
   a. Pyeloureteral obstruction causing hydro- or pyonephrosis.
   b. Diversion of urine from renal collecting system in order to heal leaks and fistulas.
   c. Decompression of renal and perirenal fluid collections (e.g., infected cysts, abscesses, urinomas).
   d. Nondilated obstructive uropathy [3].
2. Tract creation for inserting devices for stone retrieval, biopsies, stricture dilatation, and antegrade ureteral stenting [1–7].
3. Management of complications in transplanted kidneys (obstructions and leaks) [8,9].
4. Direct infusion of agents for dissolving stones; antibacterial, antitumor, or antifungal drugs [10,11].
5. To relieve urinary tract obstruction in pregnancy [12,13].

Relative Contraindications [1,2]

Clotting deficiency.

Choice of Nephrostomy Tubes

1. **Type of retention mechanism.** The tube is secured in the renal pelvis by locking the distal portion of the tube in a shape whose cross section is larger than the tract through which it was introduced. There are many variations of two basic shapes (Fig. 20-1):
   a. With a Malecot- or tulip-tip at the end, the catheter retracts slightly after being positioned and allows the sides of the catheter to flair out beyond the external diameter of the catheter. This shape is used when there is a very small renal pelvis that may not accommodate the larger loop-fixation device or when there are staghorn calculi filling the renal pelvis.
   b. The locking-loop or Cope-loop is reformed within the renal pelvis and is prevented from opening by tension applied through a monofilament suture. It has excellent retention properties but may be difficult to reform in a small renal pelvis or when the renal pelvis is filled with staghorn calculi.
2. **External diameter**. If there is no evidence of pyonephrosis then an 8 Fr. tube should be adequate for drain-

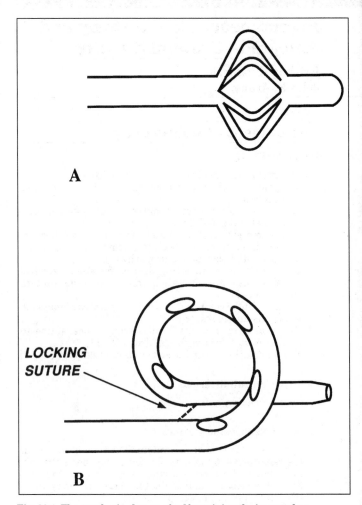

Fig. 20-1. The two basic shapes of self-retaining drainage tubes.
A. Malecot or tulip-type. B. Cope self-retaining loop.

age. If the initial sample of urine obtained during percutaneous puncture is cloudy or overtly purulent, or if there is a large crystal burden to the urine, then a tube of at least 10 Fr. should be placed to allow drainage of thicker material and prevent blockage from crystal formation within the tube.

Preprocedure Preparation [1,2]

1. Obtain informed consent.
2. Lab work: BUN/Cr, Hct/Hgb, PT, PTT, platelets; WBC, urinalysis, and urine culture and sensitivity if needed.

3. Establish IV access and ensure adequate hydration.

4. Stop oral intake, preferably about 8 hours prior to procedure.

5. Premedicate for sedation/analgesia (see Chap. 39).

6. If pyonephrosis is suspected, or if the patient has prosthetic or diseased heart valves that require endocarditis prophylaxis, appropriate antibiotic coverage is given IV, 1 hour prior to the procedure and continued as needed [14,15]. Because of the high rate of infectious complications reported when percutaneous nephrostomy (PCN) is performed on patients with struvite stones, it is recommended that all patients with a kidney stone and a history of urinary tract infections, as well as any patient with a stone that cannot be proved to be nonstruvite, should receive antibiotic prophylaxis [16] (see Antibiotics in Chap. 39).

7. Check prior available imaging studies: intravenous pyelogram (IVP), CT, US, radionuclide renography (functional assessment). If there is any question as to the existence of obstruction, a Whitaker test may be needed (see Appendix E).

8. Choose guidance system: US or fluoroscopy. Most procedures can be done with fluoroscopic guidance alone if the kidney is easily visible or if the collecting system is opacified by a small amount (50 ml) of prior IV contrast.

9. Choose an introduction system: Cope nephrostomy introduction system (Cook, Inc., Bloomington, IN), Accustick introduction system (Medi-Tech, Watertown, MA), or a sheath/needle system.

10. Prepare and drape skin entry site.

Procedure

1. Patient position. Preferably prone or prone-oblique with side to be punctured elevated 45 degrees. Prepare and drape appropriate flank (Fig. 20-2). In pregnant women, especially during the third trimester, the patient may only be comfortable lying on her side with minimal frontal obliquity. The x-ray tube should then be rotated to achieve the desired angle of obliquity for imaging the procedure.

2. Percutaneous nephrostomy approach
    a. The best path to the collecting system for a PCN in order to avoid renal hilar vessels is via an oblique posterolateral approach along what is referred to as Brödel's line (near posterior axillary line) (Fig. 20-3), about 2–3 cm below twelfth rib (in order to avoid crossing the pleural space); needle can then be directed toward an appropriate calix (usually middle or lower pole) (Fig. 20-4).
    b. Choice of calix for entry should provide optimal access to the stone if percutaneous stone removal is planned [6]; if a stent is to be placed, a higher calix is helpful.
    c. Avoid direct posterior entrance for placement of PCN, although this approach may be used for opacifying the collecting system (antegrade pyelography) with small amounts of contrast.

3. Placement of PCN (using Cope nephrostomy kit [Cook Inc.,

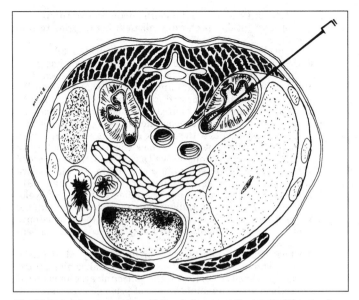

Fig. 20-2. Axial cross section of the abdomen at the level of the renal pelvis with the patient prone. A 22-gauge, 15-cm needle is shown entering a right mid-pole calix through a posterolateral approach (30–45 degrees with respect to the table surface). This approach is shown to avoid vital structures (e.g., colon) and to enter the mid-plane of the kidney avoiding major branches of the renal artery.

Bloomington, IN] or Accustick introducer system [Medi-Tech, Watertown, MA]) (Fig. 20-5).

 a. Inject local anesthesia (2% lidocaine [Xylocaine]) as deep as possible. Always aspirate prior to injection and avoid intravascular injection.

 b. Nick skin with small blade to facilitate needle entry.

 c. Ask patient to suspend respiration or limit to shallow respiration.

 d. Advance a skinny 22-gauge needle, 15-cm long, (with inner stylet in place) and direct toward the appropriate calix. In the prone-oblique position, the shaft of the needle should be parallel to the x-ray beam (must see hub end on).

 e. As soon as the renal parenchyma is entered, the tip is noted to move synchronously with respiration. At this time, suspend respiration and advance the needle in a single forward thrust by about 3–4 cm. When the collecting system is entered, there is an abrupt decrease in resistance to forward movement of the needle.

 f. Remove the stylet. If the needle tip is in a dilated collecting system, reflux of urine will be noted. Otherwise, slowly retract the needle in 2–3-mm increments while intermittently aspirating with a 20-ml plastic syringe connected to the needle hub via a long connect-

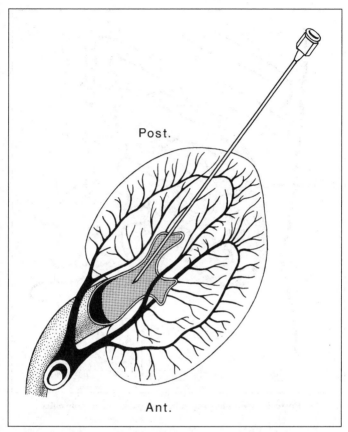

Fig. 20-3. Cross section of kidney showing needle pathway through Brödel's avascular line and cross section of kidney showing the relationship of the anterior and posterior divisions of the renal artery to the renal pelvis and infundibula. Plane of arterial division is the least vascular area of the kidney and is usually the place where nephrostomy punctures should be performed to avoid damage to large vascular structures. (Redrawn from WR Castañeda-Zúñiga, SM Tadavarthy [eds.], *Interventional Radiology* [2nd ed.]. Baltimore: Williams & Wilkins, 1992.

ing tube. When urine is aspirated, the needle tip is in the collecting system.

g. When there is no hydronephrosis, it may be difficult to aspirate urine when the needle tip is in the collecting system. Alternatively, after the needle has been passed into the renal substance, the 0.018-in. platinum-tip guidewire is used to gently probe for the collecting system. The wire will advance with minimal resistance without bending its flexible tip and arch in the direction

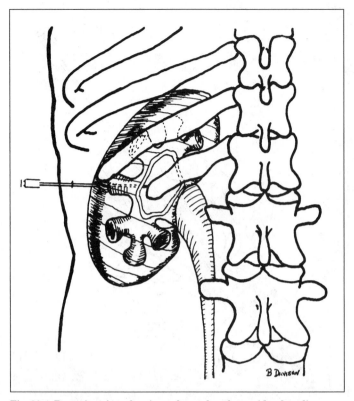

Fig. 20-4. Posterior view showing subcostal path to mid-pole calix.

    of the ureter when it is within the collecting system. This technique can work without the use of prior IV contrast media injection but is made easier by the opacification of the collecting system.

h. Remove some urine and send for cultures or cytology, or both.

i. After removing some more urine, inject contrast in order to opacify the collecting system. Do not overdecompress; this will make a new puncture difficult if present access is accidentally lost. Do not overdistend the system because this may result in bacterial seeding.

j. If a calix other than the one entered is desired, place a fine needle into the calix by a different tract if necessary. Avoid direct pelvic puncture.

k. Widen the skin nick or make 1-cm-deep skin incision, and separate the subcutaneous tissues with a hemostat in order to facilitate later passage of PCN catheter.

l. Make appropriate exchanges depending on introduction system used. With a Cope PCN set, a 0.018-in.

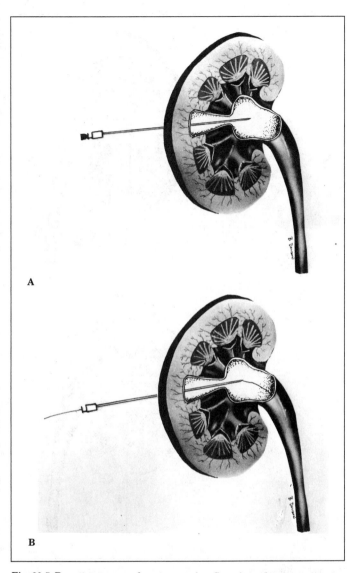

Fig. 20-5. Percutaneous nephrostomy using Cope introduction system.
A. Skinny 22-gauge (15-cm long) puncture needle tip in pelvis through
a mid-pole calix. B. A 0.018-in. J-tip wire is introduced through the
puncture needle after the stylet is removed. C. A 6 Fr. dilator with tip
tapered for a 0.018-in. wire is introduced over the wire. Dilator
has metal cannula removed. D. 0.018-in. wire is removed, and a 0.038-
in. standard J-tip guidewire is introduced through the dilator and
exits through the distal side hole. E. Tract dilation with fascial dilator
over wire. F. Catheter is introduced over wire with stiffening
cannula providing support while crossing subcutaneous soft tissues.
G. Cope PCN catheter with pigtail tip in renal pelvis.

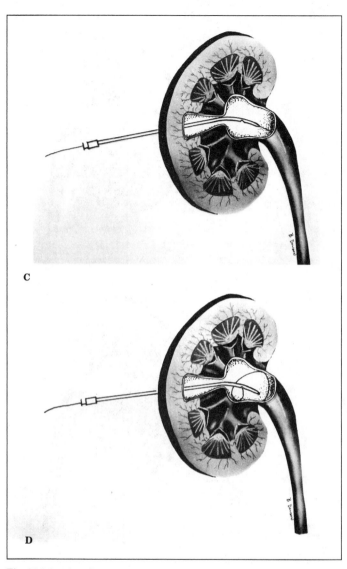

C

D

Fig. 20-5 (continued)

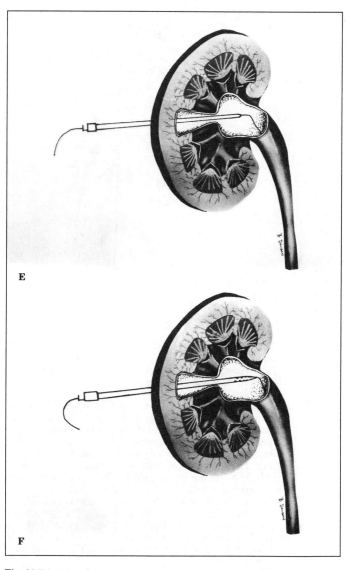

E

F

Fig. 20-5 (continued)

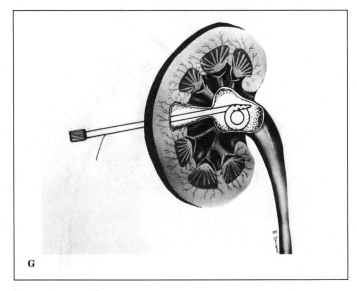

G

Fig. 20-5 (continued)

flexible platinum-tip stiff guidewire is placed through the skinny needle.

m. Introduce a 6.3 Fr. tapered dilator (end hole tapered to 0.018-in. wire) with 19-gauge stiffening cannula over the 0.018-in. guidewire.

n. Remove stiffening cannula and 0.018-in. guidewire; a standard 0.035-in. J-tip guidewire provided in the introduction set is introduced and exits through a side hole at the tip of the tapered dilator. If the guidewire does not exit the side hole on the dilator then a tight J-tip Rosen guidewire will more easily exit this side hole. Pass an adequate length 0.35-in. wire down into the ureter or coiled securely in the pelvis.

The Accustick system does not require a tight 0.035-in. J-tip guidewire to exit the dilator. The guidewire exits through the end hole (not the side hole) of the dilator, allowing the physician a choice of a 0.035- or 0.038-in. guidewire of the desired stiffness and surface coating.

o. Dilate tract up to required Fr. size.

p. Set up previously selected trocar/catheter assembly and introduce over the wire.

    (1) Do not push trocar beyond the renal parenchyma into the collecting system.

    (2) Trocar is used to facilitate passage of the PCN catheter through the extrarenal tissues.

q. Once the PCN catheter is safely within the collecting system, the trocar may be removed completely.

   r. Pull wire into the catheter with the J-tip just outside the catheter; pull on string and provide torsion to re-form the distal loop.

   s. Once satisfactory position and anchoring are attained, remove the wire.

4. Confirm catheter position by injecting a small amount of contrast after removing some urine (do not overdistend the collecting system).

5. Anchor the catheter externally (with Molnar External Retention Disk [Cook, Inc., Bloomington, IN]) and attach paraphernalia for external drainage.

Postprocedure Management

1. Bed rest for 4 hours or until hematuria begins to clear.

2. Check vital signs q30min for 4 hours, and q1h for 4 hours.

3. Monitor fluid input and output. If the nephrostomy was performed to relieve obstruction, there may be a profuse postobstructive diuresis. Monitoring urine output permits IV replacement of urine volume with half-normal saline.

4. Resume preprocedure diet.

5. Continue antibiotics if infection is present.

6. Treat pain and fever symptomatically as necessary.

7. Forward flush 5 ml of bacteriostatic normal saline and aspirate q4h if clots are persistent and obstructing flow.

8. Blood-tinged urine may be seen up to 48 hours.

   a. If gross hematuria is present, catheter position should be checked.

   b. If Hct falls without gross hematuria, check for evidence of a retroperitoneal hemorrhage.

   c. Angiogram with embolization of a bleeding branch may on rare occasions be necessary [9,10].

Follow-up

SHORT-TERM

1. If PCN is for decompression, continue external drainage until decompression is achieved or infection abates, and antegrade flow is restored.

2. If PCN is to provide tract for later stone removal, plug outside end until ready for stone removal procedure.

3. If a stent is to be placed, allow the system to drain externally for 1 week. This may facilitate manipulation through tortuous or obstructed ureters.

4. If external drainage is unsatisfactory, check tube position.

LONG-TERM

1. The patient may be discharged in 24 hours after nephrostomy tube (PCN) placement, if no complications ensue.

2. See Chap. 37, Outpatient Drainage-Catheter Care.

Results

Placement of a PCN, especially into dilated collecting systems, is usually successful (95–98%) [1,2].

Complications [1,2,16–23]

MAJOR (4.0%) OVERALL REPORTED INCIDENCE

1. Massive hemorrhage requiring surgery or transcatheter embolization: 1% [17–19].
2. Pneumothorax: 1%.
3. Death due to hemorrhage: < 0.2% [1].
4. Peritonitis: rare.

MINOR (15% OVERALL REPORTED INCIDENCE; usually no sequelae)

1. Microscopic hematuria: very common.
2. Gross hematuria (clears within 24–48 hours): rare.
3. Pain: common.
4. Perirenal bleeding (rare); clinically unsuspected retroperitoneal hematoma: 13% [11].
5. Urine extravasation: < 2.0%.
6. Catheter-related problems (obstruction, malposition, dislodgement): 12%.
7. Infectious complications: 1.4–21% (45% of patients with struvite stones will develop signs of infection following PCN placement) [16].
8. Hardening of the tube with the inability to uncoil the loop during attempted removal. (See **4.** "Removal of a failed nephrostomy tube," below).

Removal of Nephrostomy Tube

1. The Luer-Lok and locking mechanism are cut from the tube with a scissor or scalpel. This allows the locking suture to be free when the loop is uncoiled.
2. A guidewire is used to uncoil the loop and to establish access within the renal pelvis.
3. Always remove a nephrostomy tube over a wire.
    a. It is probably less uncomfortable for the patient.
    b. It helps prevent the PCN tube from catching and dragging a ureteral stent with it, if one has been placed.
    c. It allows access to the collecting system in the situation where the tube removal is accompanied by a rush of blood (iatrogenic arterial hemorrhage) through the access tract. A second tube of equal size can be rapidly inserted back into the kidney over the guidewire, to achieve tamponade of the bleeding site.
4. Removal of a failed nephrostomy tube [24]. If the tube becomes encrusted from being bathed in infected urine or left in situ for too long, the loop may not open when a guidewire is advanced within the lumen (Fig. 20-6).
    a. The hub and locking mechanism are cut off from the end of the tube and a 2-0 silk suture is sewn through the cut end of the indwelling tube and secured with several wraps of the suture around the outer portion of the tube.
    b. The suture material is brought through the lumen of the outer portion of a peel-away sheath that is the same or 1 Fr. larger than the failed nephrostomy tube.
    c. A 0.035-in. guidewire is advanced through the indwelling nephrostomy tube and coiled in the renal collecting

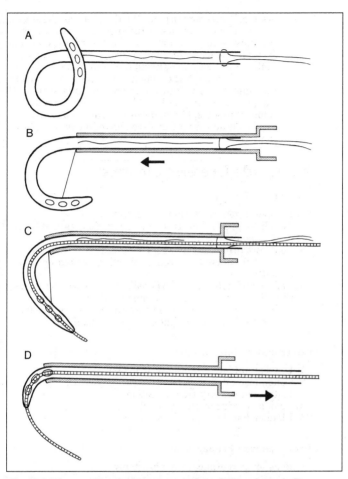

Fig. 20-6. Diagram illustrating removal of stuck Cope loop. A. Severe encrustation of urinary salts has produced binding of loop drawstring in Cope loop. Hub of catheter has been cut, and a silk suture has been passed through the blunt end of catheter. B. The silk suture has been passed into the lumen of the vascular introducer, which has then been advanced over the shaft of the Cope loop, forcing the leading edge of the introducer to release the drawstring and straighten the loop. C. Once the loop has been straightened, 0.035-in. guidewire has been passed through the lumen of the loop into the collecting system. D. While the guidewire is kept in position, the Cope loop is pulled back through the introducer. (Redrawn WR Castañeda-Zúñiga, SM Tadavarthy [eds.], *Interventional Radiology* [2nd ed.]. Baltimore: Williams & Wilkins, 1992. P. 838.)

system. With traction placed on the tube and the suture material held in one hand, the sheath is advanced over the indwelling tube until it is in the renal collecting system. The loop can then be straightened against the Teflon peel-away sheath and removed. A new tube can be placed through the lumen of the peel-away sheath that has its tip within the renal collecting system. If the peel-away sheath should become dislodged in the removal process, the guidewire should remain in place to provide access for the placement of the new nephrostomy tube.

Antegrade Ureteral Stenting

Indications [25,26]

1. Preoperative localization of the ureter.
2. To relieve ureteral obstruction from various causes (iatrogenic, neoplastic, inflammatory) [27,28].
3. To divert urine flow and relieve pressure in the management of fistulas of the renal collecting system or ureter [29,30].
4. Before and after extracorporeal shock wave lithotripsy (ESWL) in the management of stone disease.
5. Following an open or closed surgical procedure involving the ureter to maintain patency during healing.

Contraindications [25–27]

1. Untreated bladder outlet obstruction.
2. Coagulation defect.
3. Untreated urinary tract infection.
4. Spastic or noncompliant bladder.
5. Bladder fistulas.

Preprocedure Preparation

Same as for percutaneous nephrostomy.

Choice of Stent Material [31,32]

OLDER SYNTHETICS

1. Silicone. Biocompatible, nonirritating, and resistant to incrustation, making it good for long-term use. Its flexibility makes it difficult to pass through strictures or tortuous ureters. The flexibility of the material requires that the wall of the stent be thicker, and therefore the inner lumen smaller, when compared to stents made of other materials of similar outer diameter. It is also not very radiopaque, which makes its placement difficult.
2. Polyethylene. Becomes stiff and brittle resulting in a high incidence of breakage. No longer in widespread use for stents.
3. Polyurethane. Stiffer and therefore more irritating than silicone and more elastomeric than polyethylene (i.e., re-

tains its shape after a mild deforming stress.) It can be made with thinner walls than silicone, with good flow rates achieved through a larger inner lumen. These are commonly placed by urologists using a cystoscope.

NEWER COPOLYMERS

1. **C-Flex** (Cook, Inc.). A soft styrene-ethylene-butylene-styrene block copolymer with acceptably low encrustation rates. The physical properties such as stiffness and slipperiness can be modified slightly by the addition of substances such as mineral oil or silicone fluid during polymerization [32]. Memory is inferior to that of polyurethane but superior to that of silicone.

2. **Percuflex** (Medi-Tech, Watertown, MA). An olefinic copolymer that has been blended to allow production of catheter material with the largest available lumen relative to a given outside diameter [33]. These stents have good radiopacity and flexibility.

Procedure

1. Establish an antegrade access to the kidney (refer to the previous section on nephrostomy tube placement). If there is a PCN in place, pass a guidewire through the tube and direct it either into the ureter to the bladder or coiled securely in the renal pelvis. It is generally recommended that one wait at least 1 week following placement of a nephrostomy tube before placing the stent [30,33]. This decreases the risk of clot or debris occluding the lumen of the stent. However, clinical judgment should be used and stents may be placed sooner in appropriate patients.

2. Advance a peel-away type Teflon sheath over the guidewire through the skin tract into the renal pelvis to reduce frictional resistance while advancing the stent. The size of the sheath should be 0.5–1.0 Fr. larger than the anticipated diameter of the stent to be placed.

3. If the previously placed guidewire has not advanced past a point of obstruction in the ureter, advance a straight 5 Fr. or 6 Fr. catheter or an angled catheter such as a multipurpose or Berenstein catheter into the ureter over the guidewire. Use a small amount of dilute contrast to opacify the ureter, and optimize the angle of approach to the obstruction using the needed oblique angulation of the image intensifier.

4. Cross the obstruction with a similarly angled catheter loaded with an angled or straight 0.035- or 0.038-in. hydrophilic-coated guidewire. Place the catheter 5–10 mm above the obstruction and rotate while the guidewire is used to probe for the narrowed orifice. A stiff, hydrophilic-coated guidewire may be necessary to cross fibrotic obstructions. Use care, as these low-friction-surface wires may perforate the ureter.

5. Redundant ureter. If the guidewire cannot be passed across a redundant or S-shaped ureter, advance a catheter with a slight distal angle such as a Berenstein catheter to a level approximately 5 mm above the first bend and

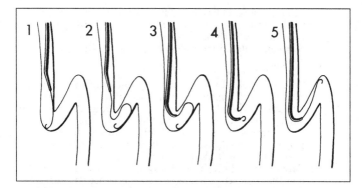

Fig. 20-7. Technique of bypassing a redundant ureter. 1. A slightly
curved tip, end-hole catheter is placed near the obstacle, and the
J guidewire is advanced until it strikes the opposite wall. 2. The
guidewire will buckle toward a new direction with continued
advancement. 3. The catheter is advanced to take advantage of the
guidewire's new direction. 4. The guidewire is retracted close to
the tip of the catheter. 5. The guidewire is advanced in a new direction,
and the procedure is repeated. (Reprinted from HM Pollack [ed.]. *Clinical
Urography: An Atlas and Textbook of Urological Imaging,* vol. 3.
Philadelphia: Saunders, 1990. P. 2769.)

    advance a floppy-tip or angled-tip hydrophilic-coated
guidewire (Glidewire, Medi-Tech, Watertown, MA.) across
the bend. Then advance the catheter over the guidewire
through the redundant segment (Fig. 20-7).

6. If further difficulty is encountered, ask the patient to perform a deep expiration, which may partially straighten
the redundant segment. Also, withdraw the catheter
slightly up the ureter; this allows the flexibility of the
guidewire to work to its best advantage to seek the lumen
and cross the redundant segment.

7. Once a guidewire is passed into the bladder, advance and
place the catheter with its tip in the bladder. Inject a small
amount of contrast material to confirm position within
the bladder.

8. Measure the length of the ureter by passing a Teflon-
coated guidewire through the catheter into the bladder.
Place the guidewire tip at the intended position of the
distal J of the stent. At the skin surface, place a bend in
the guidewire. Withdraw the guidewire tip to the intended
position of the proximal loop of the stent and place a second
bend in the guidewire at the skin surface. The distance
between the bends in the guidwire is the length of the
stent that should be placed. Stents are sized in length by
the distance between the pigtail or J curves (Fig. 20-8).

9. Coil an Amplatz Super Stiff (Medi-Tech) 0.035-in. guidewire in the bladder. Mount the stent on the guidewire and
advance through the Teflon sheath at the skin surface
down the ureter into the bladder. Depending on the type
of stent being deployed, it may be premounted on a long
delivery system or may need to be advanced by using a

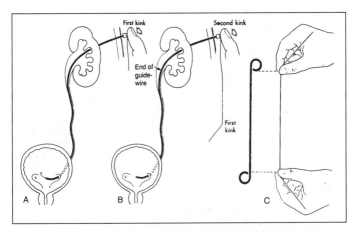

**Fig. 20-8. Measuring the ureter to determine stent catheter length.
A. The guidewire and catheter extend past the ureterovesical
junction. When the guidewire is across the midline, the guidewire that
extends from the flank is bent at the catheter hub. B. The guidewire
is retracted until the tip is located in the renal pelvis approximately
1 cm above the ureteropelvic junction. A second kink is now made in
the guidewire at the catheter hub. C. The distance between the two
guidewire bends will determine the length of the catheter between
the pigtail curves. (Reprinted from HM Pollack [ed.].** *Clinical
Urography: An Atlas and Textbook of Urological Imaging,* **vol. 3.
Philadelphia: Saunders, 1990. P. 2771.)**

stiff "pusher" mounted on the guidewire behind the stent
(Fig. 20-9).

10. When the tip of the stent is well beyond the ureteral orifice
of the bladder, retract the guidewire and the flexible stiffener, if one is employed. The distal loop of the stent will
then be coiled, resting on the floor of the bladder to give
support to the stent and help prevent distal migration. If
the stent has been measured properly the proximal loop
can then be reformed within the renal pelvis when the
guidewire and stiffener are removed. Pull the stent up
into optimal position by a loop of suture material that is
placed through the proximal side hole of the stent. Cut
one limb of the suture and pull the other limb to remove
the suture material from the stent. This should be done
under fluoroscopy to ensure that the stent is not pulled
back into the renal parenchyma or skin tract. If a peel-
away Teflon sheath is present it allows the needed coun-
tertraction against the stent to hold it in position while
the suture is being removed.

11. Place a nephrostomy tube through the existing Teflon
sheath with its loop adjacent to the proximal loop of the
ureteral stent. The peel-away sheath is then divided and
removed. Cap the nephrostomy tube so that drainage is
through the stent. The tube is fixed to the patient's skin
in the usual manner and is left in place for 24 hours, at
which time antegrade contrast is injected to ensure that

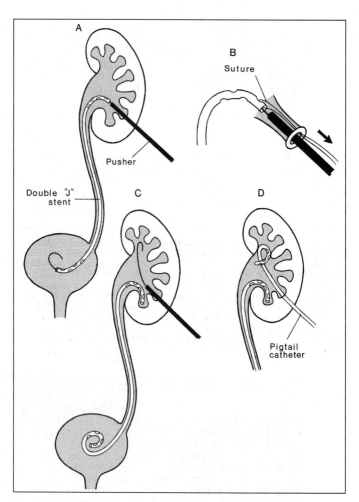

Fig. 20-9. Silastic double-J stent. A. Advancement of double-J stent over guidewire passed beyond site of obstruction. B. Close-up view of proximal end of a Silastic double-J stent with suture passed through a side hole for repositioning purposes. C. With the proximal end of the stent held in place with the pusher, the suture is removed, thus releasing the proximal loop. D. Stent has doubled back into the lower pole infundibulum, and the pusher has been replaced by a pigtail catheter for temporary external drainage. (Redrawn from WR Castañeda-Zúñiga, SM Tadavarthy [eds.], *Interventional Radiology* [2nd ed.]. Baltimore: Williams & Wilkins, 1992. P. 881.)

the stent is providing adequate drainage into the bladder.
12. Very tight or hard strictures will not allow soft ureteral stents to pass easily. An Amplatz Super Stiff 0.035-in. guidewire is passed through the crossing catheter and coiled in the bladder. The stricture may be widened by passage of a Van Andel Teflon dilator (Cook, Inc., Bloomington, IN) sized 0.5–1.0 Fr. diameter larger than the stent to be placed (usually 8 or 9 Fr.). Alternatively, advance an angioplasty balloon and use to dilate the stricture prior to stent placement. These procedures may be quite painful; adequate sedation and analgesia are necessary.
13. If a stent still cannot be passed after the stenotic ureter has been dilated, the 5 or 6 Fr. catheter is left with its tip in the bladder and the end capped at the skin surface. The catheter's presence will cause the ureter to dilate, possibly enough to pass a stent after several days. Alternatively, pass a guidewire into the bladder, snare through a cystoscope, and externalize through the urethra. With control of both ends of the guidewire a stent may be passed in an antegrade manner.

Postprocedure Management

1. Similar to that after PCN tube placement.
2. Advise patients that the loop of the stent that resides within the bladder may cause irritation and urinary frequency for a few days, but that this will resolve in most cases.
3. The patient should return for an antegrade contrast study through the nephrostomy tube in 24 hours. Do this on a tilting fluoroscopy table so that gravity can aid in the flow of contrast down the stent.
   a. If contrast is seen to traverse the stent and collect within the urinary bladder, remove the nephrostomy tube over a guidewire under fluoroscopic control to ensure that the proximal loop of the stent is not caught on the string of the nephrostomy tube and pulled out of position. Following PCN removal, an appropriate dressing is applied to the entry site.
   b. If contrast collects only within the renal pelvis or traverses only a portion of the stent, ask the patient to void urine completely or, if this not possible, place a Foley catheter, and repeat the antegrade injection through the nephrostomy tube. One cause of stent malfunction is a full bladder that cannot be emptied completely, causing high distal pressures [29].
4. All stents are a nidus for calcium formation and eventually obstruct the lumen. It is recommended that polyethylene, polyurethane, and Percuflex (Medi-Tech, Boston Scientific, Watertown, MA) stents be replaced every 6 months.

Results

1. Overall stent patency is 80%, with most failures occurring within 2 months of placement [31].

2. Stent life can be optimized by [31–33]
 a. Increasing urine flow by having the patient voluntarily drink extra fluids.
 b. Administering prophylactic antibiotics.
 c. Avoiding placement of stents into bloody or infected collecting systems.
3. Previous problems of stent brittleness and bladder irritability should be greatly reduced with the use of the newer copolymers.

Complications

24-HOURS POSTPROCEDURE

1. Perforation of the renal collecting system or ureter. This is not of significant consequence if the kidney is well drained by the stent and nephrostomy tube.
2. Improper positioning of the stent with either the upper loop placed in the proximal ureter or within the perinephric space.
3. Loss of stent patency. Most commonly from an obstructing blood clot, but transient ureteral obstruction from severe mucosal edema has been described following percutaneous stent placement [26].
4. Bladder irritation and resulting urinary frequency. In most cases this will resolve within several days. This complication is seen less frequently with the newer, softer stent materials. However, some patients may have such severe irritation and discomfort that the stent will have to be removed.

DELAYED

1. Infection with or without associated reflux of urine from the bladder.
2. Stent migration. This usually occurs secondary to improper initial stent positioning or sizing.
3. Stent fracture. Less likely with newer stent materials. The broken fragments can be retrieved with grasping forceps or baskets via the cystoscope or percutaneously if the nephrostomy access is still in place [30,33,34].
4. Erosive damage to the ureter. This occurs when a stent that is too long or too wide places continuous pressure on the ureter causing ischemic changes and erosion of the luminal surface.

References

1. Reznek RK, Talner LB. Percutaneous nephrostomy. *Radiol Clin North Am* 22:393–406, 1984.
2. Barbaric ZL. Percutaneous nephrostomy for urinary tract obstruction. *AJR* 143:803–809, 1984.
3. Naidich JB, et al. Non-dilated obstructive uropathy: Percutaneous nephrostomy performed for severe renal failure. *Radiology* 160: 653–657, 1986.
4. Bush WH, et al. Upper ureteral calculi: Extraction via percutaneous nephrostomy. *AJR* 144:795–799, 1985.

5. Leroy AJ, et al. Percutaneous removal of small ureteral calculi. *AJR* 145:109–112, 1985.
6. Coleman CC, et al. A logical approach to renal stone removal. *AJR* 143:609–615, 1984.
7. Hunter DW, et al. Percutaneous removal of ureteral calculi: Clinical and experimental results. *Radiology* 156:341–348, 1985.
8. Eklund B, et al. Percutaneous nephrostomy: A therapeutic procedure for the management of urinary leakage and obstruction in renal transplantation. *Transplant Proc* 16:1304–1307, 1984.
9. Matalon TAS, et al. Percutaneous treatment of urine leaks in renal transplantation patients. *Radiology* 174:1049–1051, 1990.
10. Bell DA, et al. Percutaneous nephrostomy for nonoperative management of fungal urinary tract infections. *J Vasc Interv Radiol* 4:311, 1993.
11. Dretler SP, Pfister RC, Newhouse JM. Renal stone dissolution via percutaneous nephrostomy. *N Engl J Med* 300:307, 1979.
12. Trewhella M, et al. Percutaneous nephrostomy to relieve renal tract obstruction in pregnancy. *Br J Radiol* 64:471, 1991.
13. Peer A, et al. Use of percutaneous nephrostomy in hydronephrosis of pregnancy. *Eur J Radiol* 15:230, 1992.
14. Cronan JJ, et al. Antibiotics and nephrostomy tube care: Preliminary observations. Part II. Bacteremia. *Radiology* 172:1043–1045, 1989.
15. Stables DP. Percutaneous nephrostomy: Techniques, indications, and results. *Urol Clin North Am* 9:15–29, 1982.
16. Cochran ST, et al. Percutaneous nephrostomy tube placement: An outpatient procedure? *Radiology* 179:843–847, 1991.
17. Cope C. Pseudoaneurysm after nephrostomy. *AJR* 139:255–261, 1982.
18. Harris RD, Walther PC. Renal arterial injury associated with percutaneous nephrostomy. *Urology* 23:215–217, 1984.
19. Cope C, Zeit RM. Pseudoaneurysms after nephrostomy. *AJR* 139:255–261, 1982.
20. Cronan JJ, et al. Retroperitoneal hemorrhage after PCN. *AJR* 144:801–803, 1985.
21. Leroy RJ, et al. Colon perforation following percutaneous nephrostomy and renal calculus removal. *Radiology* 155:83–85, 1985.
22. Chiang MS, Wise WA. Dissemination of carcinoma: unusual complication of percutaneous nephrostomy. *Urology* 25:393–394, 1985.
23. Wells AD, et al. Clostridial myositis of the psoas complicating percutaneous nephrostomy. *Br J Surg* 72:582, 1985.
24. Cope C. Replacement of obstructed loop and pigtail nephrostomy and biliary drains. *AJR* 139:1022, 1982.
25. Arsdalen KN, Pollack HM, Wein AJ. Ureteral stenting. *Semin Urol* 11:53, 1984.
26. Saltzman B. Ureteral stents: Indications, variations and complications. *Urol Clin North Am* 15:481–491, 1988.
27. Pfister RC, Newhouse JH. Interventional percutaneous pyeloureteral techniques. *Radiol Clin North Am* 17:351, 1979.
28. Smith AD, et al. Controlled ureteral meatotomy. *J Urol* 121:587, 1979.
29. Rackson ME, et al. Elevated bladder pressure: A cause of apparent ureteral stent failure. *AJR* 151:335–336, 1988.
30. Lang EK. Diagnosis and management of ureteral fistulas by percu-

taneous nephrostomy and antegrade stent catheter. *Radiology* 138:311, 1981.

31. Cardella JF, et al. Urine-compatible polymer for long-term ureteral stenting. *Radiology* 161:3133–318, 1986.

32. Mitty HA, et al. Experience with a new ureteral stent made of a biocompatible copolymer. *Radiology* 168:557–559, 1988.

33. Lang EK. Antegrade ureteral stenting for dehiscence, strictures and fistulae. *AJR* 143:795, 1984.

34. Yeung EY, Carmody E, Thurston W, Ho C-S. Percutaneous fluoroscopically guided removal of dysfunctioning ureteral stents. *Radiology* 190:145–148, 1994.

Transhepatic Cholangiography, Biliary Decompression, Endobiliary Stenting, and Cholecystostomy

John E. Aruny
Krishna Kandarpa

Transhepatic Cholangiography

Indications

1. The evaluation of the biliary ductal system in the presence of intrahepatic and extrahepatic calculi.
2. To differentiate an obstructive and surgically treatable cause of jaundice from a medically treatable cause.
3. As a prelude to percutaneous biliary decompression.
4. To evaluate the biliary ductal system in the presence of a biliary-enteric anastomosis.
5. After a failed endoscopic diagnostic procedure or to evaluate complications of a failed endoscopic stent placement.
6. To determine the site of a bile leak.

Contraindications

1. Uncorrectable bleeding disorders.
2. Totally uncooperative patient (may require general anesthesia or heavy conscious sedation).
3. Large volume of ascites (relative; procedure will be difficult with increased risk of late peritonitis).

Preprocedure Preparation

1. Assess complaints, history, physical examination, and other objective data before committing the patient to this procedure.
2. Check previous imaging workup: cholangiograms (from endoscopic retrograde cholangiopancreatography [ERCP]), abdominal CT or US, and radionuclide hepatobiliary studies.
3. Review laboratory analyses
   a. Check the liver function tests for obstructive profile (an elevated alkaline phosphatase, even in the setting of a near normal bilirubin, may indicate a low-grade obstruction).
   b. Check baseline Hct, PT, PTT, platelets. Administer fresh frozen plasma (FFP), vitamin K, and platelets as needed.
   c. Check baseline renal function: BUN and Cr, especially before administering preprocedure nephrotoxic antibiotics.
4. Explain the procedure completely and obtain informed consent.

5. Stop oral intake several hours prior to the procedure.
6. Establish a well-functioning IV and administer adequate hydration.
7. Administer antibiotics. The spectrum of coverage must include both gram-positive and gram-negative microorganisms. The incidence of infected bile is 25–36% in patients with malignant biliary obstruction and 71–90% in patients with choledocholithiasis [1,2].
   a. A suggested regimen includes ampicillin 1 g IV 6 hours prior to the procedure and gentamicin (Garamicin) 60 mg IV (adjusted to the patient's renal function—consult the latest *Physician's Desk Reference* for dosing schedule in renal insufficiency) 8 hours prior to the procedure. Repeat the dosage of both antibiotics at the beginning of the procedure.
   b. Alternatively, cefotetan (Cefotan) 1 g IV 30–60 minutes before the procedure. Adjust the dose of cefotetan for renal insufficiency, administering one-half the usually recommended dose for patients with a creatinine clearance of 10–30 ml/minute and one-quarter the usual recommended dose for patients with a creatinine clearance of less than 10 ml/minute. See Appendix F for the formula to calculate the creatinine clearance from the serum creatinine.
8. Sedation/analgesia
   a. Premedication diazepam (Valium) 5 mg PO on call to radiology, *or*
   b. Meperidine (Demerol) 50 mg IM and hydroxyzine (Vistaril) 25 mg IM on call to radiology.
9. Skin preparation. Determine the approach and prepare the appropriate skin entry site (Fig. 21-1).
   a. Right approach. 1–2 cm posterior to the right midaxillary line, eleventh intercostal space (ICS). Care must be taken to avoid transgressing the pleural space, and also to avoid directly puncturing a central hepatic duct, which is usually extrahepatic in location.
   b. Left approach to the left hepatic duct is made from a subxiphoid location.

Procedure

1. Anesthesia
   a. Local: 2% lidocaine (Xylocaine) at the puncture site.
   b. Intercostal nerve block performed with bupivacaine 0.5%, 5 ml given at the level of entry, one above and one below. Injection is made just inferior to each rib; always aspirate first in order to avoid injection into intercostal vessels.
   c. Conscious sedation/analgesia. Systemic IV administration of midazolam (Versed) and fentanyl (Sublimaze) in standard doses with close monitoring of vital signs and pulse oximetry. If placement of a drain is contemplated, some have suggested having the anesthesiologist place an epidural catheter for maximum analgesia during the procedure and for several days after the procedure.

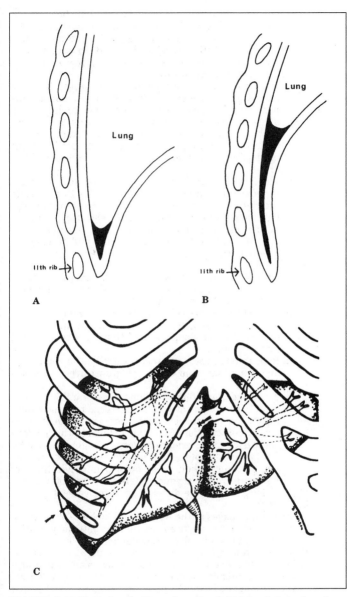

Fig. 21-1. A, B. Pleural reflections along the right lateral costophrenic angle shown in (A) inspiration and (B) expiration. Pleural transgression is avoided during a posterolateral approach by staying at or below the eleventh intercostal space. C. Correct location of skin entry site for a right posterolateral and left subxiphoid approach.

2. Make small skin nick with a sharp blade at the skin site and separate the subcutaneous tissues with a small clamp.

3. Needle introduction. A 15-cm long, flexible, 22-gauge needle with a noncutting bevel or diamond tip is most commonly used. It must be capable of accepting a 0.018-in. stiff platinum-tip guidewire.

    a. Right duct puncture is made by advancing the 22-gauge needle in a single smooth forward thrust during suspended respiration and with fluoroscopic guidance. The angle of the needle for the first pass is 30 degrees cephalad and 30 degrees ventral with respect to the table top. The target is a point just before the right paraspinal line at the level of the twelfth thoracic vertebral body.

    b. The initial approach to the left hepatic ductal system is subxiphoid with the needle angled 30–45 degrees to the right in the transverse plane. The approach to the left ductal system is usually made easier by an initial needle cholangiogram from the right intercostal approach that fills the left hepatic ducts and provides an adequate target.

4. Injection

    a. Once the needle has been advanced, remove the stylet. Connect a syringe of contrast diluted 1 : 1 with saline with a flexible plastic tube.

    b. Retract the needle a short distance (2–3 mm) and gently inject only enough contrast to leave a thin "string" of opacification along the line that has been vacated by the needle.

    c. Repeat the retraction maneuver until an adequate biliary duct is found and a cholangiogram can be safely performed.

    d. Avoid overdistention of the ductal system. However, a significant volume of contrast material may have to be injected in order to opacify the common bile duct to the point of obstruction. The biliary ducts in the left lobe of the liver are anterior to those in the right lobe. Therefore, carefully rolling the patient to the left into the left posterior oblique position will improve filling of the left intrahepatic ducts. Care must be taken not to dislodge the needle during patient movement.

5. Imaging

    a. Obtain images in the AP and both oblique projections.

    b. Review the images to ensure that the pathology or point of obstruction is adequately demonstrated.

6. If the system is to be drained, one should proceed as outlined in the section on biliary decompression. If no intervention is intended, the needle may be removed with local pressure applied over the puncture site for a short period of time.

Postprocedure Management

1. Bed rest for 4–8 hours, then activity as tolerated.

2. Continue antibiotics for 24 hours then stop if no evidence of infection.

Results

The success rate for entering a dilated ductal system approaches 100%. The ability to enter a nondilated system depends to a greater degree on the skill of the operator.

Complications

1. Mild postprocedural pain.
2. Infection
   a. Nonserious manifestations with fever, chills, and pain may be treated with a full course of antibiotics.
   b. More severe forms of cholangitis manifested by septic shock are indications for immediate biliary drainage.

Biliary Decompression

Indications [3–8]

1. To treat obstructive jaundice with associated pruritis. The etiology may be either benign or malignant.
2. To treat cholangitis and associated sepsis.
3. Failed attempt at endoscopic biliary drainage with stent placement.
4. As an access to perform endobiliary radiation brachytherapy.
5. Preoperative decompression to lower surgical morbidity (controversial). Prior to percutaneous biopsy of a pancreatic mass with common bile duct obstruction to avoid leakage of pancreatic enzymes and bile.

Contraindications

1. Same as for transhepatic cholangiography.
2. Multiple isolated intrahepatic obstructions (too numerous to drain independently). Information obtained from CT, US, previous transhepatic cholangiography, or ERCP.

Patient Preparation

1. Same as for transhepatic cholangiography.
2. When it is anticipated that transhepatic drainage will be performed following cholangiography, epidural catheter placement may be beneficial because it allows for significantly better analgesia both during and for several days following the procedure when the catheter remains in situ. This usually must be arranged and scheduled with the anesthesia department at least 24 hours prior to the procedure.

Procedure

1. Access of the biliary tree for drainage involves variations of either a single-stick or double-stick technique.
   a. Single-stick technique (Fig. 21-2; sheath-needle technique is shown) uses a small-gauge needle (22- or

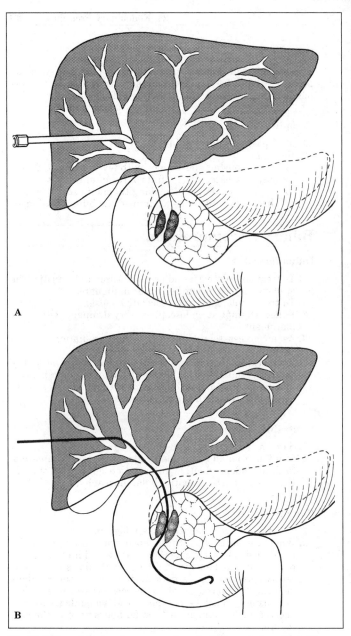

Fig. 21-2. Percutaneous decompression of a biliary system dilated by an obstructive distal common bile duct lesion. A. Teflon sheath-needle system is shown; needle is removed and tip of sheath is in a central bile duct. B. A stiff guidewire has been manipulated into the duodenum through a catheter (not shown). C. Drainage catheter pigtail tip is positioned in the duodenum with holes proximal and distal to the obstruction.

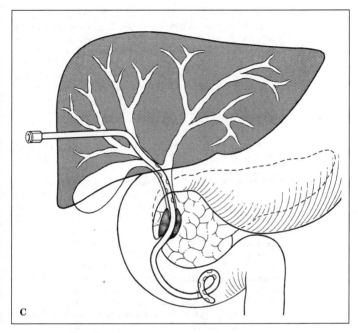

Fig. 21-2 (continued)

23-gauge) to perform the initial puncture. If, after performing a cholangiogram, the duct that has been accessed is thought to be suitable for drainage, introduce a 0.018-in. platinum-tip wire through the needle into the peripheral bile duct and direct toward the common bile duct. The needle is then removed with the wire left in place. Over the wire, place a coaxial sheath dilator with an outside diameter of approximately 6 Fr., depending on the manufacturer.

(1) The Cope one-stick system (Cook, Inc., Bloomington, IN) has a 6.3 Fr. outer Teflon sheath with an inner metal cannula. Pass this combination over the 0.018-in. wire, partially remove the metal cannula, and advance the Teflon outer sheath farther into the biliary duct. The wire and metal cannula are then removed and a 0.038-in. wire with a tight (3 mm) distal J is passed through a side port located 2 cm behind the tip of the Teflon dilator. Advance this wire as far as possible into the biliary tree.

(2) The Accustick Introduction System (Medi-Tech, Watertown, MA) is a similar system with two additional features. The 0.018-in. guidewire can be left in place as a safety wire to hold position during the introduction of the 0.035- or 0.038-in. guidewire. The larger guidewire exits the end hole next

to the 0.018-in. wire. Additionally, because it does not have to exit a side hole, this wire may be of any tip configuration or composition, including a hydrophilic-coated wire that may then pass the obstructed portion of the duct with greater ease.

(3) The small-gauge needle often enters a peripheral duct that is not of suitable caliber to place a drainage catheter. The procedure then becomes a variation of the double-stick technique with the cholangiogram performed from the peripheral position and a suitable duct chosen for catheter placement. Once the 6 Fr. dilator is in place a specimen of bile is sent for aerobic and anaerobic culture and Gram stain.

b. Double-stick technique. A skinny 22- or 23-gauge needle is used to obtain the initial cholangiogram with opacification of the right and left intrahepatic ducts. Choose a suitable caliber duct for catheter placement and with the 22-gauge needle left in place, use an 18-gauge needle that accepts a 0.038-in. guidewire to puncture that duct. The skinny needle can be used for subsequent injection of contrast material to keep the duct well opacified during attempts to puncture it. Remove both needles after placement of the 0.038-in. guidewire and continue the drainage process over this guidewire.

2. Over the 0.038-in. guidewire advance a 5 or 6 Fr. catheter into the bile duct. The catheter choice is made depending on the configuration of the ductal system to be traversed en route to the common bile duct and duodenum. Commonly a catheter with a distal curve such as a cobra or Berenstein is used. A hydrophilic-coated wire (Glidewire; Medi-Tech/Boston Scientific, Watertown, MA) can almost always be passed through a narrowed duct into the duodenum. The end-hole directional catheter is then advanced across the obstruction, over the wire, and into the duodenum. The guidewire is then removed.

3. Occasionally, the guidewire will not pass the obstruction. This usually occurs with an extremely dilated common bile duct, with edematous walls, and where a favorable approach angle to the ampula cannot be achieved. In this situation, a pigtail 8 or 10 Fr. nephrostomy tube is left coiled within the common bile duct. After several days of external drainage the system will decompress and the obstruction can then more easily be crossed.

4. If the guidewire but not the catheter passes through the obstruction, dilate with either an angioplasty balloon or Van Andel dilators.

5. Once the catheter is within the duodenum, inject contrast to confirm its position and make sure that it has not perforated into the retroperitoneum. A Teflon-coated guidewire is advanced with its tip at the estimated location of the duodenal papilla. A bend is made in the wire and the wire is then withdrawn inside the catheter. The tip is then placed, within the catheter, at the point where the most proximal side hole of the drain is to be. A second bend is

placed in the guidewire and it is completely withdrawn. The distance between the two bends is used to determine if additional side holes should be added to the drainage catheter.

6. A stiff (Amplatz Super Stiff; Medi-Tech, Watertown, MA) guidewire is advanced as far as possible into the duodenum, at least to the ligament of Treitz.

7. Introduction of the drainage catheter

  a. The Ring biliary catheter is a stiff, 8 Fr. polyethylene catheter with an inner diameter of 1.8 mm with 40 side holes in the distal 12 cm. There is a right-angle bend 3 cm from the distal pigtail loop, which, when placed at the ampulla, secures the catheter in position [9].

    (1) The previous measurement made with the guidewire (No. 4) is used to calculate the distance from the right-angle bend to where the most proximal side hole is needed. For higher drainage more side holes can easily be made with a hole punch or outer sheath of a standard 18-gauge Seldinger needle.

    (2) The Ring biliary drain has no inner stiffener but has adequate inherent axial strength to allow it to be advanced across the liver parenchyma and biliary obstruction without buckling into the space between the abdominal wall and the liver capsule.

    (3) This catheter is left in place for external drainage for 5–10 days. However, being stiff it is uncomfortable and should be replaced with a softer, larger drain at that time. This 10 or 12 Fr. drain can be placed for extended periods of internal/external drainage.

  b. The Cope loop (soft) biliary catheter is a drain made of polyvinyl chloride, Percuflex, or other soft material with a reformable distal loop and several distal side holes.

    (1) Except for the most focal distal common bile duct obstructions, extra side holes will have to be cut into the catheter. This requires some practice but can be easily done with either a hole punch or sharp suture removal scissors. Care must be taken not to cut the suture located inside the catheter when constructing the side holes. The locking mechanism should be tested after the last hole has been cut to ensure that the suture is intact.

    (2) The catheter has little inherent axial pushability and is introduced over either a plastic or metal stiffener. Advancement is facilitated by using a long (15 cm) peel-away sheath that is advanced as far as possible. The catheter-stiffener combination is advanced until the duct curves acutely toward the common bile duct. The stiffener is held stationary and the catheter advanced through the peel-away sheath over the guidewire into the duodenum as far as possible. The stiffener is removed and the sheath peeled off while the catheter is held in position.

(3) When the guidewire is removed the loop will loosely reform. The loop is more completely reformed and secured by applying tension on the intraluminal suture that pulls the loop shut. This is accomplished by a variety of locking mechanisms depending on the manufacturer.

(4) At this point the catheter will need to be pulled back into position. A rapid injection of approximately 5 ml of contrast material will identify where the highest side hole is located. The catheter is then pulled back into a position that ensures maximal exposure of the side holes for drainage, without having side holes located outside of the ductal system.

(5) A final injection of contrast confirms position of the catheter, ensuring that there is no reflux of contrast along the tract into the perihepatic space. If the catheter needs to be advanced, the guidewire will have to be reinserted.

8. Reducing pain associated with the catheter tract. 5-mg triamcinolone acetonide suspension (Kenalog 10; Squibb, Princeton, NJ) mixed with 5 ml of 0.5% bupivacaine (Marcaine; Sanofi Winthrop) is infiltrated along the track of the catheter down to the ribs and peritoneum. Aspirate prior to infiltration in order to avoid inadvertent injection into the intercostal vessels [10].

9. Securing the catheter at the skin surface. Many methods have been described. One effective method is the use of a Molnar disk (Cook, Inc., Bloomington, IN; Microvasive, Medi-Tech/Boston Scientific, Watertown, MA) and stoma-adhesive wafer combination [11]. A variation of this technique uses no suture material and allows the stoma-adhesive wafer to be changed every 2–3 weeks by the patient without disturbing the catheter [12].

With this technique the skin is cleaned with a skin prep pad that removes fat from the skin surface. We have discontinued the use of benzoin because we have seen severe skin irritation several days following its use. The Molnar disk is secured to the catheter with the serrated tie, and the end of the tie is cut off with scissors. The nipple of the Molnar disk is brought through the central hole in the stoma-adhesive wafer. The stoma-adhesive wafer is then secured to the skin which "sandwiches" the Molnar disk between the skin and the adhesive wafer.

Postprocedure Management

1. The drain is left to external gravity drainage for at least 5–7 days to allow a tract to form and prevent bile leakage causing peritonitis. Switching to internal drainage sooner invariably leads to bile leaking back along the tube and irritating the peritoneum, causing severe pain. The catheter should be flushed forward with 10 ml of sterile saline or water q6h for 24 hours if there is no hemorrhage. If there is ductal hemorrhage, the frequency of flushing should be

increased to q2h for 24 hours. After 5–7 days, if the bile is nonbloody or when the bleeding has cleared and the infection is under control, the drain may then be capped and left to internal drainage.

The patient or home health aide should be instructed on how to flush the catheter with the same 10 ml on a daily basis.

2. Check vital signs q15min × 1 hour, then q30min × 2 hours, then q1h × 5 hours.

3. Resume preprocedure diet as tolerated.

4. Monitor bile output, and fluid input and output. Normal bile output is 400–800 ml/day; if there is more, replace fluids. Evaluate for duodenal reflux. With adequate internal drainage, external port should not put out more than 200 ml/day of bile.

5. Continue antibiotics for 2–4 days depending on the clinical situation.

SHORT-TERM FOLLOW-UP

If the drainage is unsatisfactory for any reason, check the position of the tube under fluoroscopy with a contrast injection. Both the right and left hepatic ducts should fill with contrast, and no contrast should leak into the perihepatic space. Contrast should be identified outlining duodenal mucosa by the end of the study.

LONG-TERM FOLLOW-UP

1. Once the catheter has been placed to internal drainage, a connecting tube and bile bag are kept at the patient's bedside or at the nurses' station. The patient should be sent home with these items. The nurse, the patient, or the patient's family should be instructed on how to return the catheter to external drainage and to call the interventional radiologists if:

   a. The patient experiences a shaking chill.
   b. The patient develops a fever of greater than 101 degrees.
   c. The patient develops increasing abdominal pain out of proportion to what has been experienced previously.

2. Before discharge from the hospital the patient should be scheduled for an appointment to return to the interventional radiology clinic or radiology department for follow-up in 1 month.

3. Serum bilirubin values may be followed as an indicator of adequate drainage. Depending on the size and type of drain utilized, it will take on the average between 10 and 15 days for the bilirubin levels to drop 50% [13].

4. Catheters should be changed every 3–6 months depending on the buildup of obstructing bile salts within the lumen.

Results

Successful drainage in 70–97% of patients [8,14–16].

Complications [7,8,10,14–18]

Most complications are inconsequential. See Table 21-1 for methods of reducing frequency of common complications.

1. Major complications occur in about 4% of procedures [16].
2. Reports [14,15] suggest lower procedure-related deaths for benign disease (0%) compared to malignant disease (3%). This is also true of procedure-related complications (2% versus 7%).

IMMEDIATE (5–10% of patients)

1. Pericatheter bile leak: less than 16.0%
2. Hemorrhage: less than 14%. Pseudoaneurysm formation may require embolization before drainage catheter can be safely removed [16,19,20].
3. Septic shock with hypotension and positive blood cultures: 3–5% [16,21]
4. Pancreatitis: 0–4%
5. Pneumothorax, hemothorax, bilithorax: $\leq$ 1.0% [22,23]

Table 21-1. Methods of reducing frequency of common complications [9]

Sepsis	Antibiotic prophylaxis
	Minimal manipulation
	Fine-needle coaxial technique
	Restrict volume of contrast material injected
Hemorrhage	Normalize coagulation factors
	Fine-needle coaxial technique
	Peripheral-duct puncture
	Careful positioning of side holes to avoid communication with an intrahepatic vessel
Bile leak	Avoid puncture of extrahepatic ducts
	Single-puncture site in liver capsule
	Manometry to predict need for immediate percutaneous biliary drainage
	Careful positioning of side holes
Cholangitis	Ensure adequate drainage by careful positioning of side holes
	Irrigation of catheter with sterile saline
	Large-diameter catheters (12 Fr.) for long-term drainage
	Routine tube exchange every 2–3 months
Catheter dislodgement	Safety-stitch method
	Self-retaining (pigtail) catheter

Source: GR Wittich, E vanSonnenberg, JF Simeone. Results and complications of percutaneous biliary drainage. Reprinted with permission from *Seminars in Interventional Radiology* 2:39–49, 1985. Thieme Medical Publishers, Inc.

6. Contrast reaction: ≤ 2.0%
7. Hemobilia: 3.7–13.8%. Usually inconsequential and resolves spontaneously but may be fatal [16,19,20].
8. Death (procedure-related): 0–5.6%. Mortality within 30 days of percutaneous biliary drainage is about 30% [15].

DELAYED (up to 69% of patients)

1. Cholangitis: 14–25% [16,24–28]. Approximately 50% of the bile cultures will be positive when obtained at initial puncture [15]. Common organisms are enterococcus, *Klebsiella, Escherichia coli, Candida,* and *Pseudomonas* [15]. When internal-external drainage is performed with an 8 Fr. catheter, there is frequent recurrent cholangitis secondary to inadequate drainage. The rate of sepsis will decrease if this is replaced with a 10 or 12 Fr. internal-external drain [29].
2. Catheter dislodgment: < 18% [16].
3. Peritonitis: 1–3%.
4. Hypersecretion of bile: 0–5%. Can precipitate significant fluid and electrolyte imbalance and usually is seen within several days of drainage [14,30].
5. Biliopleural fistula: 2.5%.
6. Skin infection, irritation: common.
7. Intrahepatic or perihepatic abscess: rare.
8. Metastatic seeding of the serosa or tract with cholangiocarcinoma [14] and pancreatic carcinoma [16,31] has been reported.

Endobiliary Stenting

Indications

1. Palliation of symptomatic obstructive jaundice in unresectable malignant disease.
2. Benign strictures secondary to chronic pancreatitis after it is demonstrated that the strictures will persist after the disease has abated.
3. Sclerosing cholangitis (controversial) after failure of balloon dilatation or progression of fibrosis.
4. Strictures at the anastomotic site of a choledochojejunostomy.

Contraindications

1. Untreated sepsis.
2. Benign obstructive disease that has not been given sufficient time to resolve with proper therapy.

Preprocedure Preparation

1. Same as for transhepatic cholangiography and biliary drainage.
2. Some physicians prefer to have the bile ducts drained internally-externally for a short period (5–7 days) prior to the placement of a permanent endoprosthesis. However,

if the cannulation of the bile duct has been relatively atraumatic and there are no blood clots aspirated, there is no evidence of purulent material, and the diagnosis of a malignancy has been confirmed, then placement of an internal stent may be performed at the time of first intervention.

Types of Stents (see Chap. 31)

PLASTIC

1. Types
  a. Carey-Coons (Percuflex; Medi-Tech, Watertown, MA) [18].
  b. Malecot (Silastic; Cook, Inc., Bloomington, IN).
2. Advantages
  a. Easy to place.
  b. Inexpensive.
  c. May be retrieved endoscopically and replaced when occluded.
3. Disadvantages
  a. Migration: 15% [32].
  b. Cholangitis and biliary sepsis.
  c. Clogging by buildup of bile salts, blood clots, or tumor overgrowth.
  d. Questionable long-term patency (30%–100% at 1 year) [18,32].
  e. Tip of the endoprosthesis, if placed into the duodenum, may cause ulcerations.

METALLIC

1. Types
  a. Balloon-expandable. Palmaz stents (Johnson & Johnson, Warren, NJ) (Table 21-2).
  b. Self-expanding
      (1) Wallstent (Schneider USA, Minneapolis, MN) (Table 21-3).
      (2) Gianturco-Rosch Z Stent (Cook, Inc., Bloomington, IN)

Unconstrained state	6, 8, 10, or 12 mm in diameter
Unconstrained length	3, 4.5, 6, 7.5, or 9.0 cm

2. Advantages
  a. Migration unusual.
  b. Wider diameter with fewer infectious complications.
  c. All types of metal stents may be balloon dilated to approximate the diameter of the bile duct.
  d. Because of its wider diameter, a plastic stent can be inserted within it when it becomes occluded to restore patency.
  e. Wallstents are flexible and ideally suited for hilar lesions and strictures along curved portions of the ducts.
3. Disadvantages
  a. Permanent.

Table 21-2. Physical Characteristics of Palmaz and Palmaz-Schatz Balloon-Expandable Stents

Stent alone product codes	Wall thickness (in.)	Nominal length(s) available (mm)	Expanded diameter (mm)	Length at expansion diameter (mm)									Premounted stent delivery system—balloon sizes available (mm)
				4	5	6	7	8	9	10	11	12	
Medium[a] (7 Fr./0.035 in.)													
P104	.0055	10	4–9	9.9	9.7	9.4	9.0	8.5	7.8				4–7
P154	.0055	15	4–9	14.7	14.5	14.0	13.5	12.7	11.6				4–7
P204	.0055	20	4–9	19.6	19.2	18.6	17.8	16.8	15.4				4–7
P294	.0055	30	4–9	29.2	28.7	27.8	26.6	25.1	23.0				4–8
P394	.0055	39	4–9	38.9	38.2	37.0	35.5	33.4	30.6				4–7
PS204	.004	20 (articulated)	4–7	19.0	18.5	17.8	16.9						None
Large[b] (10 Fr./0.038 in.)													
P128	.005	12	8–12					11.8	11.6	11.4	11.1	10.8	8 only
P188	.005	18						17.6	17.3	17.0	16.5	16.0	8 only
P308	.005	30						28.9	28.4	27.8	N/A	26.2	8 only

[a] 2.5 mm (uncrimped) unexpanded diameter.
[b] 3.4 mm (uncrimped) unexpanded diameter.
Source: Courtesy Johnson & Johnson, Warren, NJ.

Table 21-3. Wallstent Endoprosthesis Specifications

Model number	Unconstrained diameter (mm)	Nominal unconstrained length (mm)	Constrained length (mm)	Delivery device size (Fr.)	Delivery device length (cm)
BTU7-0820-110	8	20	50	7	110
BTU7-0840-110	8	40	70	7	110
BTU7-0860-110	8	60	100	7	110
BTU7-0080-110	8	80	150	7	110
BTU7-1020-110	10	20	50	7	110
BTU7-1042-110	10	42	70	7	110
BTU7-1068-110	10	68	100	7	110
BTU7-1094-110	10	94	150	7	110
BTU7-1240-110	12	40	70	7	110
BTU7-1260-110	12	60	100	7	110
BTU7-1290-110	12	90	150	7	110

Source: Courtesy Schneider USA, Minneapolis, MN.

b. Expensive.

c. Placement of self-expanding stents not as exact since they will shorten as they increase their diameter. Metal stents are not easily seen with fluoroscopy, often making accurate placement challenging. Experience improves successful placement.

d. Tumor ingrowth will occlude stent eventually.

Procedure

1. Perform a careful cholangiogram to delineate the exact extent of the obstruction and determine where the stent is to be positioned. Malignant obstructions should be "overstented" with the stent extending well past the borders of the stricture to maintain patency as the tumor enlarges. Thus, the entry site into the bile duct must be peripheral enough to allow the stent to be placed well above the extent of the tumor.

2. A heavy duty guidewire, Amplatz Super Stiff (Medi-Tech, Watertown, MA) is placed through the transhepatic tract into the bile ducts, across the stricture, and into the duodenum.

3. In most situations, it is advantageous to balloon-dilate the stricture prior to stent placement, particularly in the self-expanding metallic stents. This will prevent uneven deployment of the device.

4. Deployment of the stent

   a. Wallstent. The stent is mounted on a 7 Fr. catheter and compressed within a sheath that is withdrawn to release the stent. The stent-catheter complex is advanced over the guidewire into position. The sheath is distended with 10 ml of sterile saline injected through the side arm. The stent is deployed by holding the metal shaft stationary in one hand and sliding the collar with the side arm outward with the other hand. The stent can be seen to expand in a distal to proximal direction under fluoroscopy.

   Radiopaque markers are located on the catheter and should be helpful for positioning. The stent will shorten by approximately one-half its length during deployment. It is advised to position the stent with the distal mark of the catheter past the point where you wish the stent to be located. When the stent is one-third to one-half deployed you can get a sense of how much the stent has shortened and how much further the stent can be expected to shorten. Then, by pulling back on the stent-catheter system, the end of the stent can be pulled back closer to its final intended location, expecting that some further shortening will occur. Remember, the stent cannot be pushed forward once the deployment process has begun.

   b. Gianturco-Rosch Z stent. The stent is manually compressed and loaded into an 8.5 or 10 Fr. sheath supplied with the unit. A pusher catheter is used to advance the stent to the tip of the sheath. The assembly is then advanced over the guidewire to the obstruction, and the stent is deployed by holding the catheter and withdrawing the sheath. The stent will tend to deploy abruptly and to move forward as it deploys. Therefore, care must be taken to ensure that the lesion is fully bridged by the stent [33].

   c. Palmaz balloon-expandable stent. This stent is manually compressed (crimped) around a polyethylene angioplasty balloon. The assembly can be passed over the guidewire through a 7 Fr. sheath (medium-sized stents: 4–9 mm expanded diameter) or an 8–10 Fr. sheath (large stents 8–12 mm expanded diameter). The selected size of the sheath depends on the type of balloon used and the quality of the crimping. The balloon-stent assembly is advanced through the diaphragm of the sheath with a plastic or metallic introducer tube supplied by the manufacturer. This prevents the sheath from being displaced off of the balloon during its introduction. The system should be tested outside of the patient to ensure compatibility of the components before attempting final introduction. When the system is ready, the sheath and its stylet are introduced so that the end of the sheath is across the narrowed portion of the duct and is where the distal edge of the sheath will be positioned. The balloon-stent assembly is introduced into the sheath and, using the radiopaque markers on the balloon, positioned over the lesion. Holding the balloon-stent assembly stationary, the sheath is pulled back over the balloon-stent assembly to expose the stent. The stent is deployed by briskly inflating the balloon, preferably by hand-injection of one-half strength contrast in a 10-ml syringe. The balloon is then deflated and withdrawn, leaving the guidewire in place. The stent, once positioned, can be further expanded by larger diameter balloons keeping in mind the shortening in length as the diameter expands (see Table 21-2).

   These stents are not flexible. They do best in straight ducts and are not suitable for hilar obstructions.

5. Once in position a cholangiogram is done through the side arm of the introducer sheath, and it is determined if other stents will be needed. If the system is adequately expanded, the guidewire and sheath are removed and the puncture site is dressed appropriately. An internal-external drainage catheter may be left across the lesion within the stent if radiation brachytherapy is planned.

Postprocedure Management

1. Continue antibiotics for 48 hours.
2. Monitor blood chemistry of liver function including bilirubin levels to confirm adequate drainage.
3. If acute blockage of stent is suspected, a hepatobiliary nuclear medicine scan will give valuable information.

Results

1. Technical success for all endobiliary stent placements approaches 100% in those patients in whom a wire can be manipulated into the duodenum.
2. The relatively poor long-term patency rates of all types of biliary stents make them a poor choice in benign biliary disease.
3. In malignant disease the main cause of failure is the growth of tumor beyond the margins of the stent. This requires initial overstenting of lesions to maximize patency.

Complications

1. The same as for percutaneous biliary decompression.
2. Migration. Uncommon in metallic stents but has been described [34–38]. Well known in plastic stents—15% [32]. It is more common in low-friction Teflon stents than in the longer Percuflex (Medi-Tech, Watertown, MA) stents.
3. Occlusion. Metallic stents: 7–15% [35,39,40]. Most often due to ingrowth of tumor above the proximal edge of the stent or between two stents that have not been adequately overlapped. Reintervention reestablishes patency in 76% of patients with Wallstents [41].

Percutaneous Cholecystostomy

Indications

1. Drainage of purulent material in patients who are critically ill or who are considered poor surgical risk for operative cholecystectomy.
2. Patients with unexplained sepsis in whom all other sites of infection except the gallbladder have been eliminated. Signs implicating the gallbladder may include distended gallbladder, sludge, cholelithiasis, or pericholecystic fluid.
3. The procedure may be considered a temporary measure to stabilize a patient until a definitive operative cholecystectomy can be performed.
4. As a conduit through which to perform lithotripsy or chemical gallstone dissolution (both controversial).

Relative Contraindication

A gallbladder packed with stones, where forming a catheter loop would be difficult or impossible.

Preprocedure Preparation

1. Obtain consent; these patients are usually critically ill and consent is obtained from family members.
2. Confirm that the patient is on adequate antibiotic coverage as explained in the section on transhepatic biliary decompression.

3. Check laboratory blood values: PT, PTT, and platelets. Correct abnormalities with FFP or transfused platelets as necessary.

Procedure

1. Most often performed under US guidance with a 5 MHz linear array transducer at the bedside in the intensive care unit.
2. The patient's skin is prepped and draped to ensure a sterile field. The US transducer is covered either with a special sterile condom or simply a large sterile surgical glove. Sterile US gel is used on the patient's skin.
3. The preferred route of puncture is through the liver and into the gallbladder. Thus, if leakage around the needle or catheter occurs, it will be extraperitoneal [42,43]. The puncture site is located with US; the patient is given local anesthesia. Lidocaine 1% is used to infiltrate the skin and course of the proposed tract. If the patient's vital signs are sufficiently stable, fentanyl and midazolam (Versed) may be administered IV in the standard doses.
4. A small nick is placed in the skin with a scalpel blade and the ostium widened with a Kelly clamp to permit introduction of the catheter.
5. We prefer trocar placement of the catheter rather than Seldinger technique because it minimizes the chances of losing access to the gallbladder during catheter and guide-wire manipulations and minimizes the amount of bile leakage. Two systems have been widely used.
   a. Hawkins accordion catheter [44].
   b. McGahan catheter set [45] (Cook, Inc., Bloomington, IN). The McGahan set is a 6.7 Fr. pigtail loop catheter that is sonographically detectable and mounted on a diamond-tip trocar needle.
6. Under US guidance the catheter-trocar system is advanced through the liver parenchyma and into the lumen of the gallbladder. The loop is reformed by removing the needle and pulling on the locking suture. If the tract is through the liver, there is no need to use an anchoring device to fix the gallbladder wall to the abdominal wall.
7. As much bile as can be aspirated is removed and sent for aerobic, anaerobic, and fungal culture and Gram stain.
8. A small amount (5 ml) of contrast is injected into the tube and portable view of the abdomen is obtained to confirm the position of the catheter. The gallbladder wall may be friable and any larger amounts of injected material may cause perforation. Also, larger volume injections may precipitate bacteremia and sepsis.
9. The catheter is fixed to the patient's skin in the usual manner with an adhesive disk. The catheter is attached to a bile bag for gravity drainage.

Postprocedure Management

1. The catheter is left to gravity drainage without flushing.
2. When the patient is able to travel to the angiography table,

a formal injection of the tube is performed. The cystic duct patency is determined. If patent, a full cholangiogram can be performed through the cholecystostomy tube. Determine if there are any stones in the gallbladder, intrahepatic ducts, or common bile duct.

3. If surgery is not contemplated but the infectious episode has resolved, the tube may be removed only after a tract has formed to prevent bile leakage and peritonitis. This usually takes at least 2–3 weeks; the clinician should realize that, once inserted, the tube must remain in place for at least this length of time.

4. The tube should be clamped for 48 hours to determine if the cystic duct will maintain its patency. If pain or fever do not return, the tube may be removed over a straight 0.035-in. guidewire. Some have advocated injecting the tract with contrast while pulling back the catheter over the guidewire to determine if the tract has formed adequately. If there is spillage outside the tract, the tube can be reinserted into the gallbladder over the guidewire [46].

Results

In a study of 82 patients with unexplained sepsis who underwent percutaneous cholecystostomy, all patients were febrile, 65 had an increased WBC count, and 37 were receiving vasopressors. Sonographic abnormalities included: distended gallbladder (71 patients), sludge (63 patients), gallstones (26 patients), wall thickening (34 patients), pericholecystic fluid (25 patients), and Murphy's sign (19 patients). After percutaneous cholecystectomy a dramatic improvement in clinical condition was observed in 48 patients (59%) within 48 hours. Signs of improvement included defervescence (41 patients), discontinuance of vasopressors (26 patients), and reduction in WBC count (33 patients) [46].

Complications

1. Bile leakage with resulting painful bile peritonitis.
2. Bradycardia and hypotension related to the vagal effect of catheter placement.
3. Hemobilia, usually transient and self-limiting.

References

1. Nichols DA, et al. Cholangiographic evaluation of bile duct carcinoma. *AJR* 141:1291, 1983.
2. Mueller PR, et al. Fine-needle transhepatic cholangiography: Reflections after 450 cases. *AJR* 136:85, 1981.
3. Oleaga JA, et al. Interventional Biliary Radiology. In Ring EJ, McClean GK (eds.), *Interventional Radiology.* Boston: Little, Brown, 1981.
4. Gobien RP, et al. Routine preoperative biliary drainage: Effect on management of obstructive jaundice. *Radiology* 152:353–356, 1984.
5. Gundry SR, et al. Efficacy of preoperative biliary tract decompres-

sion in patients with obstructive jaundice. *Arch Surg* 119:703–708, 1984.

6. Malangoni MA, et al. Effective palliation of malignant biliary duct obstruction. *Ann Surg* 201:554–559, 1985.

7. May GR, et al. Percutaneous biliary decompression. *Semin Intervent Radiol* 2:21–30, 1985.

8. Wittich GR, vanSonnenberg E, Simeone JF. Results and complications of percutaneous biliary drainage. *Semin Intervent Radiol* 2:39–49, 1985.

9. Ring EJ, et al. A multihole catheter for maintaining long-term percutaneous antegrade biliary drainage. *Radiology* 132:752, 1979.

10. Miller DL, Wall RT. Pain control after biliary drainage (letter). *AJR* 147:438, 1986.

11. Schoenfeld RB, et al. Stabilization of percutaneous catheters. *AJR* 138:972, 1982.

12. Bron KM. The non-suture skin fixation of drainage catheters. *AJR* 139:404, 1982.

13. Castañeda-Zúñiga WR, et al. Biliary Tract Intervention. Part 1. Interventional Techniques in the Hepatobiliary System. In WR Castañeda-Zúñiga, SM Tadavarthy (eds.), *Interventional Radiology*, vol. 2 (2nd ed). Baltimore: Williams & Wilkins, 1992.

14. Carrasco CH, Zornoza J, Bechtel WJ. Malignant biliary obstruction: Complications of percutaneous biliary drainage. *Radiology* 152:343, 1984.

15. Yee ACN, Ho CS. Complications of percutaneous biliary drainage: Benign vs. malignant diseases. *AJR* 148:1207–1209, 1987.

16. Hamlin JA, et al. Percutaneous biliary drainage: Complications in 118 consecutive catheterizations. *Radiology* 158:199–202, 1986.

17. McLean GK, Jordan HA: Percutaneous transhepatic biliary drainage: Comments and recommendations. *Semin Intervent Radiol* 2:69–73, 1985.

18. Coons HG, Carey PH. Large-bore, long biliary endoprosthesis (biliary stents) for improved drainage. *Radiology* 148:89–94, 1983.

19. Mintz AD, Matalon AS, Jensen DM. Iatrogenic bilovenous fistula: report of a case and its method of treatment. *J Intervent Radiol* 1:25, 1990.

20. Monden M, et al. Hemobilia after percutaneous transhepatic biliary drainage. *Arch Surg* 115:161, 1980.

21. Mudeller PR, vanSonnenberg E, Ferrucci JT Jr. Percutaneous biliary drainage: Technical and catheter related problems-experience with 200 cases. *AJR* 138:17, 1982.

22. Strange C, et al. Biliopleural fistula as a complication of percutaneous biliary drainage: Experimental evidence for pleural inflammation. *Am Rev Respir Dis* 137:959, 1988.

23. Dawson SL, et al. Fatal hemothorax after inadvertent transpleural biliary drainage. *AJR* 98:629, 1983.

24. Ferrucci JT Jr, Mueller PR, Harbin WP. Percutaneous transhepatic biliary drainage: Technique, results and applications. *Radiology* 135:1, 1980.

25. Probst P, Castañeda-Zúñiga WR, Amplatz K. Percutaneous transhepatic drainage catheter: A valuable therapeutic aid in obstructive jaundice. *ROFO* 128:443, 1978.

26. Hanson JA, et al. Clinical aspects of nonsurgical percutaneous transhepatic bile drainage in obstructive lesions of the extrahepatic bile ducts. *Ann Surg* 189:58, 1989.

27. Audisio RA, et al. The occurrence of cholangitis after percutaneous biliary drainage: Evaluation of some risk factors. *Surgery* 103: 507, 1988.

28. Cohan RH, et al. Infectious complications of percutaneous biliary drainage. *Invest Radiol* 21–705, 1986.

29. Denning D, Ellison C, Carey L. Preoperative percutaneous transhepatic biliary decompression lowers operative morbidity in patients with obstructive jaundice. *Am J Surg* 141:61, 1981.

30. Taber DS, Strohlein JR, Zornoza J. Work in progress: Hypotension and high-volume biliary excretion following external PTBD. *Radiology* 145:639, 1982.

31. Cutherell L, Wanebo HJ, Tegmeyer CJ. Catheter tract seeding after percutaneous biliary drainage for pancreatic cancer. *Cancer* 57(10):2057, 1986.

32. Mendez G, et al. Uses and misuses of biliary endoprosthesis. *Semin Intervent Radiol* 2:60, 1985.

33. Lee MJ, et al. Percutaneous management of hilar biliary malignancies with metallic endoprostheses: Results, technical problems and causes of failure. *Radiographics* 13:1249–1263, 1993.

34. Asch MR, Jaffer NM, Baron DL. Migration of a biliary wallstent into the duodenum. *J Vasc Intervent Radiol* 4:381–383, 1993.

35. Adam A, et al. Self-expandable stainless steel endoprostheses for treatment of malignant bile duct obstruction *AJR* 156:321–325, 1991.

36. Neuhaus H, et al. Percutaneous cholangioscopic or transpapillary insertion of self-expanding biliary metal stents. *Gastrointest Endosc* 37:31–37, 1991.

37. Abramson AF, et al. Wallstent migration following deployment in right and left bile ducts. *J Vasc Intervent Radiol* 3:463–465, 1992.

38. Plotner A, Lewis BS. Duodenal migration and retrieval of metallic biliary stent (letter). *Gastrointest Endosc* 37:496–497, 1991.

39. Lameris JS, et al. Malignant biliary obstruction: percutaneous use of self-expandable stents. *Radiology* 179:703–707, 1991.

40. Lee MJ, et al. Palliation of malignant bile duct obstruction with metallic biliary endoprostheses: Technique, results and complications. *J Vasc Intervent Radiol* 3:665–671, 1992.

41. Stoker J, Lameris JS. Complications of percutaneous inserted biliary Wallstents. *J Vasc Intervent Radiol* 4:767–772, 1993.

42. Cope C. Percutaneous subhepatic cholecystostomy with removable anchor. *AJR* 151:1129–1132, 1988.

43. Cope C, Burke DR, Meranze SG. Percutaneous extraction of gallstones in 20 patients. *Radiology* 176:19–24, 1990.

44. Caridi JG, Hawkins IF, Hawkins MC. Single-step placement of a self-retaining "accordion" catheter. *AJR* 143:337–340, 1984.

45. McGahan JP. A new catheter design for percutaneous cholecystostomy. *Radiology* 166:49–52, 1988.

46. Boland GW, et al. Percutaneous cholecystostomy in critically ill patients: Early response and final outcome in 82 patients. *AJR* 163:339–342, 1994.

Percutaneous Image-Guided Abdominal Biopsy

Stuart G. Silverman

The following is a practical guide for performing image-guided percutaneous biopsy in the abdomen, the most common radiologic intervention [1]. This approach to tissue diagnosis is now widely accepted for its excellent efficacy and safety [1–4], and has largely replaced costly exploratory laparotomy and the ensuing prolonged hospitalization. The general principles of a wide variety of complex biopsy techniques (more thoroughly discussed in the referenced articles) are summarized here. The more common and widely accepted methods are discussed and some recent promising techniques are introduced. Endoluminal and transvascular biopsy methods are beyond the scope of this chapter. Since every patient is different, the physician has the responsibility to choose the technique that is most appropriate for each patient.

Indications

Include, but are not limited to
1. Diagnosis of primary tumor.
2. Confirmation of suspected metastasis.
3. Determination of cancer stage.
4. Diagnosis of benign process (cysts, infection, inflammation).

Contraindications

1. Uncorrected bleeding diathesis.
2. Lesion inaccessible (e.g., surrounded by bone, no safe path).
3. Uncooperative or unwilling patient.

Preliminary Patient Evaluation and Planning of Procedure

1. **Evaluate** patient records, history, physical examination, and prior imaging studies to determine the need for and the feasibility of percutaneous biopsy.
2. **Preprocedure visit.** The benefits, risks (specific complications and their probability of occurrence), alternative procedures, and other relevant details (e.g., the planned approach) should be discussed with the patient [5]. Written **informed consent** should be obtained before all procedures.

   At this time specific **instructions** should be given to the patient on how to prepare for the procedure and how to cooperate during the biopsy (e.g., breath holding) and for the required period thereafter.

    a. All patients should have their diets temporarily adjusted. Withhold solid food for 8–12 hours; clear liquids are allowed up to 2 hours prior to procedure; **or** NPO 8–12 hours (except medications) prior to procedure [5].

    b. Many percutaneous biopsies may be performed on an **outpatient** basis.

        (1) Instruct patient on arrival time at department and expected time for starting the procedure.

        (2) The patient must have a companion to escort and drive them home.

        (3) Instruct patient on signs or symptoms of late complications of the biopsy and provide a contact telephone number.

    c. Consider **inpatient** biopsies when

        (1) Patient is in the hospital for other reasons.

        (2) Comorbid disease increases risk of biopsy.

        (3) Biopsies are high-risk.

        (4) Patient lives alone or far away.

3. Laboratory tests

    a. Tests of **hemostasis.** One suggested approach is to screen all patients with a detailed **history** (and directed physical examination), looking for symptoms and signs of a bleeding tendency or diseases (e.g., liver dysfunction), drugs (e.g., aspirin, anticoagulants) or other conditions (e.g., uremia, concurrent chemotherapy) that would affect the **coagulation cascade** or **platelet function** [5–7].

        (1) If this **screening is negative,** PTT (should be < 1.5 × control) and platelet count (should be > 100,000/ml) measurements should suffice.

        (2) If this **screening is positive** or uncertain, additional tests (e.g., PT [should be < 15 seconds], bleeding time) will be necessary.

    b. Interventions with high hemorrhagic potential. Consider Hgb/Hct (baseline should be > 10/30) in addition to all of above tests.

    c. Adrenal mass biopsy. Particularly in a hypertensive patient [8], consider: urine metanephrines, catecholamines, vanillylmandelic acid (VMA) and possibly plasma catecholamines.

    d. Liver cyst aspiration. Consider echinococcal serology in suspected cases [9].

4. Arrange for **"on site" cytopathologist** for preliminary reading of cytology; this has several advantages:

    a. Offers immediate assessment of adequacy of specimen and improves yield.

    b. Allows for altering approach or technique if preliminary tissue specimen is insufficient.

    c. Allows selective processing of specimen for special studies (e.g., culture if material suggests infection, marker studies for lymphoma; electron microscopy, cytogenetics for some soft tissue tumors, and possibly the measurement of tumor-specific markers).

    d. Limits the number of passes to no more than what is necessary, particularly in higher risk procedures.

5. Choose an **image-guidance** system [10–16].
  a. Fluoroscopy
    (1) Advantages. Readily available, allows rapid localization, real-time imaging, and identifies diaphragm.
    (2) Disadvantages. Generally requires instillation of contrast, is less precise.
  b. Ultrasound
    (1) Advantages. Rapid localization, real-time and multiplanar imaging, flexible patient positioning, no ionizing radiation.
    (2) Disadvantages. Usually does not visualize intervening bowel or pleural space.
  c. Computed tomography
    (1) Advantages. Resolves deep small lesions; depicts tissue components, vascularity, and precise anatomic relationships (e.g., bowel and pleural space).
    (2) Disadvantages. Discontinuous imaging; is time-consuming and more expensive.
  d. Magnetic resonance imaging [17]. Currently undefined clinical indications in the abdomen.

Preprocedure Preparation

1. Patient preparation [5]
  a. All patients should have an IV line placed.
  b. Sedation and analgesia. Ascertain the need for parenteral medication. Parenteral narcotics and benzodiazepines (see part **VII,** Drugs and Dosages) are used as needed by the patient at the judgment and discretion of the physician. General anesthesia is needed only in highly selected cases.
  c. Position the patient comfortably without compromising access to needle entry site.
  d. Sterilize the overlying skin (field) with iodinated scrub and alcohol.
  e. Place drapes and towels as required around field.
2. Physician preparation [18–21]
  a. Thorough handwashing is mandatory.
  b. Double gloving is recommended, as are impermeable gowns and facial shield or goggles.
  c. Protective equipment, such as needle receptacles, and specially designed biopsy trays can be used [20,21]. **Never recap needles.**

Procedure

1. Anesthetize the skin and subcutaneous tissues liberally with local 2% lidocaine [5]. Make a 3–5 mm superficial skin incision with the scalpel blade.
2. Biopsy needle selection
  a. Needle size (gauge)
    (1) Fine needles: 20–22 gauge. Ideal for cytology, safely transgresses bowel, minimal hemorrhagic potential [6,13] (e.g., if hemangioma is suspected).
    (2) Larger needles: 14–19 gauge. Increases yield [4,

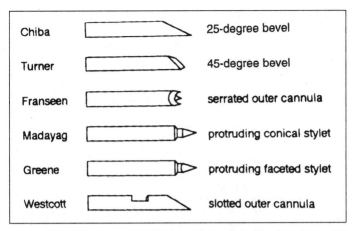

Fig. 22-1. Biopsy needles and their tip configurations. (Reprinted from GS Gazelle, JR Haaga. Biopsy needle characteristics. *Cardiov Intervent Radiol* 14:13–16, 1991.)

13,22]; helps subtype tissue, particularly in suspected lymphoma [4,23,24]; may have increased hemorrhagic potential [2] but have not been proven as an independent factor [24,25].

b. Cutting edge (Fig. 22-1) [26]

   (1) End-cutting needle types

      (a) Acute bevel: Chiba (24 degree), Turner (45 degree), Menghini (50 degree), spinal (30 degree).

      (b) Ninety-degree bevel. Greene (protruding faceted stylet), Madayag (protruding conical stylet), Franseen (serrated outer cannula).

   (2) Side-cutting needle types

      (a) Cannula-gap. Wescott (slotted outer cannula).

      (b) Stylet-gap. Inner-slotted stylet and outer-cutting cannula.

c. Spring-loaded / automated (side-cutting). Non-disposable or disposable.

d. Choose a biopsy needle [10] based on

   (1) Lesion size and depth. Small, deep lesions may require a 20-gauge needle (or larger) that is stiff enough to be directed accurately, as 22-gauge needles tend to "bow" [27].

   (2) Access route. If bowel or pleural space needs to be traversed, a fine needle (20–22 gauge) is preferred.

   (3) Suspected diagnosis

      (a) Known primary diagnosis. Requires less tissue; fine needle is often sufficient.

      (b) Unknown primary diagnosis. Fine needle aspirate equivocal or suspected lymphoma:

Larger needles (14–19 gauge) may be required.

   (c) Increased hemorrhagic potential (bleeding diathesis, hypervascular lesion). Fine needles (20–22 gauge) probably have less hemorrhagic potential [6,13]. Larger needles (14–19 gauge) may have increased hemorrhagic potential [2] but have not been proven as independent factor [24,25].

   (4) Cytopathologist preference. A preliminary "cell-layerthick" specimen for slide preparation is often preferred; hence, the first pass should be with a fine needle, but large samples may be subsequently needed.

3. Image-guidance technique
   a. US-guided biopsy
   (1) Perform full US examination of lesion and surrounding region to confirm lesion and plan biopsy. This should be done by the radiologist who will be performing the biopsy.
   (2) Localize the lesion; assess path, distance, and angle.
   (3) Free-hand technique. Real-time monitoring of biopsy may be performed with continuous imaging using a sterile transducer, particularly for small lesions; or with larger lesions, the imaging can be interrupted during needle placement. The transducer can be sterilized with iodinated scrub or alcohol before and alcohol after the biopsy, or the transducer can be covered with a sterile sheath.
   (4) Biopsy transducer guide. These are sonographic transducers with built-in needle slots that direct the needle at a predetermined angle within the plane of view of the transducer [13].
   (5) Needle-tip visualization. Demonstrate discrete echogenic complex within target lesion, preferably on two views. Some prefer scanning with the transducer perpendicular to the target [28], while others prefer scanning with a sterile transducer in close proximity to the entry site. Regardless of where the transducer is placed, the US beam should parallel the needle shaft. Needle "jiggling" or "bobbing" (in and out motion) may help. Color flow Doppler [29], use of a screw stylet (Rotex; Meadox Surgimed, Oakland, NJ) [30], and needle-tip "enhancers" (Biosponder needle; Advanced Technology Laboratories, Bothel, WA) [31,32] may aid in needle-tip visualization.

   b. CT-guided biopsy
   (1) Perform full CT examination of lesion and surrounding region **in the biopsy position** to confirm lesion and plan biopsy. This can be tailored if a prior CT is available at the time of the biopsy, and if necessary IV contrast media can be used to assess vascularity [4]. This should be done by the radiologist who will be performing the biopsy.

(2) A localizing marker grid should be placed on the skin over the lesion location before performing the control CT. The grid can be drawn with barium paste using thin lines oriented parallel to the body's long axis, 1 cm apart and at 1-cm graduated lengths. The number of visible barium dots on the imaged slice will determine the cephalocaudal plane, and can be confirmed with the CT table position. The mediolateral approach is determined by selecting the optimal barium dot as the skin entry site. The angle, distance, and structures in the path of the needle are learned by drawing a line connecting the entry site and the lesion.

(3) CT-guided needle placement. It is generally easier to direct a needle perpendicular to the floor. Without the aid of biopsy guides, angles are difficult to judge but can be mastered with experience. The trajectory should be maintained in the axial plane. If an angled approach out of the axial plane is necessary (e.g., to avoid the pleural space), US is the preferred guidance modality. But angling can be accomplished with CT, as in the biopsy of the small adrenal mass.

(4) Needle guidance aids. A number of guidance devices have been proposed including hand-held devices [33,34] to larger more fixed devices [35,36].

(5) Needle-tip visualization. The needle tip is delineated by a low-attenuation artifact (due to beam hardening) and is generally excellent. Continuous volume data acquisition, so-called spiral or helical CT may speed the process of locating the needle tip, particularly in cases with angled needle paths or in patients who breathe inconsistently [37,38].

4. Biopsy technique

  a. General principles

   (1) Have the patient suspend respiration during needle placement or other movement.

   (2) Choose shortest path possible.

   (3) The first, **localizing needle** should be placed using the thinnest gauge needle that can be accurately directed into the lesion. A 22-gauge caliber needle can usually be accurately directed into superficial targets (less than 10-cm deep); 20-gauge needles may be required in deeper lesions.

   (4) Use the least number of needle placements to obtain diagnostic tissue.

   (5) **Structures to avoid** during needle placement:

     (a) Lung. (Be sure that the position of the lung is known in the biopsy position, and at the level of inspiration used at the time of the needle insertion.)

     (b) Pleura.

     (c) Gallbladder.

     (d) Small and large bowel. (The colon and small intestines should not be transgressed if a fluid-containing structure is accessed; however, they can be safely transgressed with a fine needle, if absolutely necessary, to biopsy a solid lesion.)

  (e) Pancreas.

  (f) Dilated duct (biliary, pancreatic).

  b. Single-needle technique. Many interventionalists biopsy with a single needle and make multiple separate passes [13,38]. If multiple samples are needed, however, and the lesion is small and difficult to localize, multiple localizations could prolong the procedure.

  c. Two-needle technique. This technique requires only one precise needle placement, which serves as a reference (tandem technique) or a conduit (coaxial technique) guide for all subsequent needle placements. Hence, precise needle placement is required only once.

  (1) Tandem technique [39]

  (a) Mandatory short (3–5 mm) superficial blade incision.

  (b) Place initial 20 or 22-gauge reference needle.

  (c) Image and confirm needle tip within most desirable biopsy location of lesion.

  (d) Insert a second tandem 20 or 22-gauge needle alongside reference needle via **same incision site.**

  (e) Biopsy with the second needle for cytology smear.

  (f) Obtain additional (typically two or three) tandem passes, using larger gauge needles if necessary.

  (g) Complete procedure using reference needle for final biopsy.

  (2) Coaxial technique [4,40] is most helpful with small lesions requiring greater precision.

  (a) Place initial 18 or 19-gauge reference needle.

  (b) Image needle within lesion to confirm optimal location for biopsy.

  (c) Obtain multiple biopsies with 20 or 22-gauge needles **through reference needle.**

  (d) Complete biopsy with reference needle in selected cases

5. Sampling technique

  a. Use corkscrew drilling motion, maintaining continuous suction on a small-volume syringe. Transgress the most optimal portion of the lesion with each insertion and retraction. Release suction before withdrawing needle.

  b. Automatic spring-loaded firing devices may be used to consistently obtain a core of tissue. They appear to be reliable and safe in selected cases [41,42].

  c. Cytology smears are obtained dry. Subsequent specimens are obtained with syringes preloaded with 2 ml of sterile saline, which may be heparinized.

  d. Specimen preparation, a crucial step, is usually properly done if a cytologist is present during the procedure.

  (1) Gently spread aspirated material onto a glass slide and fix it immediately in 95% ethanol for later staining. Ethanol fixation may be continued for up to 24 hours.

(2) Residual material in the syringe and needle can be placed in sterile nonbacteriostatic saline or a 50-50 mixture of Ringer's lactate and ethanol for cell block examination.

(3) Tissue cores and larger fragments should be fixed in 10% formalin for histologic examination.

(4) Gram stains and cultures are obtained as necessary.

6. Organ-specific approaches

a. Liver. Use a transparenchymal route by interposing normal "cuff" of liver tissue. This should decrease the risk of hemorrhage into the peritoneal space when sampling a suspected hypervascular lesion [4,43] and help prevent peritoneal spillage in suspected echinococcal disease [9].

b. Adrenal gland. CT approaches are given (consider using US for large lesions).

(1) Right (lateral) transhepatic [4,44].

(2) Left (anterior) transhepatic [4,44].

(3) Alternative approaches (all designed to avoid or minimize pleural space transgression).

(a) Prone position, angle needle superiorly, caudal to the posterior sulcus [4,44].

(b) Lateral decubitus (dependent diaphragm is elevated) offers a direct posterior approach with a path caudal to posterior sulcus [45].

(c) Triangulation method [46,47] may be used to determine optimal angle and to calculate distance to lesion.

(d) Gantry tilt technique (maintains needle in imaging plane) [48].

c. Retroperitoneum. Although anterior and posterior approaches can be used, the latter is preferred when employing needles 19-gauge or larger (e.g., suspected lymphoma). Also, an anterior approach necessitates transgressing the bowel (see **(d)** under Structures to avoid).

d. Presacral / pelvic mass.

(1) Transgluteal. Posterior half of greater sciatic notch, horizontal path to avoid sacrum posteriorly and sciatic nerve anteriorly [49].

(2) More recent approaches include transvaginal [50] and transrectal [51] biopsy using transabdominal US, as well as using both transrectal US [52] and transvaginal US to guide these routes.

Postprocedure Management

The following should follow all biopsies:

1. Consider chest x ray or expiratory chest CT to rule out pneumothorax if pleural space transgression is suspected.

2. Bed rest for 1–2 hours; bathroom use with assistance; lounge chair thereafter as tolerated.
3. Monitor vital signs in recovery area: q15min × 1h; q30min × 2h; then qh × 2h.
4. Clear liquid diet for first hour; regular diet thereafter as tolerated.
5. Specimen brought to appropriate lab(s).
6. Postprocedure note and orders written on records.
7. Verbal reports to referring physicians and nursing staff.
8. If vital signs are stable and no complications are noted, the patient may be discharged, usually after 2–4 hours.
9. Give instructions to outpatients regarding follow-up for potential late complications.

Results

1. Positive tissue should be recovered in at least 80–95% of cases [1–4].
2. Obtaining inadequate material is the usual cause of a false-negative biopsy. Diagnostic yield is improved by sampling multiple and different sites.
3. Biopsy of the periphery of a large lesion avoids the necrotic center and related confusing results.

Complications

1. Are variable, **overall** estimate: **< 2%** [53–55].
2. Hemorrhage. Most common complication, but clinically significant hemorrhage occurs in less than 2% of all nonrenal biopsies (there is a slightly greater risk in core renal biopsies); however, hemorrhagic death is extremely rare [53].
3. Infection: probably < 2%.
4. Organ injury needing surgery or other intervention (primary organ or adjacent organ [e.g., viscous or duct perforation], often depends on route): < 2%.
5. Pneumothorax: Variable, depending on access route, probably < 1% for nonlung biopsies.
6. Pancreatitis (depends on access route): 2–3% if normal pancreas is biopsied; less if normal pancreas not transgressed [53,54].
7. Needle-tract tumor seeding. Reported with most tumors, but overall extremely rare. Approximate frequency: 0.003–0.009% [53].
8. Mortality rate: 0.006–0.031% [53,55].

References

1. Mueller PR, vanSonnenberg E. Interventional radiology in the chest and abdomen. *N Engl J Med* 322:1364–1374, 1990.
2. Welch TJ, et al. CT-guided biopsy: Prospective analysis of 1,000 procedures. *Radiology* 171:493–496, 1989.
3. Reading CC, et al. Sonographically guided percutaneous biopsy of small (3 cm or less) masses. *AJR* 151:189–192, 1988.
4. Gazelle GS, Haaga JR. Guided percutaneous biopsy of intraabdominal lesions. *AJR* 153:929–935, 1989.

5. Barth KH, Matsumoto AH. Patient care in interventional radiology: A perspective. *Radiology* 178:11–17, 1991.

6. Silverman SG, Mueller PR, Pfister RC. Hemostatic evaluation before abdominal interventions: An overview and proposal. *AJR* 154:233–238, 1990.

7. Silverman SG, et al. Current use of screening laboratory tests before abdominal interventions: A survey of 603 radiologists. *Radiology* 181:669–673, 1991.

8. Casola G, et al. Unsuspected pheochromocytoma: Risk of blood-pressure alteration during percutaneous adrenal biopsy. *Radiology* 159:733–735, 1986.

9. Bret PM, et al. Percutaneous aspiration and drainage of hydatid cysts in the liver. *Radiology* 168:617–620, 1988.

10. Charbonneau JW, et al. Radiologically Guided Needle Biopsy. In JM Taveras, JT Ferrucci (eds.), *Radiology: Diagnosis—Imaging—Intervention,* vol. 4. Philadelphia: Lippincott, 1991. Pp.1–9.

11. Wittenberg J, Ferrucci JT. Radiographically guided needle biopsy of abdominal neoplasms—Who, how, where, why? *J Clin Gastroenterol* 1:273–284, 1979.

12. Ferrucci JT, et al. Diagnosis of abdominal malignancy by radiologic fine-needle aspiration biopsy. *AJR* 134:323–330, 1980.

13. Charbonneau JW, et al. CT and sonographically guided needle biopsy: Current techniques and new innovations. *AJR* 154:1–10, 1990.

14. Haaga JR, Alfidi RJ. Precise biopsy localization by computed tomography. *Radiology* 118:603–607, 1976.

15. Sundaram M, et al. Utility of CT-guided abdominal aspiration procedures. *AJR* 139:1111–1115, 1982.

16. Harter LP, et al. CT-guided fine-needle aspirations for diagnosis of benign and malignant disease. *AJR* 140:363–367, 1983.

17. Mueller PR, et al. MR-guided aspiration biopsy: Needle design and clinical trials. *Radiology* 161:605–609, 1986.

18. Wall SD, Olcott EW, Gerberding JL. AIDS risk and risk reduction in the radiology department—perspective. *AJR* 157:911–917, 1991.

19. Williams DM, Marx MV, Korobkin M. AIDS risk and risk reduction in the radiology department—commentary. *AJR* 157:919–921, 1991.

20. Mueller PR, et al. New universal precaution aspiration tray. *Radiology* 173:278–279, 1989.

21. vanSonnenberg E, Casola G, Maysey M. Simple apparatus to avoid inadvertent needle puncture. *Radiology* 166:550, 1988.

22. Martino CR, et al. CT-guided liver biopsies: Eight years' experience. *Radiology* 152:755–757, 1984.

23. Zornosa J, et al. Percutaneous needle biopsy in abdominal lymphoma. *AJR* 136:97–103, 1981.

24. Erwin BC, et al. Percutaneous needle biopsy in the diagnosis and classification of lymphoma. *Cancer* 57:1074–1078, 1986.

25. Haaga JR, et al. Clinical comparison of small- and large-caliber cutting needles for biopsy. *Radiology* 146:665–667, 1983.

26. Gazelle GS, Haaga JR. Biopsy needle characteristics. *Cardiovasc Intervent Radiol* 14:13–16, 1991.

27. Bernardino ME. Percutaneous biopsy. *AJR* 142:41–45, 1984.

28. Matalon TAS, Silver B. US guidance of interventional procedures. *Radiology* 174:43–47, 1990.

29. Hamper UM, Savader BL, Sheth S. Improved needle-tip visualization by color Doppler sonography. *AJR* 156:401–402, 1991.

30. Reading CC, et al. US-guided percutaneous biopsy: Use of a screw biopsy stylet to aid needle detection. *Radiology* 163:280–281, 1987.

31. Winsberg F, et al. Use of an accoustic transponder for US visualization of biopsy needles. *Radiology* 180:877–878, 1991.

32. Perrella RR, et al. A new electronically enhanced biopsy system: Value in improving needle-tip visibility during sonographically guided interventional procedures. *AJR* 158:195–198, 1992.

33. Palestrant AM. Comprehensive approach to CT-guided procedures with a hand-held guidance device. *Radiology* 174:270–272, 1990.

34. Reyes GD. A guidance device for CT-guided procedures. *Radiology* 176:863–864, 1990.

35. Onik G, et al. CT-guided aspirations for the body: Comparison of hand guidance with stereotaxis. *Radiology* 166:389–394, 1988.

36. Magnusson A, Akerfeldt D. CT-guided core biopsy using a new guidance device. *Acta Radiol* 32:83–85, 1991.

37. Silverman SG, et al. Needle-tip localization during CT-guided abdominal biopsy: Comparison of conventional and spiral CT. *AJR* 159:1095–1097, 1992.

38. Bernardino ME. CT-Guided Biopsy and Needle Selection. In PR Mueller, E vanSonnenberg, G Becker (eds.), *Syllabus: A Diagnostic Categorical Course in Interventional Radiology*. Oak Brook, IL: RSNA Publications, 1991. Pp. 17–21.

39. Ferrucci JT, Wittenberg J. CT biopsy of abdominal tumors: Aids for lesion localization. *Radiology* 129:739–744, 1978.

40. Haaga JR, et al. Interventional CT scanning. *Radiol Clin North Am* 15:449–456, 1977.

41. Parker SH, et al. Image-directed percutaneous biopsies with a biopsy gun. *Radiology* 171:663–669, 1989.

42. Bernadino ME. Automated biopsy devices: Significance and safety. *Radiology* 176:615–616, 1990.

43. Solbiati L, et al. Fine needle biopsy of hepatic hemangioma with sonographic guidance. *AJR* 144:471–474, 1985.

44. Bernadino ME, et al. CT-guided adrenal biopsy: Accuracy, safety, and indications. *AJR* 144:67–69, 1985.

45. Heiberg E, Wolverson MK. Ipsilateral decubitus position for percutaneous CT-guided adrenal biopsy. *J Comput Assist Tomogr* 9:217–218, 1985.

46. Axel L. Simple method for performing oblique CT-guided needle biopsies. *AJR* 143:341–342, 1984.

47. van Sonnenberg E, et al. Triangulation method for percutaneous needle guidance: The angled approach to upper abdominal masses. *AJR* 137:757–761, 1981.

48. Yueh N, et al. Gantry tilt technique for CT-guided biopsy and drainage. *J Comput Assist Tomogr* 13:182–184, 1989.

49. Butch RJ, et al. Drainage of pelvic abscesses through the greater sciatic foramen. *Radiology* 158:487–491, 1986.

50. Graham D, Sanders RC. Ultrasound directed transvaginal aspiration biopsy of pelvic masses. *J Ultrasound Med* 1:279–280, 1982.

51. Nosher JL, et al. Transrectal pelvic abscess drainage with sonographic guidance. *AJR* 146:1047–1048, 1986.

52. Savader BL, et al. Pelvic masses: Aspiration biopsy with transrectal US guidance. *Radiology* 176:351–353, 1990.

53. Smith EH. Complications of percutaneous abdominal fine-needle biopsy. *Radiology* 178:253–258, 1991.
54. Mueller PR, et al. Pancreatitis after percutaneous tumor biopsy. *AJR* 151:493–494, 1989.
55. Livraghi T, et al. Risk in fine-needle abdominal biopsy. *J Clin Ultrasound* 11:77–81, 1983.

Percutaneous Drainage
of Abdominal Abscesses
and Fluid Collections

Krishna Kandarpa
Sanjay Saini

Indications [1–9]

In general, radiologic signs are unable to distinguish among various types of fluid collections or to predict utility of therapeutic catheter drainage [1,2].

1. For needle aspiration. To determine nature (infected versus noninfected) of any abnormal intraabdominal fluid collection (differential diagnosis: abscess, hematoma, urinoma, bileoma, seroma, loculated ascites).
2. For catheter drainage
   a. To treat or palliate sepsis (e.g., diverticular abscess) associated with an infected fluid collection.
   b. To alleviate symptoms that may be caused by fluid collections by virtue of their size or location (e.g., noninfected pancreatic pseudocyst, lymphocele).

Contraindications [1–9]

ABSOLUTE

Absence of safe access route (avoiding major blood vessels) to the collection. In addition, transgression of solid organs and bowel should be avoided. However, selected solid organs (e.g., liver, kidney) and small bowel may be transgressed during diagnostic needle aspiration [4,10–12]. Catheter drainage requires a safe access route with the possible exception of pelvic collections that can be drained via a transrectal or transvaginal approach [13–17]. Prior to catheter drainage, use of "nonsafe" routes should be discussed with the consulting surgeon.

RELATIVE

1. Coagulopathy (should be corrected).
2. If possible, avoid transgressing pleural space. Pleural reflections lie at the twelfth rib anteriorly and posteriorly, and at the tenth rib along the midaxillary line.
3. Intrahepatic echinococcal cyst (leakage of contents may cause fatal anaphylactic reaction or dissemination of scoleces; mural calcification of the cyst or presence of daughter cysts should alert one to this diagnosis).

Preprocedure Preparation

1. Check prior imaging studies to plan the procedure (e.g., CT versus US). For guidance, choose the most efficient imaging system that allows demonstration of location, extent, and relationship of fluid collection to vital structures.

Occasionally, procedures may require more than one modality. Remember to exclude vascular aneurysms mimicking fluid collections.

   a. Real-time US is preferred if the fluid collection is clearly visualized and a safe access route can be identified.

   b. CT guidance is more time-consuming but is preferred for deep-seated fluid collections with overlying vital structures.

   c. Fluoroscopy is seldom used as the primary guidance method except in combination with US or CT when Seldinger technique is used to place a catheter. Fluoroscopy is useful for determining reduction in cavity size from healing, the presence of internal communications, and for catheter exchanges and repositioning.

2. Check history (especially for aspirin use) and laboratory results; need PT (< 15 seconds), PTT (< 1.5 control), platelets (> 75,000/ml).

3. Stop oral intake (except medication), preferably several hours prior to the procedure. For CT-guided procedures, oral contrast is necessary to identify bowel. In some cases, rectal contrast may be needed.

4. Obtain informed consent (prior to administration of sedatives) for aspiration and possible drainage. Breathing instructions also are given at this time. In general, scanning is performed during quiet breathing and needles and catheters are placed at end-expiration.

5. Obtain IV access for hydration, medication, and contrast administration (20-gauge or larger). Patients for abscess drainage should be on antibiotics to prevent septicemia associated with drainage (see Chap. 40 regarding antibiotics).

Procedure

GENERAL COMMENTS [1–9,18,19]

1. Position the patient for optimal access to the collection while keeping patient's comfort in mind.

2. Adequate local anesthesia and conscious sedation is mandatory. Vital-signs should be monitored (BP, heart rate, oxygen saturation). The procedure should not be unnecessarily painful.

3. Rescan the patient and mark skin entry site. Rescanning must be done with the patient breathing such that needle/catheter placement can be performed under similar conditions.

4. Determine angle of needle/catheter placement and depth of insertion. Shortest safe route is preferred. Note that for catheter drainage, it is preferable to have an entry site that allows the patient to lie comfortably in bed.

DIAGNOSTIC NEEDLE ASPIRATION [9,18]

1. Prepare and drape skin puncture site in a sterile fashion.

2. Administer local anesthesia (2% lidocaine [Xylocaine]) and IV sedation.

3. Use 22- or 20-gauge needle of adequate length (e.g., spinal needle) for initial localization and aspiration. Note or mark the length of needle to be inserted (with a sterile adhesive strip).

4. Insert the needle during suspended respiration, generally at end-expiration. It may be necessary to check if the needle is following the desired route.

5. Withdraw 5 ml of fluid for Gram stain, culture, and special chemistry tests (e.g., amylase for suspected pancreatic leak). Additional fluid (>20–100 ml) may be necessary for cytologic analysis. Volume of fluid aspirated should be minimized in case percutaneous catheter placement is required.

6. If no fluid can be aspirated, rescan to check position of needle tip. If needle tip position is acceptable, the fluid may be too viscous (e.g., pus, hematoma) and a larger (18-gauge) needle should be used. If difficulty with aspiration persists, perform a biopsy.

7. Do not remove this diagnostic needle. In the event that catheter drainage is needed, it serves as a guide for catheter insertion.

THERAPEUTIC CATHETER DRAINAGE [1–9,18–27]

1. Diagnostic needle aspiration usually precedes catheter placement. The needle also will serve to guide the placement of a "tandem" drainage catheter.

2. Catheter selection [9]. Use the largest catheter (usually between 10 and 14 Fr.) that can be safely placed; choose one with an adequate number of side holes to facilitate drainage. The more viscuos the fluid, the larger the catheter which will be needed. Drainage of cysts, seromas, and noninfected abscesses may be accomplished with a 7–9 Fr. catheter. However, removal of necrotic debris may require 16–20 Fr. catheters. Multiple catheters may be needed for large collections.

3. Technique for catheter placement
   a. Direct trocar technique is used most often.
      (1) The assembled catheter (needle-stylet + metal stiffener + plastic catheter) is inserted alongside the diagnostic needle already in place.
      (2) Once the tip is at the desired depth, the inner stylet is removed and fluid aspirated. Fluid aspiration confirms that the catheter tip is appropriately positioned.
      (3) The catheter is advanced over the metal stiffener which is held stationary. Catheter should slide easily; difficulty with deployment or sudden patient pain suggests improper placement.
   b. Sheath-needle technique is used only if the access route is limited and there may be risk of injury to vital structures (see Fig. 21-2). The technique involves placement of an 18-gauge needle with a plastic sheath through which 0.038-in. guidewires can be inserted. After dilation of the tract with angiographic fascial dilators, catheters are positioned within the collection. Dilation without fluoroscopic guidance must be done carefully

because inadvertent kinking of the guidewire will cause difficulties with catheter placement.

4. Initial drainage and irrigation
   a. Irrigating the cavity with normal saline until the return is clear of pus and particulate debris facilitates evacuation and prevents subsequent catheter occlusion. Do not overdistend the cavity as this may cause hematogeneous seeding and sepsis.
   b. Near-complete evacuation of the collection at the time of initial catheter placement is desirable, but often does not occur. This should be confirmed by immediate rescanning. If indicated, further manipulation or placement of an additional catheter should be performed immediately.

5. Anchor the catheter externally with an adhesive-backed locking device. Attach a bag for gravity drainage and place a stopcock at the catheter's external end for routine irrigation.

Postprocedure Management

1. Daily ward rounds must be made by the radiologist to monitor patient's response, catheter function, need for follow-up imaging, or timing of catheter removal.

2. Continue systemic antibiotics, covering for specific organism(s) (see section on antibiotics in Chap. 40), until all signs and symptoms of infection abate (reduced fever and leukocytosis).

3. Gently irrigate the catheter to maintain patency, q8–24h (frequency depending on viscosity of fluid), with 5 ml saline using sterile technique. Monitor catheter output daily. Frequency of irrigation can be slowed or stopped altogether as drainage volume decreases and the patient has a successful clinical response. Low suction is often applied to drainage catheters [9].

4. Patient conditions
   a. With adequate drainage, defervescence is prompt (24–48 hours).
   b. Persistent fever suggests undrained pus, which should be evaluated with a repeat CT scan. If necessary, catheter manipulation under fluoroscopy may be needed for better positioning, or additional catheter(s) may be required, or intracavitary urokinase (UK) may be administered to break loculations [20].
   c. With adequate drainage and good patient response, catheter output should decrease progressively over several days (2–7 days depending on the cavity size and nature of fluid). A sudden decrease or cessation may mean the catheter is obstructed or kinked. A sudden increase or change in character of fluid should alert one to fistulous communications [28]. In case of a fistula-to-bowel, biliary tree, or urinary collecting system, longer-term (3–4 weeks) drainage may be needed; and the bile or urine may need to be diverted by independent external drainage. Drainage of unresectable infected tumors requires "permanent" drainage [29].

  d. Therapy of loculated collections and hematomas may
  be enhanced with use of intracavitary fibrinolytic
  agents such as UK [30].
 5. Catheter removal is based on
  a. Successful therapy as determined by abatement of clinical symptoms and signs of infection, and less than 10
  ml of drainage per 24 hours. Corroborative radiographic evidence (sinogram) of cavity closure and healing of communications is useful.
  b. Sterile collection (e.g., hematoma, seroma), even if in-
  completely drained. Early catheter removal is recommended in order to prevent introducing an infection.
  c. Failed percutaneous drainage requiring surgery.

Results

See Table 23-1 [1,2,7,19].

Complications

See Table 23-2 [1,2,5,7,9,19,31].

Table 23-1. Results of percutaneous drainage of abdominal abscesses [1,2,7,9,19]

Success[a]	Partial success[b]	Recurrence[c]	Failure[d]	Duration[e]
70–90%	7–18%	8%	8–20%	1–2 weeks

[a]Cure without surgery (rate depends on location and type of abscess).
[b]Successful drainage with surgical repair of fistula or other complicating factors.
[c]Causes of recurrence: abnormal communication or leak, early catheter removal, infected tumor [7].
[d]Cause of failure: failure to recognize multiloculation, phlegmon, immature abscess membrane, associated fistula, organized hematoma, improper catheter position, or premature catheter removal [2,6,19].
[e]For pyogenic abscess, results of surgical drainage are as follows: success 70%, complications 16%, mortality 21%, duration of drainage 29 days [1].

Table 23-2. Complications of percutaneous drainage of abdominal abscesses [1,2,5,7,9,19]

Total	Major[a]	Minor[b]	Mortality (30 days)
5–10%	5–7%	3%	1–6%

[a]Major: septicemia (with associated disseminated intravascular coagulation, or hypotension), infection of initially sterile collection, small-bowel fistula, death (usually due to sepsis or hemorrhage).
[b]Minor: bacteremia, catheter back-bleeding (usually resolves spontaneously, but may need angiographic investigation on occasion [31]), pleural transgression without pneumothorax or infection, entry-site skin infection.

References

1. Gerzof SG, et al. Percutaneous catheter drainage of abdominal abscesses: A five-year experience. *N Engl J Med* 305:653–657, 1981.

2. Jacques P, et al. CT features of intraabdominal abscesses: Prediction of successful percutaneous drainage. *AJR* 146:1041–1045, 1986.

3. Lambiase RE, et al. Percutaneous drainage of 335 consecutive abscesses: Results of primary drainage with 1-year follow-up. *Radiology* 184:167–179, 1992.

4. Lang EK. Renal, perirenal, and pararenal abscesses: Percutaneous drainage. *Radiology* 174:109–113, 1990.

5. Mueller PR, vanSonnenberg E, Ferrucci JT Jr. Percutaneous drainage of 250 abdominal abscesses and fluid collections. Part II: Current procedural concepts. *Radiology* 151:343–347, 1984.

6. Mueller PR, vanSonnenberg E. Interventional radiology in the chest and abdomen. *N Engl J Med* 322:1364–1374, 1990.

7. vanSonnenberg E, Mueller PR, Ferrucci JT Jr. Percutaneous drainage of 250 abdominal abscesses and fluid collections. Part I: Results, failures, and complications. *Radiology* 151:337–341, 1984.

8. vanSonnenberg E, et al. Temporizing effect of percutaneous drainage of complicated abscesses in critically ill patients. *AJR* 142:821–826, 1984.

9. vanSonnenberg E, et al. Percutaneous abscess drainage: Current concepts. *Radiology* 181:617–626, 1991.

10. Ho CS, Taylor B. Transgastric drainage of pancreatic pseudocyst. *AJR* 143:623–625, 1984.

11. Mueller PR, et al: Inadvertent percutaneous catheter gastroenterostomy during abscess drainage: Significance and management. *AJR* 145:387–391, 1985.

12. Mueller PR, et al. Lesser sac abscesses and fluid collections: Drainage by transhepatic approach. *Radiology* 155:615–618, 1985.

13. Abbitt PL, Goldwag S, Urbanski S. Endovaginal sonography for guidance in draining pelvic fluid collections. *AJR* 154:849–850, 1990.

14. Butch RJ, et al. Drainage of pelvic abscesses through the greater sciatic foramen. *Radiology* 158:487–491, 1986.

15. Gazelle GS, et al. Pelvic abscesses: CT-guided transrectal drainage. *Radiology* 181:49–51, 1991.

16. Nosher JL, et al. Transrectal pelvic abscess drainage with sonographic guidance. *AJR* 146:1047–1048, 1986.

17. vanSonnenberg E, et al. US-guided transvaginal drainage of pelvic abscesses and fluid collections. *Radiology* 181:53–56, 1991.

18. vanSonnenberg E, et al. Percutaneous drainage of abscesses and fluid collections: Technique, results and applications. *Radiology* 142:1–10, 1982.

19. Lang EK, et al. Abdominal abscess drainage under radiologic guidance: Causes of failure. *Radiology* 159:329–336, 1986.

20. Lieberman RP, et al. Loculated abscesses: Management by percutaneous fracture of septations. *Radiology* 161:827–828, 1986.

21. Johnson RD, et al. Percutaneous drainage of pyogenic liver abscesses. *AJR* 144:463–467, 1985.

22. Mueller PR, et al. Iliopsoas abscess: Treatment by CT-guided percutaneous catheter drainage. *AJR* 142:359–362, 1984.

23. Mueller PR, et al. Sigmoid diverticular abscesses: Percutaneous drainage as an adjunct to surgical resection in 24 cases. *Radiology* 164:321, 1987.

24. Steiner E, et al. Complicated pancreatic abscesses: Problems in interventional management. *Radiology* 167:443–446, 1988.

25. Tyrrel RT, Murphy FB, Bernardino ME. Tubo-ovarian abscesses: CT-guided percutaneous drainage. *Radiology* 175:87–89, 1990.

26. vanSonnenberg E, et al. Percutaneous drainage of infected and noninfected pancreatic pseudocysts: experience in 101 cases. *Radiology* 170:757–761, 1989.

27. vanSonnenberg E, et al. Periappendiceal abscesses: Percutaneous drainage. *Radiology* 163:23, 1987.

28. Papanicolaou N, et al. Abscess-fistula association: Radiologic recognition and percutaneous management. *AJR* 143:811–815, 1984.

29. Mueller PR, et al. Infected abdominal tumors: Percutaneous catheter drainage. *Radiology* 173:627, 1989.

30. Vogelzang RL, et al. Transcatheter intracavitary fibrinolysis of infected extravascular hematomas. *AJR* 148:378–380, 1987.

31. Routh WD, et al. Tube tamponade: Potential pitfall in angiography of arterial hemorrhage associated with percutaneous drainage catheters. *Radiology* 174: 945–949, 1990.

Percutaneous Gastrostomy and Gastrojejunostomy Tube Placement

Kathleen Reagan
Krishna Kandarpa

Percutaneous radiologic placement of gastrostomy and gastro-jejunostomy tubes is generally considered to be safer than surgical placement [1–3]. No general anesthesia is required; therefore, associated morbidity is eliminated. Endoscopic placement may result in temporarily delayed gastric emptying. The latter procedure is also associated with an increased incidence of aspiration and wound infection. Feedings can be started much sooner following radiologic placement.

Indications [1–3]

1. Nutritional support in a debilitated patient with inadequate oral intake (e.g., patients with neurologic disorders, head and neck lesions, or esophageal lesion).
2. Decompression in chronic small-bowel obstruction.
3. Decreased gastric motility (e.g., diabetic gastropathy, scleroderma).

Contraindications

ABSOLUTE

1. Uncorrectable bleeding diathesis.
2. Presence of a ventriculoperitoneal shunt (risk of infection is unacceptable).
3. Unsatisfactory percutaneous access to stomach (e.g., massive hepatomegaly or interposed colon).

RELATIVE

1. Massive ascites.
2. Abdominal varices from portal hypertension.
3. Prior gastric surgery per se is not a contraindication to percutaneous gastrostomy (PG) [4]. However, access to the stomach will be difficult if the patient has had a partial gastrectomy and the gastric remnant is above the costal margin [2]. If a patient has had a Witzel gastrostomy without gastropexy, the seromuscular tunnel is directed toward the gastric fundus and conversion to a percutaneous gastrojejunostomy (PGJ) tube will be extremely difficult, if not impossible [4,5].
4. Inflammatory, neoplastic, or infectious involvement of the gastric wall (may result in poor wound healing and tract formation).
5. Gastric feeding should be avoided if severe gastroesophageal reflux is present (feedings should be in jejunum via a gastrojejunostomy tube [1,6,7]).

Preprocedure Preparation

1. Review type of prior gastric surgery, if any, to determine if the intended procedure can be successfully completed; this will also allow planning of needed modifications to the procedure. Review prior barium studies, if available.
2. A preliminary CT or US examination can be used to rule out a left hepatic lobe that may overlie the stomach. A transhepatic puncture may result in significant hemorrhage or extravasation of bile, or both. Localization of the transverse colon is important in order to avoid inadvertent puncture (Fig. 24-1). If difficulties with fluoroscopic guidance are anticipated, a gastrostomy tube may be placed under CT guidance [8].
3. Obtain consent from patient or responsible person.
4. Stop all oral intake overnight.
5. Check CBC, PT, PTT, platelet count, and bleeding time.
6. It is helpful to have the nasogastric (NG) tube placed the evening before the procedure for adequate suction of gastric contents. If there is difficulty placing the NG tube, it may be done with fluoroscopic guidance using a multipurpose or curved catheter over a guidewire, immediately prior to the percutaneous procedure. If this is also impossible, CT guidance should be considered [8].
7. Preprocedural conscious sedation should be given judiciously in patients with head and neck malignancies or respiratory compromise or both.

Procedure [1–3,9–12]

1. Sterile preparation of the left subcostal area and epigastrium.
2. Glucagon 0.5–1.0 mg IV may be administered to diminish peristalsis.
3. Insufflate air into the stomach via NG tube, usually 500–1000 cc or until adequate gastric distention is achieved. It is often necessary to continue air insufflation during the procedure, particularly at the time of needle puncture and tract dilatation, to keep the stomach distended so as to oppose the anterior gastric wall against the anterior abdominal wall.
   a. Effervescent granules may be used in some patients who are able to swallow.
   b. Alternative methods for PG/PGJ tube placement and maintenance include:
      (1) Use of an intragastric, contrast-filled balloon for gastric distention and support of the anterior wall of the stomach against the anterior wall of the abdomen during puncture [13].
      (2) Use of four T-fasteners to fix the anterior gastric wall to the abdominal wall (gastropexy) during PG tube placement and subsequent manipulation [5,14]. The intention is to prevent tube dislodgment and leakage of gastric contents into the peritoneum. However, the need for these fixation devices remains controversial [15].

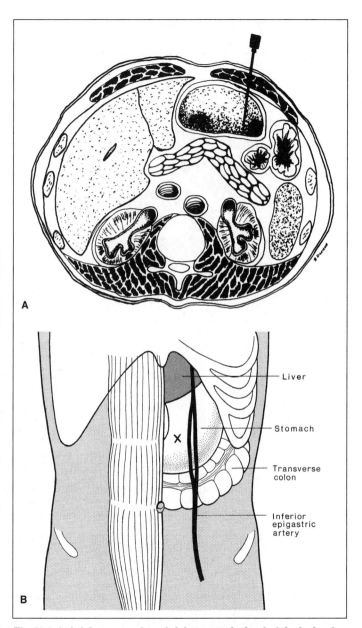

Fig. 24-1. A. Axial cross-section of abdomen at the level of the body of the stomach with patient supine. No liver or colon noted anteriorly. **B.** Frontal cut-away view shows window to body of stomach, avoiding the inferior epigastric artery, left lobe of the liver, and transverse colon. **C.** Sagittal view demonstrating superficial location of the anterior wall of a distended stomach. Liver is cephalad to, and lumen of transverse colon is caudal to, the stomach.

Labels in figure B: Liver, Stomach, Transverse colon, Inferior epigastric artery

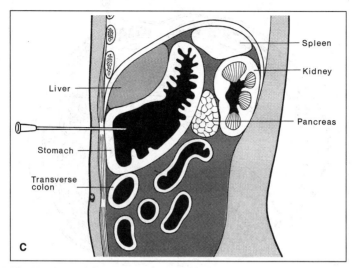

Fig. 24-1 (continued).

(3) Use of a single temporary suture anchor (in place for 7 days), which simplifies initial tract dilatation and tube placement, and prevents tube dislodgment [16].

4. After air insufflation, frontal and lateral views of the upper abdomen are helpful to determine the depth to the anterior gastric wall (Fig. 24-2). The puncture site is chosen (with fluoroscopic guidance) to overlie the distal body of the stomach below the costal margin and above the transverse colon. The risk of hemorrhage should be diminished if one avoids the inferior epigastric artery that courses at the junction of the medial two-thirds and lateral one-third of the rectus muscle [9]. Care must be taken not to advance the puncture needle too deeply, in order to avoid puncturing the posterior gastric wall, pancreas, left kidney, aorta, or spleen.

5. Anesthetize the puncture site with liberal local injection of 1% lidocaine down to the peritoneal surface (distance from skin to the anterior gastric wall is usually 4–5 cm) [11,12]; a small skin incision (5 mm) is made and a subcutaneous tract is created with a blunt-nosed hemostat.

6. A Seldinger needle may be used for gastric puncture in thin or cachectic patients. A 22-gauge needle (Cope Introduction Set; Cook, Inc., Bloomington, IN) may be used in larger patients. Puncture with either needle should be made with a brief, deliberate thrust so as not to push the anterior gastric wall away from the anterior abdominal wall, if gastropexy has not been performed. The needle should be directed toward the pylorus, if conversion to a PGJ tube is anticipated. If the procedure is for simple gastric drainage, the needle may be directed vertically down or slightly toward the fundus [1].

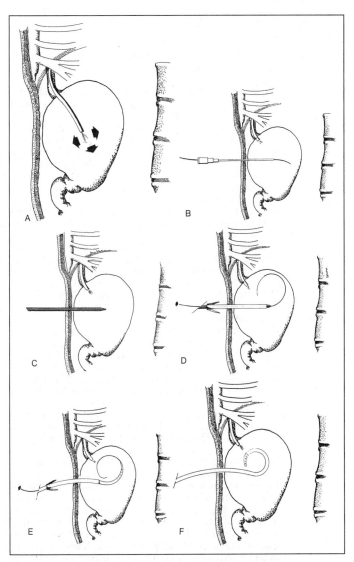

Fig. 24-2. Alternative method for placement of a percutaneous gastrostomy tube. A. The stomach is inflated with air through the nasogastric tube to bring the gastric wall close to the abdominal wall. B. The puncture is made with a 16-gauge needle/catheter pointing vertically down, and a 0.035-in. J guidewire is advanced through it. C, D. Before inserting the peel-away introducer sheath, fascial dilators are advanced over the guidewire until an adequate diameter is reached. E. The catheter is advanced over the guidewire through the peel-away sheath. F. After the catheter is in place, the guidewire is removed and the sheath is peeled away. (Reprinted from M Maynar et al. Gastrointestinal Tract Intervention. In WR Castañeda-Zúñiga, SM Tadavarthy [eds.], *Interventional Radiology* [2nd ed.]. Baltimore: Williams & Wilkins, 1992. Pp. 1218–1219.)

7. Once the gastric lumen is entered, the needle position is confirmed by injection of contrast, outlining gastric rugal folds
    a. When the Seldinger needle tip is within the stomach, a standard 0.038-in. J-tipped guidewire is inserted and looped in the stomach.
    b. When a 22-gauge needle is used (Cope Introduction Set, Cook), a 0.018-in. guidewire is passed into the stomach, the needle is withdrawn, and a 6.3 Fr. tapered dilator is introduced over the wire. The 0.018-in. wire is then replaced with the standard 0.038-in. J-tipped guidewire, which exits through the distal side hole of the 6.3 Fr. dilator.
8. Fascial dilators are exchanged over the 0.038-in. guidewire and a tract of adequate diameter to accommodate the catheter is created.
9. For placement of a gastrojejunostomy tube, a curved catheter, such as a Cobra-1, is used over the guidewire to direct and advance it into the pylorus and small bowel. Occasionally, use of a torquable Ring A or B guidewire or guidewire M (Terumo, Medi-Tech/Boston Scientific Corp., Watertown, MA) is helpful in directing the catheter.
10. Tube placement
    a. Gastrostomy. A 10 Fr. Cope loop nephrostomy tube (Cook, Inc., Bloomington, IN) is placed in the gastric body or fundus [17]. Larger self-retaining gastrosotomy tubes (16 Fr.) also may be introduced directly and safely when the proper techniques are employed [15]. Foley catheters have a higher reported incidence of complications [17].
    b. Gastrojejunostomy. An 8–12 Fr. Flexiflo enteral feeding tube (114 cm) (Ross Laboratories, Columbus, Ohio) is placed over the guidewire, with its distal tip beyond the ligament of Treitz.
    Note: Pureed foods will not pass easily through a 10 Fr. catheter but less viscous foods will [12].
    c. Conversion of a gastrostomy to a gastrojejunostomy tube. Can be accomplished in 80% of cases, regardless of how the gastrostomy tube was placed. Failures (and difficulties with successfully converted tubes) are due to an unfavorable fundal angulation during initial (surgical or endoscopic) entry into the stomach. When the initial angulation is unfavorable, a new puncture directed towards the pylorus is suggested so as to avoid later proximal migration and recoil of a successfully placed PGJ tube [6]. Gastrosotomy tubes themselves do not cause gastroesophageal reflux. However, patients may be selected for conversion to a PGJ tube, if gastroesophageal reflux is detected on scintigraphy [7].
11. Following tube placement, repeat frontal and lateral films of the upper abdomen after injection of contrast are obtained.
12. The PG or PGJ tube is secured to the skin by suturing the taped tube to a Stomadhesive disk (Drain/Tube attachment device, Hollister, Inc., Libertyville, IL) at the skin site.

13. Feedings through the gastrostomy tube leave the patient with a sense of satiety due to gastric distention. However, if gastroesophageal reflux is present (reported in about half of the cases studied [7,10]), the PG tube may be converted to a PGJ tube at any time after placement with gastropexy [5,16], or after the tract matures (usually in 7–10 days) if a fixation device is not used [3].

Postprocedural Management

1. Vital signs and serial abdominal examination must be closely followed, looking for signs of peritonitis that may indicate leakage of gastric contents. Pneumoperitoneum is not unexpected and slowly resolves over 24–72 hours.

2. The PG tube should remain clamped, or put to low, intermittent suction for the 24 hours following placement before attempting feedings. The NG tube may remain clamped overnight; if the patient does well, it may be removed the next morning. If the PG or PGJ tube is placed for chronic small-bowel obstruction, low, intermittent suction should be begun early and continued. A successfully placed or converted PGJ feeding tube may be used within hours of insertion.

3. Feeding. A consultation with a nutritionist is suggested. If the abdominal exam remains benign, dilute tube feedings may begin via the PG tube the day after placement—after a contrast study is done to rule out leakage. If a PGJ tube is placed, the stomach can be decompressed for 24 hours through the NG tube, but feeding can be started immediately via the PGJ tube since the nutrients are delivered to the jejunum [2].

4. The Stomadhesive disk (Hollister, Inc., Libertyville, IL) secures the tube to the skin; therefore, it must remain dry.

5. Dressing-changes over the tube and disk are on a prn basis—at least daily.

6. If leakage of gastric contents results in skin breakdown at the insertion site, a liquid antacid may be applied topically to the area.

Results

Technical success of percutaneous fluoroscopic placement of gastrostomy tubes approaches 100% [2,11,12,17].

Complications

1. Thirty-day mortality ranges from 8% [3] to 12% [15] but may be higher depending on the severity of the underlying illness [17]. Procedure-related mortality is less than 1% [1].

2. Major morbidity (hemorrhage, peritonitis, tube migration, aspiration, and sepsis): 3–6% [3,15,17]. Minor morbidity: 1–12% [3,15,17]. Surgical mortality and complications rates are statistically significantly higher, and percutaneous radiologic placement is considered to be the safer and preferred approach [3].

3. Aspiration secondary to gastroesophageal reflux with gastric or duodenal (NG or ND) tube feedings: incidence approaches 38%. PG tube placement itself will not significantly alter this risk, yet gastric reflux can be minimized by placing a PGJ tube (distal to the ligament of Treitz) [7,10].

4. Gastric bleeding following PG or PGJ tube placement has an incidence of 0.7%—however, it is 0.9–1.4% with surgically placed gastrostomy and gastrojejunostomy tubes [18].

5. Other potential complications: laceration of the liver, pancreas, or spleen; gastroenteric fistula.

References

1. Ho CS. Percutaneous Gastrostomy and Transgastric Jejunostomy. In S Kadir (ed.), *Current Practice of Interventional Radiology.* Philadelphia: B.C. Decker, 1991. Pp. 444–449.

2. Ho CS, et al. Percutaneous gastrostomy for enteral feeding. *Radiology* 156:349–351, 1985.

3. Ho CS, Yee AC, McPherson R. Complications of surgical and percutaneous nonendoscopic gastrostomy: Review of 233 patients. *Gastroenterology* 95:1206–1210, 1988.

4. Stevens SD, et al. Percutaneous gastrostomy and gastrojejunostomy after gastric surgery. *J Vasc Intervent Radiol* 3:679–683, 1992.

5. Saini S, et al. Percutaneous gastrostomy with gastropexy: Experience in 125 patients. *AJR* 154:1003–1006, 1990.

6. Lu DS, et al. Gastrostomy conversion to transgastric jejunostomy: Technical problems, causes of failure, and proposed solutions in 63 patients. *Radiology* 187:679–683, 1993.

7. Olson DL, Krubsack AJ, Stewart ET. Percutaneous enteral alimentation: Gastrostomy versus gastrojejunostomy. *Radiology* 187:105–108, 1993.

8. Sanchez RB, et al. CT guidance for percutaneous gastrostomy and gastroenterostomy. *Radiology* 184:201–205, 1992.

9. vanSonnenberg E, et al: Percutaneous gastrostomy and gastroenterostomy: II. Clinical experience. *AJR* 146:581–586, 1986.

10. Alzate GD, et al. Percutaneous gastrostomy for jejunal feeding: A new technique. *AJR* 147:822–825, 1986.

11. Wills JS, Oglesby JT. Percutaneous gastrostomy. *Radiology* 154:71–74, 1985.

12. Wills JS, Oglesby JT. Percutaneous gastrostomy. *Radiology* 162:41–43, 1988.

13. vanSonnenberg E, et al. Percutaneous gastrostomy: Use of intragastric balloon support. *Radiology* 152:531–532, 1984.

14. Brown AS, Mueller PR, Ferrucci JT Jr. Controlled percutaneous gastrostomy: Nylon T-fastener for fixation of the anterior gastric wall. *Radiology* 158:543–545, 1986.

15. Deutsch LS, et al. Simplified percutaneous gastrostomy. *Radiology* 184:181–183, 1992.

16. Coleman CC, et al. Percutaneous enterostomy with the Cope suture anchor. *Radiology* 174:889–891, 1990.

17. Hicks ME, et al. Fluoroscopically guided percutaneous gastrostomy and gastroenterostomy: Analysis of 158 consecutive cases. *AJR* 154:725–728, 1990.
18. Rose DB, Wolman SL, Ho CS. Gastric hemorrhage complicating percutaneous transgastric jejunostomy. *Radiology* 161:835–836, 1986.

Transvaginal Fallopian Tube Recanalization

Michael F. Meyerovitz

Indications

Infertility due to proximal fallopian tube occlusion (20–40% of female infertility is due to tubal disease).

Contraindications

1. Active pelvic inflammatory disease.
2. Previous tubal surgery.
3. Severe tubal or peritubal pathology on laparoscopy.
4. Distal tubal occlusion.
5. Intrauterine adhesions (severe).

Preprocedure Preparation

1. Schedule procedure during first 10 days of menstrual cycle, in the follicular phase, after menstrual bleeding has stopped. This is an outpatient procedure.
2. Prophylactic antibiotics, doxycycline 100 mg PO bid, started on evening prior to procedure and continued for 3 days postprocedure.
3. Obtain informed consent.
4. Start peripheral IV.
5. Premedicate with midazolam (Versed) 1–2 mg IV (make sure someone can drive the patient home following the procedure). Fentanyl 25 µg IV as needed.

Procedure [1–6]

1. Place patient in dorsal lithotomy position.
2. Utilize sterile technique for preparation of perineum (Betadine scrub) drape.
3. Insert vaginal speculum.
4. Perform paracervical block utilizing 20 ml 0.5% lidocaine without adrenaline at 4 and 7 o'clock positions.
5. Cannulate cervix with introducing catheter and perform hysterosalpingogram.
6. If hysterosalpingogram confirms proximal tubal occlusion, insert curved 5 Fr. catheter coaxially through introducing catheter and selectively catheterize ostium of occluded tube. Inject contrast medium selectively into the tubal ostium.
7. If selective ostial injection confirms proximal tubal occlusion, insert a 3 Fr. Teflon catheter coaxially through the 5 Fr. catheter, and probe the obstruction with a 0.015-in. guidewire. Once the 0.015-in. guidewire is successfully manipulated past the obstruction, the 3 Fr. catheter is gently passed over the guidewire, the guidewire is with-

drawn, and contrast medium is injected through the 3 Fr. catheter to check distal tubal patency.

8. An alternative technique instead of a 3 Fr. Teflon catheter and 0.015-in. guidewire is to use a 0.035-in. Glidewire (Medi-Tech, Inc., Watertown, MA) to probe and recanalize the tubal occlusion. After this wire is successfully manipulated past the tubal obstruction, it is removed, and distal tubal patency is checked by ostial injection through the 5 Fr. catheter.

9. Alternatively (to 7 and 8 above), a 2 mm balloon catheter can be used to dilate the proximal fallopian tube.

10. After manipulations are completed on one side, the procedure is repeated in the contralateral occluded fallopian tubes.

11. A final hysterosalpingogram is performed through the introducing catheter in the cervix, to document tubal patency.

Postprocedure Management [1–3]

1. Observe patient for 30–60 minutes and discharge, if stable, to a responsible adult who can drive her home.

2. Continue antibiotics for 3 days (e.g., doxycycline 100 mg PO bid).

3. Advise patient that vaginal spotting may occur for up to 3 days.

Results [2–4,7–9]

1. Overall, successful recanalization of at least one fallopian tube is achieved in 79–83% of patients, and intrauterine pregnancy is achieved in 26–33% of patients [2–4,7]. The results are less encouraging as the blockage gets more distal from the uterus [8].

2. In a small series of patients (n = 20) with proximal tubal occlusion, successful recanalization of at least one fallopian tube was achieved in 95% of patients, and intrauterine pregnancy was achieved in 47% of patients [2]; mean time to pregnancy is about 4 months [2,4].

3. If pregnancy has not occurred within 6 months of successful tubal recanalization, repeat hysterosalpingography demonstrates that in approximately 50% of patients, one or both fallopian tubes will have reoccluded [2].

Complications [2,4,9,10]

1. Tubal perforation 5% (however, no clinical sequelae).
2. Ectopic pregnancy 1–5%.
3. Low-grade fever.

References

1. Rosch J, et al. Selective transcervical fallopian tube catheterization: Technique update. *Radiology* 168:1–5, 1988.
2. Thurmond AS, Rosch J. Nonsurgical fallopian tube recanalization for treatment of infertility. *Radiology* 174:371–374, 1990.

3. Thurmond AS, Uchida BT, Rosch J. Device for hysterosalpingography and fallopian tube catheterization. *Radiology* 174:571–572, 1990.

4. Confino E, et al. Transcervical balloon tuboplasty: A multicenter study. *JAMA* 264:2079–2082, 1990.

5. LaBerge JM, Ponec DJ, Gordon RL. Fallopian tube catheterization: Modified fluoroscopic technique. *Radiology* 176:283–284, 1990.

6. Meyerovitz MF. Hysterosalpingography and fallopian tube cannulation: Use of a double-balloon introducing catheter. *Radiology* 181:901–902, 1991.

7. Hovsepian DM, et al. Fallopian tube recanalization in an unrestricted patient population. *Radiology* 190:137–140, 1994.

8. Hayashi N, et al. Fallopian tube disease: Limited value of treatment with fallopian tube catheterization. *Radiology* 190:141–143, 1994.

9. Thurmond AS. Pregnancies after selective salpingography and tubal recanalization. *Radiology* 190:11–13, 1994.

10. Isaacson KB, et al. Transcervical fallopian tube recanalization: A safe and effective therapy for patients with proximal tubal obstruction. *Int J Fertil* 37:106–110, 1992.

Complementary Noninvasive Vascular Evaluation

Noninvasive Vascular Studies

John E. Aruny
Joseph F. Polak

Venous Ultrasound of the Lower Extremity

Indications

1. Acute onset of lower extremity swelling or pain, raising suspicion of acute deep venous thrombosis (DVT).
2. Early pregnancy or other contraindications for contrast phlebography in cases that suggest DVT.
3. The evaluation of high-risk, asymptomatic patients (controversial). The definition of "high-risk" is extensive and includes the elderly, bedridden, postsurgery (especially those who have had hip replacement), or posttrauma patients [1].
4. To establish a baseline study following the completion of anticoagulation. This will permit the detection of any venous changes that may cause confusion in future studies.
5. Preoperative mapping of the saphenous vein.
6. Detection and segmental analysis of venous reflux in patients with:
   a. Obesity with varicose veins.
   b. Recurrent varicose veins after surgery.
   c. Cutaneous ulceration.
   d. Serious venous stasis complaints with or without subcutaneous induration.

Relative Contraindications

1. Difficulty of the examination is a function of body habitus and the transducer used (5.0 MHz or 7.5 MHz).
2. Recent surgical or skin wounds along sites to be surveyed.
3. Painful extremity that does not permit adequate compression of the skin surface over the vein being examined.

Preprocedure Preparation

1. No patient preparation is needed.
2. Intensive care patients can be examined with portable units.
3. Equipment
   a. Below the inguinal ligament. High-resolution B-mode imaging with 5.0 MHz or 7.5 MHz linear array transducer with pulsed Doppler capability. The flat face of the linear array transducer is an excellent surface to compress the vein without it rolling from under the transducer [1] (Fig. 26-1). Color-assisted duplex Doppler mapping is used for detection and segmental evaluation venous reflux.

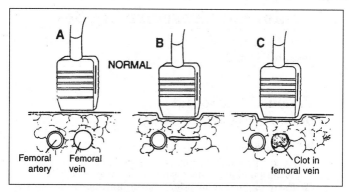

Fig. 26-1. A. The flat surface of the linear array transducer is an excellent surface with which to perform venous compression. **B.** With compression, the normal vein completely collapses with the opposite walls coapted. **C.** With DVT, the vein resists compression and the lumen persists. Chronic venous changes may mimic the inability to perform complete coaptation as seen in acute DVT. (Reprinted from JJ Cronan. Venous thromboembolic disease: The role of US. *Radiology* 186:619–630, 1993.)

    b. Above the inguinal ligament in the iliac veins and inferior vena cava (IVC) a 3.5–5.0 MHz sector scanner is used. The gain is set so that the lumen of a normal vessel will be free of internal echoes. The accompanying artery may be used as a reference to set the gain appropriately.

    c. Color Doppler US may be helpful in the thigh and popliteal regions where it is used in a complementary manner to the compression maneuver. In the IVC and iliac veins, color-assisted Doppler is useful to demonstrate prograde flow and the detection of nonobstructive thrombus. It is also helpful and timesaving in the evaluation of the postphlebitic syndrome. It is essential when evaluating the calf veins.

    d. The use of a tilt table or reclining stretcher may help in distending veins of poorly mobile patients (reverse Trendelenburg position).

Procedure

DETECTION OF THROMBOEMBOLIC DISEASE

1. **Clot visualization** within the lumen of the vein is the most specific criteria for DVT. However, this is not efficient because of the variable acoustic density of fresh thrombus, which may be close to that of blood. Therefore, fresh clot may escape detection.
2. **Compressibility** of the vein walls is the most important and reproducible part of the examination to detect acute thrombus.
       a. Interrogation of the vein should begin at the inguinal ligament and continue to the distal popliteal vein.

b. For examination of the femoral veins, the patient is positioned supine with the leg to be examined in slight external rotation. The patient's head may be elevated 15–20 degrees (reverse Trendelenburg) to facilitate venous filling. The examination includes interrogation of the common femoral and superficial femoral veins including the proximal portion of the greater saphenous vein at the saphenofemoral junction, just below the inguinal ligament.

c. With the vein beneath the midportion of the US transducer, pressure is applied with the transducer in the transverse imaging position to compress the vein (see Fig. 26-1). A normal vein without clot within its lumen will coapt its walls completely with minimal pressure, which causes the skin to pucker. If the accompanying artery compresses and the walls of the vein are still separated, this is regarded as a positive finding.

d. The compression maneuver is performed in a continuous manner with the operator "walking" the transducer along the vein and compressing every few centimeters.

e. The area where the superficial femoral vein passes through the adductor canal is problematic. Here the normal vein may be difficult to compress. Identifying this area as the only positive site in a study should be done with caution.

f. A second area is the saphenofemoral junction, which may be difficult to compress. This area should be carefully examined as clot in the greater saphenous vein at its junction with the femoral vein may propagate into the femoral vein and increase its potential for embolization to the lung.

g. In the mobile patient, the popliteal vein is examined with the patient prone and the legs elevated at 30 degrees, with a towel or pillow beneath the shin to prevent spontaneous collapse of the vein [2]. Alternatively, in those who are unable to assume this position, the patient may be examined in the decubitus position.

h. Using the compression technique, the popliteal vein is examined from the adductor hiatus to the level of the trifurcation of the calf veins.

3. Pulsed Doppler is used to evaluate:

a. Spontaneous flow. Doppler signal is easily detected in large veins but may require blood flow augmentation in smaller veins [1].

b. Respiratory phasicity. Cyclical variation in venous blood flow that parallels the respiratory cycle. Continuous, nonphasic flow is compatible with venous outflow obstruction.

c. Increase in venous blood flow with augmentation with distal limb compression. The momentary increase in blood flow velocity indicates the absence of occlusion between the point of compression and the location of the transducer.

4. Color Doppler flow imaging may be helpful when results of compression US are indeterminate or the examination is compromised by technical factors such as large patient size, previous episodes of DVT, or pain with compression [3].

   a. The color gain and sensitivity are set to enhance the detection of low velocity blood flow.

   b. Evaluation of the lower extremity veins is performed in the longitudinal plane and begins at or just above the inguinal ligament and extends to the popliteal trifurcation.

   c. The study is considered positive if thrombus is identified within the color signal of the vessel lumen and negative if the color column extends from one wall of the vein to the other.

   d. It has been proposed that chronic DVT can be identified by a narrowed, irregular color column or the detection of numerous venous collateral channels [3].

5. Evaluation of calf vein thrombosis

   a. Use the highest frequency transducer that will permit adequate depth penetration (7.0 MHz or 5.0 MHz). Color assistance is essential.

   b. The anterior tibial veins are identified by placing the transducer in the transverse orientation anterolateral over the lower leg and angled 30 degrees toward the foot. Color will identify the pulsating anterior tibial artery on the hyperechoic interosseous membrane, and the veins can be identified on both sides of the artery [4]. The posterior tibial and peroneal veins can be found by placing the transducer medial to the tibia and angled 30 degrees toward the foot. The posterior tibial artery and associated paired veins are identified, lying medial and posterior to the tibia. The peroneal artery and veins are found lying deep to the posterior tibial artery. Gentle calf compression will accentuate the flow in the veins, making their identification easier [4].

   c. Compression requires somewhat more force than in the popliteal and femoral regions. Compression is performed in the transverse and longitudinal orientation. The presence of thrombus is diagnosed when a dilated noncompressing vein is demonstrated.

Postprocedure Management

Patients with positive calf vein thrombosis and who are not treated with anticoagulation should be followed at 2-day intervals to identify the propagation of clot into the popliteal vein [5]. Twenty percent of calf vein thrombus will eventually extend upward.

Results

   1. Combined series of over 1600 patients comparing compression US with ascending venography (not including calf veins) indicated a 95% sensitivity and a 98% specificity [1].

   2. Calf vein US will require at least an additional 20 minutes examination time, and longer during the initial learning period. Calf veins can be successfully evaluated in approximately 60–90% of patients [6,7]. The sensitivity for detecting thrombus approaches 85% [7].

Complication (Rare)

Dislodgment of blood clot during compression causing pulmonary embolism has been reported [8–10].

SAPHENOUS VEIN MAPPING PRIOR TO INFRAINGUINAL
BYPASS PROCEDURES

1. Equipment. Linear array 7.5 MHz or 10.0 MHz transducer with color assistance.
2. Place the limb to be scanned in a dependent position to maximize distention. The examination is performed with the patient standing or in 30-degree reverse Trendelenburg position with the knee slightly flexed.
3. Begin the examination at the saphenofemoral junction just below the inguinal ligament with the transducer in transverse orientation and color Doppler used to identify the vein.
4. Keep the vein centrally beneath the transducer, which is kept perpendicular to the skin surface. Follow the course of the vein and use a marker to draw the path of the vein on the skin surface. Note the vein diameter, any duplication or bifurcations, and any abnormal appearing valves. Compression examination is performed to confirm the vein patency.
5. The same procedure may be used for the lesser saphenous vein that originates laterally at the ankle and joins the popliteal vein at the popliteal fossa.

Results

1. Mapping of the greater saphenous vein reveals several anatomic variations [11]. Complete double venous system 8%, branching double system 25%, and the standard single medial dominant trunk in the thigh with an anterior dominant vein in the calf in only 67%.
2. Adequacy of the vein for use as a graft is unsuitable in approximately 10% and questionable in another 10% of patients studied [12].

DETECTION AND SEGMENTAL EVALUATION OF VENOUS REFLUX

1. Equipment. A 10.0 MHz or 7.5 MHz transducer with color-assisted pulsed Doppler.
2. The examination is performed with the patient standing and using a chair or orthopedic walker for support. If the patient cannot stand, use a radiographic fluoroscopy table with a block under the foot of the leg not being examined so that the leg being examined can dangle without bearing weight.
3. The saphenofemoral junction is identified and the range-gate sample volume placed on the femoral vein at least 4 cm distal to the saphenofemoral junction.
4. The calf muscles are compressed by hand so that antegrade flow is demonstrated within the vein. The compression is suddenly released, and the degree of retrograde flow is recorded. Retrograde flow will exist for approximately 0.45 second until the valves close completely. Longer periods of retrograde flow are abnormal [13].

5. The study is repeated over the greater saphenous vein 4 cm from the saphenofemoral junction. Other veins that may be studied, depending on the clinical situation, are the lesser saphenous vein just below the saphenopopliteal junction and the veins of the gastrocnemius muscles.

6. Segmental evaluation is performed with color-assisted duplex spectral analysis [13]. Standardized pressure cuffs are placed around the leg at various points:

Sample Cuff Placement	Cuff Size (cm)	Inflation Pressure (mm Hg)	Location of Volume
Thigh	24	80	Superficial femoral v. Proximal greater saphenous v. Profunda femoral v.
Calf	12	100	Popliteal v Lesser saphenous v.
Ankle	12	100	Post-tibial v. Peroneal v. Greater saphenous v. Lesser saphenous v.
Foot	7	120	Post-tibial v. Greater saphenous v.

Each segment is evaluated separately. The cuff is inflated for 3 seconds; reflux is noted during rapid cuff deflation.

Postprocedure Management
None.

Results
1. The upper normal limit for maximum duration of reflux is 0.45 second.
2. The detection of segmental venous incompetence can guide surgical therapy decreasing the length of vein to be removed and lessening the risk of associated cutaneous nerve injury.
3. Although controversial, it appears that superficial vein incompetence does contribute to the pathogenesis of venous ulceration [14]. Identification of these incompetent veins may be important information for therapy.
4. The volume flow at peak reflux (VFPR) can be calculated. The diameter of the vein (measured with electronic calipers) is used to calculate the cross-sectional area. This is multiplied by the average velocity at peak reflux to obtain the VFPR. The prevalence of liposclerosis and ulceration is high when VFPR is greater than 15 ml/second in either a superficial or deep vein.
5. Color flow duplex scanning has been used to identify injection sites for venous sclerotherapy and to evaluate the success of sclerotherapy treatment of the greater saphenous vein [15].

Complications
None.

Segmental Pressure Measurements of the Lower Extremity: Ankle-Brachial Index and Stress Testing

Indications

1. History of claudication.
2. Clinical findings of arterial insufficiency.
3. As a prognostic indicator for the healing of skin lesions of the toes or feet [16,17].
4. Postoperative surveillance of infrainguinal bypass grafts (traditional).
5. Short- and long-term follow-up of endovascular interventions including thrombolysis, balloon angioplasty, and endovascular stenting.

Contraindications

1. Open wounds.
2. Recent surgery.

Preprocedure Preparation

None.

Procedure

1. Pressure cuffs are positioned around the upper and lower thigh and the upper and lower calf. The segments have been designated high thigh (HT), above-knee (AK), below-knee (BK), and ankle (A).
2. Doppler signals are detected in either the dorsalis pedis or the posterior tibial artery.
3. Each BP cuff is inflated in turn and the systolic pressure determines when a Doppler signal is detected in the dorsalis pedis or posterior tibial branch.
4. A systolic BP measurement is taken from both arms at the brachial artery. By convention, the higher of the two systolic pressure values is used to calculate the pressure index for both legs. A difference of greater than 10 mm Hg in the systolic pressures should prompt an investigation of the upper extremities.
5. A ratio is constructed from the peak systolic pressure measured during deflation of the ankle cuffs to the systolic brachial pressure, the **ankle-brachial index** (ABI).
6. **Stress testing** is performed on patients when the ABI indicates claudication.
   a. Stress testing is performed with the patient walking on a treadmill with a 12-degree incline, moving at 2 miles per hour. BP cuffs are placed on the ankles. ECG monitoring is performed during stress.
   b. The patient exercises for 5 minutes or until the symptoms are reproduced. Sequential ankle pressures are measured at 30 second intervals for the first 4 minutes

and then every minute until the pressure measurement returns to normal or to the preexercise level [18].

Postprocedure Management

None.

Results

1. Ankle-brachial index

Normal   ABI = 1.0 or slightly greater
Claudication (moderate   ABI = 0.6–0.9
  stenosis or occlusion)
Rest pain (severe   ABI = ≤ 0.5
  occlusive disease)

2. Prognosis for healing skin lesions of toes and feet [16].

Pressure	Probability of Healing (%)	
(ankle) (mm Hg)	Nondiabetic	Diabetic
Below 55	0	0
55–90	85	45
Above 90	100	85

3. A drop of 30 mm Hg or greater in peak systolic pressure between the different segments is considered abnormal.
4. An HT pressure greater than 20 mm Hg above the brachial pressure is considered abnormal. This is consistent with:
   a. Stenosis or occlusion of the aorta, iliac artery, or common femoral artery.
   b. Superficial femoral artery disease combined with stenosis or occlusion of the profundus femoral artery. The pulse volume recordings (PVR) should help in the differential diagnosis (see section on PVR).
5. Normal response to exercise is unchanged, or there is slight elevation of the pressure measurement. Any decline in pressure is a marker for significant arterial disease. The severity of the disease is indicated by the time it takes for the pressures to return to the pretest level.

Single level of disease   2–6 minutes
Multiple levels of disease   6–12 minutes
Severe occlusive disease   up to 30 minutes or longer

6. Ankle pressures during exercise and rest are used as objective criteria for the clinical categories of chronic limb ischemia (Table 26-1) [19].
7. A decrease in the ABI of 0.15 or greater is considered a significant change.
8. An increase in the ABI of greater than 0.15 as a stand-alone criteria is defined as hemodynamic improvement. An increase of 0.10 if associated with categoric clinical improvement (see Table 26-1) is also defined as hemodynamic improvement [20].

Complications

None.

Table 26-1. Clinical categories of chronic limb ischemia [36]

Grade	Category	Clinical description	Objective criteria
	0	Asymptomatic, no hemodynamically significant disease	Normal results of treadmill* stress test
I	1	Mild claudication	Treadmill exercise completed, postexercise AP > 50 mm Hg but more than 25 mm Hg less than normal
	2	Moderate claudication	Symptoms between those of categories 1 and 3
	3	Severe claudication	Treadmill exercise cannot be completed, postexercise AP < 50 mm Hg
II	4	Ischemic rest pain	Resting AP of ≤ 40 mm Hg, flat or barely pulsatile ankle or metatarsal plethysmographic tracing, toe pressure < 30 mm Hg
III	5	Minor tissue loss: nonhealing ulcer, focal gangrene with diffuse pedal ischemia	Resting AP of ≤ 60 mm Hg, ankle or metatarsal plethysmographic tracing flat or barely pulsatile, toe pressure < 40 mm Hg
	6	Major tissue loss: extending above transmetatarsal level, functional foot no longer salvageable	Same as for category 5

AP = Ankle pressure.
*Five minutes at 2 mph on a 12-degree incline.

Limitations and Artifacts

1. Diabetic patients typically can have a high ABI despite significant stenoses of their arteries. This occurs because of the noncompressibility of the vessel. In some cases, the arteries are so rigid that no pressure measurements can be obtained.
2. Pulsatile venous signals present in patients with congestive heart failure may be mistaken for arterial signals [18].
3. Extreme obesity may distort pressure measurements.
4. Absence of Doppler signal because of severely diminished flow or complete occlusion may prevent measurements.

Pulse Volume Recording

Indications

1. To complement pressure measurements in the evaluation of arterial disease.
2. In the evaluation of compression syndromes such as the thoracic outlet syndrome and the popliteal entrapment syndrome.
3. In the evaluation of arterial disease when noncompressible calcified arteries do not permit the meaningful interpretation of pressures.
4. To perform anatomic localization of hemodynamically significant peripheral vascular lesions.

Contraindications

1. Open wounds.
2. Recent surgery.

Preprocedure Preparation

None.

Procedure

1. Studies may be performed at rest or before and after exercise.
2. PVR cuffs are placed around both thighs, calves, and ankles.
3. The cuffs are inflated with a measured quantity of air (75 ± 10 cc) until a determined pressure (65 mm Hg) is achieved.
4. The cuffs are calibrated so that a 1 mm Hg pressure change in the cuff provides a 20-mm chart deflection.
5. Cuff pressure changes are proportional to cuff volume changes, which are related to instantaneous limb volume changes.

Results

1. Normal and abnormal pulse volume waves are shown in Figure 26-2.

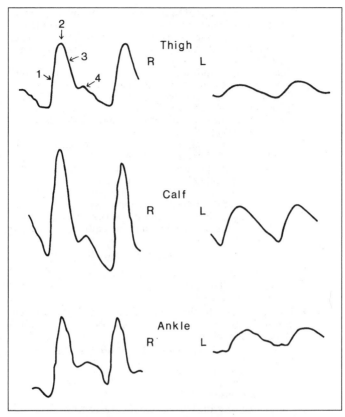

Fig. 26-2. Pulse volume recording of a patient with a left common iliac artery stenosis. Right leg with normal pulse volume wave demonstrating: (1) anacrotic rise, (2) pulse crest, (3) catacrotic decline, (4) reflected diastolic wave. The left pulse crest is rounded with absence of the reflected diastolic wave at the thigh, calf, and ankle. (Study courtesy of the Vascular Laboratory of Virginia Beach General Hospital. Virginia Beach, VA.)

2. PVR data has been classified into 5 categories [17]:

	Chart Deflection (mm)	
PVR Category	**Thigh and Ankle**	**Calf**
1	> 15[a]	> 20[a]
2	> 15[b]	> 20[b]
3	5–15	5–29
4	< 5	< 5
5	Flat	Flat

[a]With reflected wave.
[b]Without reflected wave.

3. Pulse volume amplitudes have been found to remain highly reproducible in the same patient if constant cuff volumes and pressures are used [21]. Significant changes correlate well with the appearance of significant occlusive vascular lesions.

4. Pulse volume amplitudes will vary with alterations in ventricular stroke volume, BP, vasomotor tone, and volume.

5. Exercise. The normal response to exercise is an increase in amplitude. Patients with occlusive arterial disease uniformly show a decrease in pulse volume at the ankle following exercise [22].

6. Other indications of significant arterial disease as indicated by the PVR contour include
   a. Decrease in the rise of the anacrotic limb.
   b. Rounding and delay in the pulse crest.
   c. Decreased rate of fall of the catacrotic limb.
   d. Absence of the reflected diastolic wave.

7. PVR categories in the evaluation of **rest pain** [17]. The results are the likelihood that the pain is of vascular etiology.

	Unlikely	Probable	Likely
Ankle PVR category: diabetic and nondiabetic	1,2,3	3,4	4,5

8. PVR categories in the evaluation of **limiting claudication** [17]. The results are the likelihood that the pain is of vascular etiology.

	Unlikely	Probable	Likely
Ankle PVR category: postexercise	2,3	4	4,5

9. PVR categories in the prediction of **lesion healing** [15]:

	Unlikely	Probable	Likely
Ankle PVR category: diabetic and nondiabetic	4,5	3	1,2,3

Complications

None.

Color-Assisted Duplex Venous Ultrasound of the Upper Extremity

Indications

1. Unexplained swelling of the upper extremity.
2. Suspicion of venous thrombosis associated with a central venous catheter.

Contraindications

None.

Preprocedure Preparation

None.

Procedure

1. Patient positioned supine or in slight Trendelenburg position to distend the upper extremity veins. The jugular and subclavian veins are examined with the patient's arm at his or her side; axillary and brachial veins are examined with the patient's arm extended 90 degrees. The examiner is positioned either at the patient's head or at his or her side.
2. Equipment. 5.0 MHz and 7.0 MHz color linear array transducer with Doppler capability. We switch the color on and off frequently during the examination as the vein is examined for the presence of thrombus that may deflect color flow around it.
3. We begin the examination at the jugular vein in the mid- to upper-neck. Here the vein is easily identified next to the carotid artery. Compression examination is performed here as in the lower extremity. Color flow confirms flow. Doppler velocity waveform is generated and the increased velocity in response to inspiration is confirmed. We image the vein in both longitudinal and transverse orientations.
4. In the transverse orientation, the transducer is swept down the jugular vein to the clavicle. The common carotid artery-brachiocephalic artery junction is encountered first. Then caudad to the artery, the junction of the jugular vein-brachiocephalic vein-subclavian vein is found. To reach this level, the transducer may have to be acutely angled caudad and pressed into the supraclavicular fossa. The patient is told that firm pressure may be needed and to expect some discomfort. This area is examined for the presence of thrombus, and a color flow image is recorded.
5. The medial aspect of the upper arm is scanned with color flow and gray scale. Compression examination is performed as far into the axilla as can be reached. An infraclavicular approach is used to image the segment of the axillary and subclavian vein not seen in the previous orientations.
6. While imaging over the subclavian vein in transverse orientation, the patient is asked to sniff vigorously. Electronic calipers are used to measure the change in diameter of the vein.

Postprocedure Management

None.

Results

1. Compression examination, augmentation, and respiratory variation are similar to the evaluation of the lower extremity.
2. The sniff maneuver will normally produce a mean decrease of 61% in the diameter of the subclavian vein [23].

3. In a small group of patients with symptomatic effort-thrombosis in the upper extremity color Doppler flow US correlated closely with venography to permit its use in the follow-up of patients with this disease [24].

Complications

None reported.

Color-Assisted Duplex Ultrasound of Lower Extremity Venous Bypass Grafts

Indications

1. Routine periodic evaluation of saphenous vein bypass grafts to detect early failure and allow for salvage procedures.
2. Symptomatic ischemic changes following bypass grafting to evaluate the graft for area(s) of intragraft or anastomotic stenosis.
3. To detect persistent venous fistulas following in situ vein graft placement.

Contraindications

Open surgical wounds or ulcerations.

Preprocedure Preparation

None.

Procedure [25]

1. Equipment. 5.0 MHz color-assisted Doppler linear array transducer.
2. The transducer is held parallel to the graft while the proximal anastomosis is imaged. Blood flow is confirmed by both color Doppler imaging and by pulsed Doppler waveform analysis.
3. The transducer remains oriented longitudinally. The transducer is advanced in successive increments equal to the length of the probe. The color window is kept at a 20-degree angle to the graft lumen in order to enhance flow sensitivity. The color scale is set to a maximal mean velocity between 0.68 and 0.92 m/second in order to keep the color flow signals from the lumen within the range of the red color map. The distal graft anastomosis is identified with color Doppler imaging and examined by using pulsed Doppler sonography.
4. Any areas with loss of normal color signals are examined with pulsed Doppler spectral analysis. Pulsed Doppler measurements are made every 10 cm if no zones of abnormal color are detected.
5. If the color signal of the graft is lost, the transducer is reoriented transversely to ascertain if the course of

the graft has taken a sudden curve or if the graft is thrombosed.

6. Particular note is made of the peak systolic velocity at the point of the graft with the smallest diameter.

7. Reactive hyperemia may be used with 3 minutes of cuff compression placed just below the knee, measuring the peak systolic velocity in the distal bypass [26]. The graft that doubles its peak systolic velocity is unlikely to be developing a critical stenosis.

Postprocedure Management

None.

Results

1. A complete examination takes 10–20 minutes.

2. Doubling of the peak systolic velocities measured with pulsed Doppler at a site of abnormal color signal is considered indicative of a greater than 50% narrowing of the lumen [27]. This method has a sensitivity of 95% and a specificity of 100%.

3. A peak systolic velocity of greater than 45 cm/second or a decrease of greater than 30 cm/second compared to earlier evaluations should prompt further investigation for a stenotic lesion. These grafts usually fail within 3–9 months [28]. However, this method is subject to variation in velocities with grafts of different luminal diameters.

4. Reactive hyperemia with measurement of distal graft velocities should normally produce a ratio of hyperemic to resting flow of greater than 2.5. A ratio of less than 2.5 is significantly correlated with occlusion and stenosis [26].

5. A measured inner diameter of 3.0 mm or less has been correlated with graft failure [26].

Complications

None.

Color-Assisted Duplex Imaging of Peripheral Arterial Disease

Indications

1. To differentiate a stenosis from occlusion in symptomatic patients.

2. To grade a stenosis.

3. To determine the extent of an occlusion.

4. To evaluate iatrogenic arterial injuries [29–31].

5. To confirm the short-term technical adequacy of percutaneous transluminal balloon angioplasty (PTA). For the long-term follow-up of lesions following endovascular intervention.

6. To evaluate peripheral aneurysms.

Contraindications

Open wounds or ulcerations.

Preprocedure Preparation

None.

Procedure [32]

1. Equipment. 5-MHz linear array color Doppler transducer.
2. Examination performed with patient supine.
3. The transducer is placed longitudinally, parallel to the artery. The color Doppler window is angled 20 degrees caudad.
4. The examination begins at the common femoral artery and ends at the distal popliteal artery. The transducer is moved along the course of the superficial femoral artery, and all areas of abnormal color signal (increased velocity) are sampled with Doppler spectral analysis. A ratio is calculated from the peak systolic velocity at the point of increased velocity divided by the systolic velocity measured in a segment 2–4 cm proximal to the site of flow abnormality.
5. Aneurysms are evaluated with and without color imaging. The diameter of the aneurysm and estimation of the amount of thrombus is made with gray scale images. The proximal and distal extent of the aneurysm is documented and the diameters of the vessel recorded with electronic calipers. Color flow and Doppler spectral analysis are used to confirm flow within the aneurysm.
6. Pseudoaneurysms formed from iatrogenic injury are evaluated in a similar fashion. The channel from the artery to the aneurysm should be evaluated with Doppler spectral analysis to confirm the bidirectional flow in and out of the pseudoaneurysm sac, the "to-and-fro" sign [33].
7. Iatrogenic arteriovenous (AV) fistulas are evaluated with color flow to confirm the connection between the artery and vein and with Doppler spectral analysis to demonstrate the pulsatility in the draining vein and the low resistance diastolic flow in the feeding artery. Pseudoaneurysms may be associated with AV fistulas [34].

Postprocedure Management

None.

Results

1. The criteria for a vessel segment that does not have a significant focal lesion within the femoropopliteal arterial system are normal color Doppler flow lumen signals or the absence of any focal zones showing a peak systolic velocity ratio greater than 1.8. An increase in peak systolic velocity ratio of greater than 2.2 is considered evidence of lesions causing greater than 60% luminal diameter narrowing

that are amenable to angioplasty if the lesion is shorter than 7 cm [32].

2. Popliteal aneurysms can be successfully evaluated with color-assisted duplex sonography. Information regarding size, extent, and presence of thrombus as well as the patency of tibial vessels can be obtained.

3. Ultrasound examination of iatrogenic arterial injury can demonstrate the presence of a pseudoaneurysm, AV fistula, or a complex combined lesion.

Complications

None.

Iatrogenic Arterial Injuries: Ultrasound-Guided Compression Repair

Indication

Uncomplicated catheterization arterial injuries such as pseudoaneurysm or AV fistulas—ideally less than 1 month in duration. Lesions may be in the femoral artery [35] or brachial artery [36].

Contraindications

ABSOLUTE

1. Demonstrated compression of the adjacent artery so that flow distal to the lesion is occluded. This can be determined with color flow imaging during a period of preliminary compression.
2. Infected hematoma.
3. Coexisting very large hematomas with impending compartment syndrome or overlying skin ischemia.
4. Injuries above or near the inguinal ligament.
5. Pseudoaneurysms originating at vascular surgical anastomoses.

RELATIVE

1. Severe discomfort, unrelieved by adequate local anesthesia and IV sedation.
2. Obesity preventing adequate compression of the lesion.
3. Lesions more than 1 month old. These have tracts that have decreased thrombogenicity and seem to resist closure.

Preprocedure Preparation

1. Preliminary color-assisted duplex Doppler US examination confirming the presence of abnormal blood flow within the pseudoaneurysm or fistula.
2. Equipment. 5-MHz linear array color transducer. Adequate monitoring of the patients vital signs in anticipation of IV sedation and analgesia as needed.

3. Obtain informed consent and have appropriate lab work performed in case of rupture and the need for emergency surgery.

Procedure

1. The procedure is performed with the patient in the supine position.
2. The area is scanned with the transducer perfectly vertical. An image that best displays the tract to the pseudoaneurysm or the draining vein of an AV fistula is obtained with the abnormal connection at the center of the color flow image.
3. Straight downward force is applied with the transducer until flow through the abnormal connection is eliminated. Pressure is applied for 10 minutes, or 20 minutes if the patient is being treated with anticoagulants. Compression is released slowly.
4. If color flow imaging shows persistent flow, the compression is immediately reapplied and continued for 10 additional minutes. The cycle is repeated until the abnormal channel is occluded or operator fatigue prevents further compression.
5. Compression repair of a pseudoaneurysm in a brachial artery with the operator's finger has been reported where the transducer could not compress the lesion without obstructing flow in the artery [36]. Compression was applied under US guidance for two 20-minute sessions.
6. Successful compression repair of a pseudoaneurysm in the brachial artery with a transducer has also been reported. Echogenic clot formed and there was cessation of Doppler flow within 10–15 minutes [37].

Postprocedure Management

1. Bed rest for 6 hours with the affected leg straight.
2. Withhold anticoagulants if possible.
3. Follow-up scan in 24–72 hours to confirm closure.
4. Usual postsedation precautions if IV analgesia / sedation was used.

Results

1. US-guided compression repair in the initial series had an overall success rate of 74% (26/35) [35].
2. Compression times in successful cases ranged from 10–60 minutes (mean: 30.2 minutes).
3. Case reports of successful compression repair of the brachial artery have been published [35,36].
4. A case report of uncomplicated duplex-directed manual occlusion of a traumatic false aneurysm of the extracranial vertebral artery has also been reported [38].

Complications

Acute arterial thrombosis has been reported in one case [35].

References

1. Cronan JJ. Venous thromboembolic disease: The role of US. *Radiology* 186:619–630, 1993.
2. Lensing AWA, et al. Detection of deep-vein thrombosis by real-time B-Mode Ultrasonography. *N Engl J Med* 320:342–345, 1989.
3. Lewis BD, et al. Diagnosis of acute deep venous thrombosis of the lower extremities: Prospective evaluation of color Doppler flow imaging versus venography. *Radiology* 192:651–655, 1994.
4. Polak JF, Cutler SS, O'Leary DH. Deep veins of the calf: Assessment with color Doppler flow imaging. *Radiology* 171:481–485, 1989.
5. Huisman MV, et al. Serial impedance plethysmography for suspected deep venous thrombosis in outpatients. *N Engl J Med* 314:823–828, 1986.
6. Rose SC, et al. Symptomatic lower extremity deep venous thrombosis: Accuracy, limitations, and role of color duplex flow imaging in diagnosis. *Radiology* 175:639–644, 1990.
7. Yucel EK, et al. Isolated calf venous thrombosis: Diagnosis with compression US. *Radiology* 179:443–446, 1991.
8. Schroder WB, Bealer JF. [letter to the editor] *J Vasc Surg* 15:1082–1083, 1992.
9. Perlin S. Pulmonary embolism during compression US of the lower extremity. *Radiology* 184:165–166, 1992.
10. Yedlicka JW, Hunter DW, Letourneau JG. Pulmonary embolism after femoral vein compression during sonography: Case report. *Semin Intervent Radiol* 7:24–26, 1990.
11. Leather RP, Kupinski AM. Preoperative evaluation of the saphenous vein as a suitable graft. *Semin Vasc Surg* 1:51, 1988.
12. Kupinski AM, et al. Preoperative Mapping of the Saphenous Vein: In EF Bernstein (ed.), *Vascular Diagnosis* (4th ed.). St. Louis: Mosby–Year Book, 1993.
13. van Bemmelen PS, et al. Quantitative segmental evaluation of valvular reflux with duplex ultrasound scanning. *J Vasc Surg* 10:425–431, 1989.
14. Hanrahan L, et al. Distribution of valvular incompetence in patients with venous stasis ulceration. *J Vasc Surg* 13:805–812, 1991.
15. Bishop CC, et al. Real-time color duplex scanning after sclerotherapy of the greater saphenous vein. *J Vasc Surg* 14:505–510, 1991.
16. Sumner DS. Noninvasive Assessment of Peripheral Arterial Disease. In RD Rutherford (ed.), *Vascular Surgery* (3rd ed.). Philadelphia: Saunders, 1989.
17. Raines JK, et al. Vascular laboratory criteria for the management of peripheral vascular disease of the lower extremities. *Surgery* 79:21, 1976.
18. Gerlock AJ, Jr, Giyanani VL, Krebs C. Noninvasive Vascular Examinations of the Lower Extremity Arteries. In *Applications of Noninvasive Vascular Techniques*. Philadelphia: Saunders, 1988. Pp. 299–322.
19. Rutherford RB, Becker GJ. Standards for evaluating and reporting the results of surgical and percutaneous therapy for peripheral arterial disease. *J Vasc Interv Radiol* 2:169–174, 1993.
20. Ahn SS, et al. Reporting standards for lower extremity arterial endovascular procedures. *J Vasc Surg* 17:1103–1107, 1993.
21. Darling RC, et al. Quantitative segmental pulse volume recorder: A clinical tool. *Surgery* 72:873, 1972.

22. Raines JK. The Pulse Volume Recorder in Peripheral Arterial Disease. In EF Bernstein (ed.). *Vascular Diagnosis* (4th ed.). St. Louis: Mosby–Year Book, 1993. Chap. 59.

23. Hightower DR, Gooding GAW. Sonographic evaluation of the normal response of subclavian veins to respiratory maneuvers. *Invest Radiol* 30:517–520, 1985.

24. Grassi CJ, Polak JF. Axillary and subclavian venous thrombosis: Follow-up evaluation with color Doppler flow US and venography. *Radiology* 175:651–654, 1990.

25. Polak JF, et al. Early detection of saphenous vein arterial bypass graft stenosis by color-assisted duplex sonography: A prospective study. *AJR* 154:857–861, 1990.

26. Chang BB, et al. Hemodynamic characteristics of failing infrainguinal in situ vein bypass. *J Vasc Surg* 12:596–600, 1990.

27. Jager KA, et al. Noninvasive mapping of lower limb arterial lesions. *Ultrasound Med Biol* 11:515–521, 1985.

28. Bandyk DF, et al. Monitoring functional patency of in situ saphenous vein bypasses: The impact of a surveillance protocol and elective revision. *J Vasc Surg* 9:286–296, 1989.

29. Igidbashian VN, et al. Iatrogenic femoral arteriovenous fistula: Diagnosis with color Doppler imaging. *Radiology* 170:749–752, 1989.

30. Mitchel DG, et al. Femoral artery pseudoaneurysm: Diagnosis with conventional duplex and color Doppler US. *Radiology* 165:687–690, 1987.

31. Sheik KH, et al. Utility of Doppler color flow imaging for identification of femoral arterial complications of cardiac catheterization. *Am Heart J* 117:623–628, 1989.

32. Polak JF, Karmel MI, Meyerovitz MF. Accuracy of color Doppler flow mapping for evaluation of the severity of femoropopliteal arterial disease: A prospective study. *J Vasc Interv Radiol* 2:471–479, 1991.

33. Abu-Yousef MM, Wiese JA, Shammer AR. Case report: The "to-and-fro" sign: Duplex Doppler evidence of femoral artery pseudoaneurysm. *AJR* 150:632–634, 1988.

34. Digman KE, Pozniak MA. Ultrasound case of the day. *Radiographics* 13:962–964, 1993.

35. Fellmeth BD, et al. Postangiographic femoral artery injuries: Nonsurgical repair with US-guided compression. *Radiology* 178:671–675, 1991.

36. Skibo L, Polak JF. Case report: Compression repair of a postcatheterization pseudoaneurysm of the brachial artery under sonographic guidance. *AJR* 160:383–384, 1993.

37. Kehoe ME. US-guided compression repair of a pseudoaneurysm in the brachial artery. *Radiology* 182:896, 1992.

38. Feinberg RL, et al. Successful management of traumatic false aneurysm of the extracranial vertebral artery by Duplex-directed manual occlusion: A case report. *J Vasc Surg* 18:889–894, 1993.

Radionuclide Vascular Evaluation

Joseph F. Polak
John E. Aruny

Ventilation-Perfusion Pulmonary Scintigraphy

Indications

1. Acute episode of chest pain (cardiac etiology ruled out).
2. Clinical suspicion of pulmonary embolism.
3. Baseline and follow-up scanning in patients at high risk for pulmonary embolism.
4. To determine the need for pulmonary angiography and direct the angiographic study toward a specific lung and lobe [1,2].

Contraindications

ABSOLUTE

Anatomic right-to-left shunt.

RELATIVE

1. Severe pulmonary hypertension (the only reported instances of death have occurred in such cases). The dose (number of particles) should be appropriately reduced.
2. Pregnancy.

Preprocedure Preparation

A chest x ray (CXR) should be taken within several hours of performing the lung scan.

Procedure

1. Labeling of technetium, Tc 99m macro-aggregated albumin (MAA) or Tc 99m albumin microspheres (HAM).
2. Injection of 3–5 mCi and 200,000–1,000,000 particles (10–60 μ diameter).
3. Images performed in the anterior, posterior, right lateral, left lateral, left posterior oblique, right posterior oblique, right anterior oblique, and left anterior oblique projections.
4. When xenon-133 is the ventilation agent used, this study should precede the perfusion study because of the low photopeak (80 keV) which will interfere with the 140 keV photopeak of technetium. The patient is asked to inhale for a single breath image, followed by a rebreathing period of 3–5 minutes and a washout of the gas.
5. Ventilation studies in the Prospective Investigation of Pulmonary Embolism Diagnosis (PIOPED) study were performed with 5.6×10^8 to 11.1×10^8 Bq of xenon-133 with

a 20% symmetric window set over the 80-keV energy peak. A 100,000 count, posterior view, first-breath image, and posterior equilibrium images for two consecutive 120-second periods. Washout consisted of three serial 45-second posterior views, 45-second left and right posterior oblique views, and a final 45-second posterior view. Then perfusion scans were obtained [1].

6. When Tc 99m aerosols are used as a ventilatory agent, this scan also should precede the perfusion scan.

7. Scans with krypton (Kr) 81m gas may be performed after the perfusion scan since the 190 keV photopeak of Kr is higher than the 140 keV photopeak of Tc and causes little interference.

8. Ventilation imaging with Tc 99m aerosols and Kr allows multiple matching images to compare side by side with the perfusion images. Krypton imaging is usually limited to an AP or PA and one view of either both anterior or posterior obliques performed during the equilibrium phase.

Postprocedure Management

No special management is needed.

Results

1. Revised PIOPED $\dot{V}/\dot{Q}$ scan interpretation criteria [1]

   a. High probability

   (1) Two or more large (> 75% of a segment) segmental perfusion defects without corresponding ventilation or CXR abnormalities.

   (2) One large segmental perfusion defect and two or more moderate (25–75% of a segment) segmental perfusion defects without corresponding ventilation or CXR abnormalities.

   (3) Four or more moderate segmental perfusion defects without corresponding ventilation or CXR abnormalities.

   b. Intermediate probability

   (1) One moderate to less than two large segmental perfusion defects without corresponding ventilation or CXR abnormalities.

   (2) Corresponding $\dot{V}/\dot{Q}$ defects and CXR parenchymal opacity in lower lung zone.

   (3) Corresponding $\dot{V}/\dot{Q}$ defects and small pleural effusion.

   (4) Single moderate matched $\dot{V}/\dot{Q}$ defects with normal CXR findings.

   (5) Difficult to categorize as normal, low, or high probability.

   c. Low probability

   (1) Multiple matched $\dot{V}/\dot{Q}$ defects, regardless of size, with normal CXR findings.

   (2) Corresponding $\dot{V}/\dot{Q}$ defects and CXR parenchymal opacity in upper or middle lung zone.

(3) Corresponding V̇/Q̇ defects and large pleural effusion.
(4) Any perfusion defects with substantially larger CXR abnormality.
(5) Defects surrounded by normal perfused lung (stripe sign).
(6) Single or multiple small (< 25% of a segment) segmental perfusion defects with normal CXR.
(7) Nonsegmental perfusion defects (cardiomegaly, aortic impression, enlarged hila).

d. Normal
No perfusion defects; perfusion outlines the shape of the lung seen on CXR.

2. Correlation of V̇/Q̇ scan category (PIOPED) with the clinical likelihood of PE [1].

3. The Biello categorization of V̇/Q̇ scans for the probability of PE [3]

a. High probability
(1) Single large (> 90% of a segment) V̇/Q̇ mismatch.
(2) Perfusion defect substantially larger than density on CXR.
(3) Multiple medium (25–90% of a segment) or large V̇/Q̇ mismatches without matched density on CXR.

b. Intermediate probability
(1) Severe diffuse obstructive pulmonary disease with perfusion defects.
(2) Perfusion defect same size as change on CXR.
(3) Single medium V̇/Q̇ mismatch.

c. Low probability
(1) Small (≤ 25% of an anatomic segment) V̇/Q̇ mismatch(es).
(2) V̇/Q̇ mismatches without corresponding changes on CXR.
(3) Perfusion defect substantially smaller than CXR density.

d. Normal
Normal perfusion.

4. The McNeil categorization of V̇/Q̇ scans for the probability of PE [4]

a. High probability
(1) Single V̇/Q̇ mismatch, lobe or larger, with normal CXR.
(2) Multiple V̇/Q̇ mismatches, segmental or larger; CXR normal.

b. Intermediate probability
(1) Mixed V̇/Q̇ match and mismatch.
(2) Perfusion defect with matched density on CXR.

c. Low probability
(1) Single V̇/Q̇ mismatch, segmental or subsegmental; CXR clear.
(2) V̇/Q̇ perfusion match(es) alone.
(3) Multiple V̇/Q̇ mismatches, subsegmental; CXR clear.

d. Normal. Normal perfusion.

5. The three criteria were compared in 96 patients who underwent V̇/Q̇ scans with technetium perfusion and aerosol ventilation, CXR, and pulmonary angiography [5].

   a. The **PIOPED** criteria had the most favorable likelihood ratio for predicting an angiogram showing pulmonary emboli. However, it also had the most intermediate studies.

   b. The **McNeil** criteria had the least favorable likelihood for predicting pulmonary emboli on an angiogram.

   c. The **Biello** and **McNeil** criteria showed the most favorable likelihood ratio for predicting an angiogram not showing pulmonary emboli.

Complications

1. The potential for embolization of albumin particles to sensitive small-vessel areas such as the brain exists when there is an unsuspected, anatomic right-to-left shunt.

2. Inadvertent intraarterial injection of a large number of albumin particles could cause digital ischemia in the hand or foot by blocking the capillary bed.

Gastrointestinal Bleeding Studies

Indications

1. Acute gastrointestinal hemorrhage distal to the gastric antrum (nasogastric [NG] tube aspirate negative for blood).

2. Suspected episodic gastrointestinal hemorrhage.

3. To determine the need for visceral angiography.

Relative Contraindications

1. Multiple prior transfusion and chronic dialysis (since in both cases there is poor red blood cell (RBC) labeling).

2. Pregnancy.

3. Patients with bright red blood aspirated from the NG tube or with large and frequent hematochezia. These patients who are actively bleeding on a clinical basis should go directly to angiography for localization of the bleeding site and embolization or vasoconstrictor therapy.

Preprocedure Preparation

None needed.

Procedure [6,7]

1. In vivo labeling of the patient's RBCs with 20 μg/kg IV of stannous pyrophosphate and 20 minutes later, 20 mCi IV (740 MBq) of Tc 99m pertechnetate.

2. Dynamic flow study following a bolus injection of the radiopharmaceutical with images obtained at 1 frame/second for 60 seconds.

3. Cine scintigraphy, performed by acquiring 60 consecutive images (15 minutes) at 15 seconds/frame (average 350,000 counts/15-second frame), is performed. While the first 15 minutes worth of images are reviewed, a subsequent, identical set of 60 images (15 minutes worth) is acquired. This sequence is performed for four 15-minute image sequences. Cine scintigraphy has been shown to improve localization and detection of gastrointestinal bleeding [8].
4. Alternatively, static images are obtained q5–10min for 1 hour.
5. If the initial imaging sequence is negative or equivocal in a symptomatic patient, delayed images at 3, 6, or as late as 24 hours are obtained to improve sensitivity.

Results [6]

1. Sensitive for acute bleeding at rates above 0.1 ml/minute; can estimate bleeding rates and identify those patients who are at higher risk for developing massive gastrointestinal hemorrhage, which requires more aggressive therapy [9].
2. Detection of foci of hemorrhage in symptomatic cases (hematochezia, melena, chronic anemia) in up to 64% of cases [6]. Subacute hemorrhage often is confirmed on delayed (12–24 hours) scintigrams [10]. Scintigraphic localization of a site of bleeding was correct in 77% of cases.
3. Angiography is likely to be negative if the bleeding scan fails to show the bleeding focus.

Captopril-Enhanced Renal Scintigraphy for Diagnosis of Hypertension

Indications

1. To uncover an anatomic cause of hypertension.
2. To obtain an estimate of the differential renal function.
3. To stratify hypertensive patients into those who will benefit from revascularization—either surgical or with balloon angioplasty (controversial).

Relative Contraindications

1. Inability to discontinue the use of angiotensin-converting enzyme (ACE) inhibitor drugs in sufficient time prior to the study.
2. Inability of the patient to lie flat on the imaging table without movement for at least 30 minutes.

Preprocedure Preparation

1. Patients should be instructed to discontinue the use of ACE inhibitors for at least 48 hours [11,12] if a baseline and ACE-inhibition study is to be performed.
2. If the patient cannot stop taking the ACE inhibitor, the patient should hold their morning dose and take it in

the nuclear medicine section 1 hour before the study. If the examination is positive, the patient may either return 48 hours after stopping the medicine, be admitted to the hospital for monitoring of BP while the medicine is discontinued, or be referred directly to angiography.

3. All other non–ACE-inhibitor antihypertensive medication should be discontinued (at least overnight) if possible to prevent a hypotensive response to captopril when it is administered before the test. Unfortunately, this is often difficult to achieve on a practical basis.
4. Stop oral intake at 3 A.M. the night before the procedure.
5. Establish IV access with normal saline running at a slow rate (15 to 20 ml/minute). The IV should be 18–20 gauge to allow for urgent volume expansion if a hypotensive response to captopril occurs.
6. A Foley catheter is used in patients with bladder emptying problems or renal transplants.

Procedure

There are several protocols for performing ACE-inhibition scintigraphy. Some are performed with the glomerular agent Tc 99m DTPA and some with tubular agents such as iodine 131 Hippuran (I 131 HIP) or Tc 99m mertiatide (MAG_3). Some investigators perform the baseline and ACE-inhibited scintigram on different days and some on the same day. We present two protocols, one with a tubular agent and one with a glomerular agent. Each is performed on the same day.

TUBULAR AGENT (Tc 99m MAG-3) [13]

1. A baseline study is performed with bolus IV injection of 1 mCi MAG-3.
2. An ACE-inhibition scintigram is then performed immediately. Enalaprilat (Vasotec, Merck Sharp and Dohme, West Point, PA) 2.5 mg (0.04 mg/kg) is given over 5 minutes by slow IV drip. BP is monitored q5min. Ten minutes after the infusion, give 40 mg IV of furosemide (80 mg in renal insufficiency). The dose of MAG_3 is 9 mCi given as a bolus IV injection.
3. Alternatively, 50 mg PO of captopril may be given and the patient waits for 1 hour before injection of the radiopharmaceutical.
4. If the patient has a systolic BP of less than 140 mm Hg, we would not administer IV enalaprilat and would consider decreasing the oral dose to 25 mg of captopril. There is no consensus on exactly how this decreased dose will influence the sensitivity of the exam.
5. A 60-second, rapid sequence flow image of 1 frame/second is acquired following injection, beginning when activity is seen in the abdominal aorta on the persistence scope. A 20–30 minute acquisition is performed at a frame rate of 20–30 seconds/frame. Whole kidney and cortical regions of interest are constructed and time-activity curves constructed. Curves are analyzed for time to peak and residual cortical activity (RCA) [14].

$$RCA = \frac{\text{Cortical counts at 20 minutes}}{\text{Cortical counts at peak}} \times 100$$

GLOMERULAR AGENT (DTPA) [15]

1. The preparation of the patient is similar to that with tubular agent. Twelve mCi of Tc 99m DTPA is administered intravenously. Images are acquired in the posterior view at a rate of one frame/20 seconds for 20–30 minutes with the patient supine.
2. Regions of interest over each kidney are defined and held constant for both the pre- and post-captopril studies.
3. Three hours following the completion of the baseline study, 50 mg PO of captopril is administered. One hour later, a repeat scintigram is performed. Renal pelvic activity is substracted from that of the renal parenchyma utilizing the computer, and then the renogram curves are plotted.
4. Time to peak activity is determined from the time-activity curves and a split function index calculated from the radionuclide uptake between the second and third minute of the study.

Postprocedure Management

1. Check the patient's BP in the supine and sitting positions. If there is an orthostatic drop in systolic BP, the patient should receive IV hydration—and not be discharged—until this is corrected.
2. Advise the patient to resume all medications as previously prescribed.

Results

1. Proposed grading system for the renogram curves [16]

   Grade 0   Normal (Fig. 27-1)
   Grade 1   Mild delay in upslope, maximal activity, T_{max} ($6 \leq T_{max} \leq 11$), or excretory phase (Fig. 27-2)
   Grade 2   Delay in upslope and T_{max} with evidence of an excretory phase (Fig. 27-3)
             Delay in upslope and T_{max} without evidence of an excretory phase
   Grade 3   Marked reduction or absence of uptake (Fig. 27-4)

2. Schematic of renogram grade before and after captopril challenge [16]; Table 27-1 shows the likelihood of critical renal artery stenosis (RAS).
3. Using the tubular agent I-131 HIP, an RCA of 30% or greater had a sensitivity of 96% and a specificity of 95% for the detection of renovascular hypertension in patients with normal renal function (serum creatinine $\leq$ 1.5 mg/dl) [14]. It appears that the criteria for I 131 HIP may be applied to studies performed with Tc 99m MAG$_3$ [17].
4. In patients with RAS, the captopril-enhanced renogram has prognostic value in predicting which patients will have a reduction in BP (cure or improvement) after percutaneous transluminal angioplasty [18]. The sensitivity of the

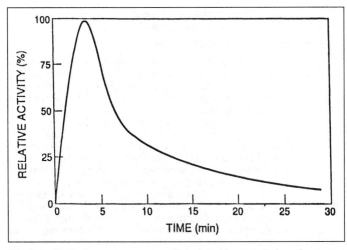

Fig. 27-1. Grade 0 renogram curve. (Reprinted by permission of
Elsevier Science Inc. from JV Nally et al. Diagnostic criteria of
renovascular hypertension with captopril renography. *Am J
Hypertens* 4:749S–752S. Copyright 1991 by American Journal of
Hypertension, Inc.)

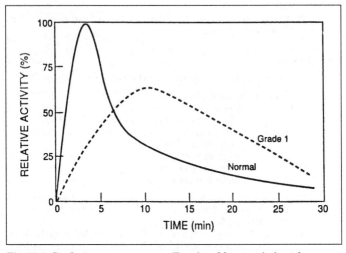

Fig. 27-2. Grade 1 renogram curve. (Reprinted by permission of
Elsevier Science Inc. from JV Nally et al. Diagnostic criteria of
renovascular hypertension with captopril renography. *Am J
Hypertens* 4:749S–752S. Copyright 1991 by American Journal of
Hypertension, Inc.)

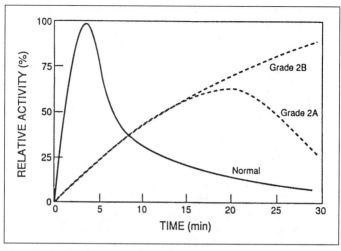

Fig. 27-3. Grade 2A and 2B renogram curves. (Reprinted by permission of Elsevier Science Inc. from JV Nally et al. Diagnostic criteria of renovascular hypertension with captopril renography. *Am J Hypertens* 4:749S–752S. Copyright 1991 by American Journal of Hypertension, Inc.)

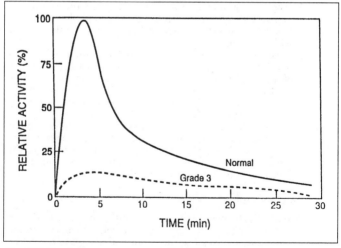

Fig. 27-4. Grade 3 renogram curve. (Reprinted by permission of Elsevier Science Inc. from JV Nally et al. Diagnostic criteria of renovascular hypertension with captopril renography. *Am J Hypertens* 4:749S–752S. Copyright 1991 by American Journal of Hypertension, Inc.)

Table 27-1. Probability table: Predicting the likelihood of RAS following baseline and captopril-enhanced renal scintigraphy

| Baseline | Postcaptopril | | | | |
	Grade 0	Grade 1	Grade 2A	Grade 2B	Grade 3
Grade 0	L	H	H	H	H
Grade 1	L	I	H	H	H
Grade 2A	L	L	I	H	H
Grade 2B	L	L	L	I	H
Grade 3	L	L	L	I	I

RAS = renal artery stenosis; L = low probability of RAS; I = indeterminant probability of RAS; H = high probability of RAS.
Source: Reprinted by permission of Elsevier Science, Inc., from JV Nally et al. Diagnostic criteria of renovascular hypertension with captopril renography. *Am J Hypertens* 4:749S–752S. Copyright 1991 by American Journal of Hypertension, Inc.

test was 91% (53/58 patients) for all patients, 95% in patients with unilateral RAS (35/37 patients), and 86% in patients (18/21) with bilateral RAS, bilaterally treated. In 18 patients with a negative captopril renogram, the BP improved in 5 and did not change in 13 patients.

5. Hypotension during the exam may create the artifactual appearance of bilateral RAS. This renographic diagnosis in a patient who was rendered hypotensive should be made with caution.

6. False-positive scans may be caused by a full urinary bladder from any cause. The full bladder delays the emptying of the renal collecting system, causing prolonged elevation of the renogram curve. Patients with bladder-emptying problems should have a Foley catheter during the study to avoid false-positive results.

7. Patient motion artifact can cause spurious points on the renogram curve and can be a cause of a false-positive scan. This is easily checked by comparing the position of the kidneys at 3 minutes and at 20 minutes in a composite image to determine motion artifact.

Complications

Profound hypotension may be induced with the use of ACE inhibitors. This usually occurs in the volume-contracted patient and emphasizes the importance of adequate hydration and BP monitoring during this exam.

References

1. The PIOPED investigators. Value of the ventilation/perfusion scan in acute pulmonary embolism: Results of the prospective investigation of pulmonary embolism diagnosis (PIOMED). *JAMA* 263:2753–2759, 1990.

2. Worsley DF, Alavi A, Palevsky HI. Role of radionuclide imaging in patients with suspected pulmonary embolism. *Radiol Clin North Am* 31:849–858, 1993.

3. Biello DR. Radiological (scintigraphic) evaluation of patients with suspected pulmonary embolism. *JAMA* 257:3257–3259, 1987.

4. McNeil BJ. Ventilation-perfusion studies and the diagnosis of pulmonary embolism: Concise communication. *J Nucl Med* 21: 319–323, 1980.

5. Webber MM, et al. Comparison of Biello, McNeil, and PIOPED criteria for the diagnosis of pulmonary emboli on lung scans. *AJR* 154:975–981, 1990.

6. McKusick KA, et al. Tc-99m red blood cells for detection of gastrointestinal bleeding: Experience with 80 patients. *AJR* 137:1113–1118, 1981.

7. Bunker SF, et al. Detection of gastrointestinal bleeding sites: Use of in vitro technetium Tc99m-labeled RBCs. *JAMA* 247:789–792, 1982.

8. Maurer AH, et al. Gastrointestinal bleeding: Improved localization with cine scintigraphy. *Radiology* 185:187–192, 1992.

9. Smith R, Copely DJ, Bolen FH. 99mTc RBC scintigraphy: Correlation of gastrointestinal bleeding rates with scintigraphic findings. *AJR* 148:869–874, 1987.

10. Alavi A. Scintigraphic detection of acute gastrointestinal bleeding. *Gastrointest Radiol* 5:205–208, 1980.

11. Sfakianakis GN, et al. Fast protocols for obstruction (diuretic renography) and for renovascular hypertension (ACE inhibition). *J Nucl Med Tech* 20:193–208, 1992.

12. Balufox MD. The role and rationale of nuclear medicine procedures in the differential diagnosis of renovascular hypertension. *Nucl Med Biol* 18:583–587, 1991.

13. Sfakianakis GN, et al. Diagnosis of renovascular hypertension with ACE inhibition scintigraphy. *Radiol Clin North Am* 31:831–848, 1993.

14. Erbsloh-Moller B, et al. Furosemide I-131-Hippuran renography after angiotensin-converting enzyme inhibition for the diagnosis of renovascular hypertension. *Am J Med* 90:23–29, 1991.

15. Setaro JF, et al. Captopril renography in the diagnosis of renal artery stenosis and the prediction of improvement with revascularization: The Yale vascular center experience. *Am J Hypertens* 4:698S-705S, 1991.

16. Nally JV Jr, et al. Diagnostic criteria of renovascular hypertension with captopril renography: A consensus statement. *Am J Hypertens* 4:749S–752S, 1991.

17. Sfakianakis GN, Bourgoignie JJ. Renographic diagnosis of renovascular hypertension with angiotensin converting enzyme inhibition and furosemide. *Am J Hypertens* 4:706S-710S, 1991.

18. Geyskes GG, de Bruyn AJG. Captopril renography and the effect of percutaneous transluminal angioplasty on blood pressure in 94 patients with renal artery stenosis. *Am J Hypertens* 4:685S-689S, 1991.

Materials, Methods, and Safety

Angiographic Contrast Media

Michael A. Bettmann

Patient Evaluation: Areas for Specific Attention

1. Obvious but essential: Determine that the procedure to be performed is optimal for the patient and his or her current clinical status (i.e., can US, MRI/MRA, or CT, with or without a contrast agent, be substituted?).
2. There are no absolute contraindications to the use of an iodinated contrast agent. Several cautions, however, are important, in regard to
   a. Should a contrast agent be administered?
   b. What class of agent should be given?
3. Relevant history
   a. Has there been prior contrast administration? If so, did a reaction occur and what type?
   b. Are there any active, serious allergies (e.g., anaphylactoid responses to *multiple* medications)?
   c. Is there active asthma?
   d. Is there significant cardiac disease (e.g., pulmonary hypertension, class III-IV congestive heart failure [CHF], class III-IV angina)?
   e. Is there a history of renal disease, paraproteinemia, diabetes mellitus?
4. Physical
   a. Assess level of hydration.
   b. Assess ability to understand, cooperate with examination.
   c. Assess level of anxiety.
5. Laboratory assessment
   a. BUN, Cr if concern about renal function (e.g., diabetes mellitus).
   b. CBC, urinalysis (for proteinuria) if concern about hydration, general status.
6. Informed consent
   a. Tailor to examination, not necessarily to type of contrast.
   b. Physician should be available to answer questions.

Principles for Angiographic Contrast Agent Administration [1–4]

1. Minimize volume of contrast/iodine as much as possible, without compromising image quality and diagnostic information. Increase in volume and iodine content may increase image quality, but may obscure certain lesions (i.e., prevent observation of detail through a vessel) or may add nonuseful information. Increased volume may add risk in patients with limited cardiac output or renal failure. Increased iodine concentration increases osmolality, which may increase risk as well.
2. When possible, use intraarterial digital subtraction angiography (DSA), with diluted contrast (e.g., Conray 43 or

Hypaque 60 diluted 1 : 1 or 2 : 1 with normal saline) or smaller volumes of full-strength contrast.

3. Low-osmolality contrast agents decrease discomfort (as does use of dilute high-osmolality contrast) and may decrease adverse reactions. **They do *not*, however, eliminate severe or fatal reactions.**

4. Emergency equipment to treat reactions as severe as cardiopulmonary arrest and personnel fully trained to use this equipment (Advanced Cardiac Life Support [ACLS] certification or the equivalent), must be readily available.

Reactions to Intravascular Contrast Agents [5–10]

1. Incidence varies with route of administration, presence or absence of specific risk factors, and the type of agent. Incidence also depends on definition used for "reaction."

2. Overall incidence of reactions is lower with low- than with high-osmolality agents. The difference, however, is primarily due to differences in minor reactions (nausea, vomiting, urticaria). There does not appear to be a difference in mortality, and there may or may not be one in the incidence of severe reactions.

3. Risk factors for reactions
   a. General reactions: prior contrast reaction, active asthma, significant allergies, impaired cardiac function/limited cardiac reserve, blood-brain barrier breakdown, marked anxiety.
   b. Renal reactions: renal failure, with or without diabetes mellitus.

Steps to Prevent Contrast Reactions

1. **Obtain a good history** (general health, prior contrast administration, renal status).

2. **Minimize patient anxiety** [11,12]
   a. Explain procedure clearly. Note likely occurrences (e.g., discomfort, heat). Obtain fully informed consent, but attempt to minimize unfounded/unlikely concerns.
   b. Ensure patient comfort before and during procedure.
   c. Use anxiolytic (e.g., midazolam, diazepam) and analgesic (e.g., fentamyl) medications prophylactically as necessary, with careful monitoring.

3. **Select appropriate contrast agent** (Tables 28-1, 28-2)
   a. For patients without specific risk factors, in general use a high-osmolality agent.
   b. For peripheral angiography (upper or lower extremity study), use DSA and a dilute high-osmolality agent. If a cut-film study is necessary, use a low-osmolality agent.
   c. If there is history of a prior minor reaction (nausea, limited urticaria), use a different high-osmolality agent (e.g., Conray instead of Hypaque). If prior agent is not known, use a low-osmolality contrast agent.
   d. In patients with specific risk factors (see Table 28-2) use a low-osmolality contrast agent.
   e. If **documented prior severe reaction** (e.g., cardiopulmonary collapse, laryngeal edema)

Table 28-1. Intravascular iodinated contrast agents

Class	Generic name	Trade name (company)	Iodine content (mg iodine/ml)	Osmolality (mOsm/kg)
High osmolality	Sodium and/or meglumine diatrizoate	Hypaque (Nycomed, New York, NY)	141	633
			282	1415
			370	2016
		Renografin (Bracco, Princeton, NJ)	141	644
			282	1404
			370	1940
		MD (Mallinckrodt, St. Louis, MO)	292	~1500
		Angiovist (Berlex, Wayne, NJ)	370	1800
	Sodium and/or meglumine lothalamate	Conray (Mallinckrodt)	202	~1000
			282	~1400
			400	~2100
Low osmolality Ionic dimer	Sodium meglumine Ioxaglatte	Hexabrix (Mallinckrodt)	320	~602
Nonionic	Ioversol	Optiray (Mallinckrodt)	160	355
			320	680
			350	702
	Iohexol	Omnipaque (Nycomed)	240	520
			300	672
			350	844
	Iopamidol	Isovue (Bracco)	200	413
			300	616
			370	796
	Iopromide	Optivist (Berlex)	300	~650
			370	~780

Table 28-2. Indications for use of low-osmo¹ality contrast agents in angiography

1. Painful procedure (e.g., upper- or lower-extremity angiograms)
2. True prior reaction to contrast agent (e.g., symptomatic urticaria, prolonged vomiting, true bronchospasm, periorbital edema)
3. Active, treatment-requiring allergies (not merely seasonal rhinitis)
4. Active, treatment-requiring asthma
5. Significant cardiac disease (pulmonary hypertension, aortic stenosis, class III–IV angina, class III–IV CHF)
6. Situations in which a minor reaction might be hazardous (e.g., suspected cervical spine injury, recent open neurosurgical procedure)
7. Marked patient anxiety

CHF = congestive heart failure.

        (1) Reassure the patient that such a reaction is un-likely to recur [11].
        (2) Ensure patent IV access.
        (3) Ensure the availability of personnel trained in resuscitation; consider anesthesia standby.
        (4) Use a low-osmolality contrast agent (value, al-though not proved, is widely accepted).

  4. Prophylactic treatment
    a. There is no clear evidence that any regimen prevents severe reactions.
    b. Low-osmolality (specifically nonionic) contrast agents reduce risk of recurrence of mild reactions, but there is no evidence to suggest that they prevent severe reactions [7,8].
    c. Reassurance is paramount.
    d. Only regimen found effective to date (overall, but stud-ies too limited to address severe or clinically significant reactions) is methylprednisolone 32 mg PO 12 and 2 hours prior to contrast use [13]. **Note:** This study dealt only with IV infusion. Concurrent use of specific H_1-, and H_2-blockers has also been recommended [14,15].

  5. Renal failure (see Chap. 30 for a more comprehensive dis-cussion)
    a. Clinically significant renal dysfunction due to the use of a radiographic contrast agent is essentially limited to patients with preexisting renal compromise.
    b. In such patients, risk is increased with
      (1) Diabetes mellitus.
      (2) Increasing age.
      (3) Increasing volume of contrast.
    c. Multiple myeloma and other paraproteinemias lead to renal failure through a combination of dehydration and protein precipitation in tubules, a different mechanism from contrast-related failure.

d. Preventive considerations
  (1) Ensure adequate hydration (before, during and after procedure).
  (2) Limit volume of contrast.
  (3) Use low-osmolality agent, especially for patients over 70 with Cr $\geq$ 2 mg/dl.
  (4) Consider alternative imaging examinations.
  (5) Avoid other risk factors (e.g., surgery, gentamicin).

References

1. Korn WT, Bettmann MA. Low-osmolality versus high-osmolality contrast material. *Curr Opin Radiol* 4:9–15, 1992.
2. Smith DC, et al. Three new low osmolality contrast agents: A comparative study of patient discomfort. *AJNR* 9:157–159, 1988.
3. Shehadi WH. Contrast media adverse reactions: Occurrence, recurrence and distribution patterns. *Radiology* 143:11–17, 1982.
4. Lalli AF, Greenstreet R. Reactions to contrast media: Testing the CNS Hypothesis. *Radiology* 138:47–49, 1981.
5. Caro JJ, Trindade E, McGregor M. The risks of death and of severe nonfatal reactions with high vs. low-osmolality contrast media: A meta-analysis. *Am J Roentgenol* 156:825–832, 1991.
6. Katayama H, et al. Adverse reactions to ionic and nonionic contrast media: A report from the Japanese committee on the Safety of Contrast Media. *Radiology* 175:621–628, 1990.
7. Lawrence V, Matthai W, Hartmaier S. Comparative safety of high-osmolality and low-osmolality radiographic contrast agents: Report of a multidisciplinary working group. *Invest Radiol* 27:2–28, 1992.
8. Steinberg EP, et al. Safety and cost effectiveness of high-osmolality as compared with low-osmolality contrast material in patients undergoing cardiac angiography. *N Engl J Med* 326:425–430, 1992.
9. Barrett BJ, et al. A comparison of nonionic low-osmolality radiocontrast agents with ionic, high-osmolality agents during cardiac catheterization. *N Engl J Med* 326:431–436, 1992.
10. Bettmann MA. The evaluation of contrast-related renal failure. *AJR* 157:66–68, 1991.
11. Padrid PJ. Role of higher nervous activity in ventricular arrythmia and sudden cardiac death: Implications for alternative antiarrythmic therapy. *Ann NY Acad Sci* 432:296–313, 1985.
12. Samuel MA. Neurogenic heart disease: A unifying hypothesis. *Am J Cardiol* 60:15J–19J, 1987.
13. Lasser EC, et al. Pretreatment with corticosteroids to alleviate reactions to intravenous contrast material. *N Engl J Med* 317:845–849, 1987.
14. Greenberger PA, Patterson R. The prevention of immediate generalized repeated reactions to radiocontrast media in high-risk patients. *J Allergy Clin Immunol* 87:867–872, 1991.
15. Cusmano J. Premedication regimen eases contrast reaction. *Diagn Imaging* 181–182, 185–186, 1992.

Treatment of Contrast Media Reactions

Michael A. Bettmann
John E. Aruny

General Principles

1. The radiologist should have the knowledge and equipment to treat most contrast media reactions without assistance.
2. It is the responsibility of the radiologist performing the procedure to have the necessary medications and equipment readily available and in working order.
3. The response time to treatment should be minimized. All contrast reactions do not present with a classical complex of signs and symptoms. Failure to consider and recognize that a patient is indeed having an adverse reaction may delay appropriate treatment [1].
4. Three rules to remember
   a. Know the patient.
   b. Recognize that there is a problem.
   c. Be prepared to deliver treatment quickly and know when to call for help.

KNOW THE PATIENT

1. Before procedure, inquire about any allergic **history,** prior exposure to iodinated contrast material, and previous adverse reactions.
   a. Does the patient have a history of coronary artery disease or other significant cardiac problem? Contrast material can compromise cardiac function.
   b. Is the patient being treated for congestive heart failure? Contrast material will increase the effective circulating volume and may cause pulmonary edema in the poorly compensated patient.
   c. Does the patient have a history of asthma? If yes, is the patient actively wheezing? Contrast media can provoke bronchospasm and worsen preexisting airway constriction.
2. The radiologist performing the procedure should have a knowledge of the **medications** that a patient is taking before the procedure. Some medications may mask the symptoms of a contrast reaction.
   a. **Beta blockers** slow the heart rate and block its acceleration response to physiologic stress. They may therefore interfere with a tachycardiac response, which may presage severe reactions.
   Beta blockade blunts the effects of epinephrine, requiring increased doses to achieve similar physiologic effect. Once the beta effect is overcome, there is an unopposed alpha-adrenergic effect of epinephrine that predominates with a marked increase in peripheral vascular resistance and a subsequent hypertensive re-

sponse. Beta blockers may increase the rate of moderate to severe anaphylactoid reactions caused by contrast media [2].

b. Calcium channel blockers are frequently prescribed for hypertension, coronary insufficiency, and arrhythmias. They are peripheral vasodilators; correction of hypotension by fluid replacement may be more difficult due to persistent peripheral vasodilation.

RECOGNIZE THAT THERE IS A PROBLEM

Look for the classical and more subtle signs that the patient is having an adverse reaction. Dermal: urticaria, pruritus, and skin flushing. Mucosal edema may present with increased production of tears, difficulty in swallowing, nasal congestion, severe bronchoconstriction, or laryngeal edema with hoarseness. Generalized edema may present with edematous eyelids or perioral edema. All patients in the angiography suite should have continuous BP monitoring. Patients who receive contrast for CT-guided procedures or IV urography may be less closely monitored. The person in attendance will have to depend on physical signs and the patient's symptoms to determine if the patient is having an adverse reaction. A patient who is becoming hypotensive may display a change in mental status, becoming restless or confused. This may be related to analgesic or sedative medications, or indicate a vasovagal reaction. This should prompt the radiologist to check the patient's vital signs.

BE PREPARED TO DELIVER TREATMENT QUICKLY AND
KNOW WHEN TO CALL FOR HELP

Evaluate the situation, categorize the type of adverse reaction, and determine if it is mild or severe. After treatment is given reevaluate the patient frequently and decide if the situation is improving or becoming worse.

Treatment of Adverse Reactions (Table 29-1)

1. Mild or Minor
   a. Definition. Minor symptoms or signs which are not life-threatening and require no treatment.
   b. Types. Nausea, mild or isolated episode of vomiting, upper respiratory congestion, limited urticaria.
   c. Action. Observe carefully to ensure that symptoms do not worsen. Monitor vital signs.

2. Moderate/Intermediate
   a. Definition. Symptoms or signs requiring limited treatment or observation, not hospitalization, which are transient and not imminently life-threatening.
   b. Types. Symptomatic urticaria, bronchospasm (shortness of breath), vasovagal reaction.
   c. Action. Treat symptoms or signs for comfort (antihistamine for urticaria, oxygen for dyspnea) or to prevent progression/worsening (leg elevation, fluids for hypotension/bradycardia). A vasovagal reaction must be observed until complete resolution; treatment is necessary if spontaneous resolution does not occur rapidly.

Table 29-1. Treatment of major adverse reactions

Symptoms	Treatment (in order of increasing severity)
Symptomatic urticaria	25–50 mg diphenhydramine IM
Bronchospasm	1. Nasal oxygen, IV access, monitor ECG and oxygen saturation 2. Beta-agonist inhaler (metaproterenol, terbutaline, albuterol) 3. Epinephrine 0.1–1.0 ml, 1 : 1000 SC 4. Epinephrine 1.0–3.0 ml, 1 : 10,000 IV
Laryngotracheal edema; symptomatic facial edema	1, 3, then 4, as above
Pulmonary edema	1. Oxygen, IV access, monitor ECG and oxygen saturation 2. Elevate head; rotating extremity tourniquets 3. Furosemide 40 mg slow IV push 4. MSO_4 1–10 mg slow IV push
Vagal reaction (hypotension and bradycardia)	1. Monitor vital signs, ensure IV access 2. Elevate legs; Trendelenburg position 3. Push IV fluids 4. As needed to stabilize BP and pulse, atropine 0.3–2.0 mg IV push (0.3–0.5-mg increments)
Toxic convulsions	1. Diazepam 1–10 mg IV push, in 1-mg increments 2. Monitor vital signs 3. Obtain neurologic consultation
Cardiopulmonary arrest	1. Monitor vital signs and ECG 2. Ensure IV access 3. Ensure functional airway 4. Begin resuscitation 5. Call code team 6. Epinephrine 0.1–1.0 ml, 1 : 1000 SC; or 1–3 ml, 1 : 10,000 IV

MSO_4 = morphine sulfate.

3. Major/Severe

a. **Definition.** Symptoms or signs which are life-threatening or may rapidly progress to such status.

b. **Types.** Laryngospasm, facial and glottic edema, respiratory difficulty, cardiorespiratory collapse/arrest (many etiologies), generalized seizures.

c. **Action**

(1) Respiratory: Nasal oxygen, beta-agonist (metaproterenol or similar) inhaler or epinephrine SC or IV if needed.

(2) Cardiovascular

(a) Vasovagal. Fluids, leg elevation, atropine 0.3–1.0 mg IV.

(b) Other. Fluids, epinephrine (1 : 1000) 0.1–1.0 ml, SC; if necessary, 1.0–3.0 ml (1 : 10,000) IV. Call cardiac arrest team.

(3) Seizures. Diazepam 1 mg IV increments as needed, with careful monitoring of respiratory status.

4. Remember

a. **Hypotension + bradycardia = vagal reaction.**

b. **Hypotension + tachycardia = anaphylactoid or cardiac reaction.**

c. Respiratory distress with a wet cough and pink frothy sputum = pulmonary edema. Think: Is this patient having an acute **myocardial infarction** (MI)?

References

1. Siegle RL, Lieberman P. A review of untoward reactions to iodinated contrast material. *J Urol* 1119:581–587, 1978.

2. Lang DM, et al. Increased risk for anaphylactoid reaction from contrast media in patients on β-adrenergic blockers or with asthma. *Ann Intern Med* 115:270–276, 1991.

Iodinated Contrast Media in Patients with Renal Dysfunction

Albert A. Maniscalco
Susan Grossman

Contrast-Induced Nephropathy

Contrast-induced nephropathy is a diagnosis of exclusion. It usually manifests as an acute deterioration of renal function after the administration of radiographic contrast material. It can be seen with intravenous, intraarterial, or rarely after oral administration of iodinated contrast. The incidence of acute renal failure after iodinated contrast administration is difficult to assess because the degree of rise in creatinine used to define renal failure varies from study to study (e.g., 0.5–1.0 mg/dl rise, or 25–50% increase over control value [1]. The incidence also depends on variables such as the clinical status of the patient.

1. **Normal renal function.** The rate of renal failure in people with normal renal function is very low (approximately 0.6%) after intravenous pyelography (IVP) but has been reported to be as high as 5.8% after abdominal angiography [2].

2. **Preexisting renal insufficiency.** Prior renal insufficiency is the most important predisposing factor to developing acute renal failure after contrast. One study shows that 5.6% of nondiabetic patients who had prior renal disease developed deterioration of renal function after an IVP [3]. After abdominal or cardiac angiography, the incidence of acute renal failure in patients with preexisting renal disease has been reported to be as high as 23–40% [4]. In general, there is a strong correlation between the degree of prior renal insufficiency and the severity of post-contrast renal failure, that is, the greater the degree of preexisting renal disease, the more severe the renal failure after contrast injection. Notably, most patients with acute renal failure following contrast administration, including those with preexisting renal insufficiency, experience only a transient rise in serum creatinine (Cr). Renal function almost always returns to baseline within 5–10 days of the radiographic procedure. An incidence of 2.5% of patients requiring permanent dialysis after contrast has been reported [4]. More recent studies, however, have failed to show any case of clinically important acute renal failure in patients with chronic renal insufficiency who are not diabetic.

3. **Diabetes mellitus.** Diabetics deserve special consideration. A diabetic patient with normal renal function (Cr < 1.5 mg/dl) does not appear to be at risk. Diabetics with Cr between 1.5 and 4.5 mg/dl are more at risk than nondiabetics with similar degrees of renal insufficiency. It is generally agreed that diabetics with Cr greater than

4.5 mg/dl will develop severe and at times permanent renal damage when given contrast. The incidence has been reported to be as high as 90%. Some authors have observed that type I diabetics who have retinopathy, neuropathy, and nephropathy carry the highest risk for contrast-induced renal insufficiency [4].

4. **Dehydration.** In older studies, dehydration appeared to be a major risk factor. This has not been substantiated in more recent studies, perhaps because current practice is for patients to be well-hydrated before contrast administration [1].

5. **Other factors**
   a. Patients with **multiple myeloma**, in the setting of renal failure, dehydration, or hypercalcemia may be at greater risk, especially in those who excrete free light chains (positive Bence-Jones protein) in the urine.
   b. It would appear that patients with **low cardiac output** and **congestive heart failure** (CHF) are at increased risk. In one study, patients with class IV cardiac disease had a 71% incidence of renal failure after injection of contrast [4].
   c. Historically, **age, hypertension, dose,** and **site** of contrast material injection (intravenous versus intraarterial), and **proteinuria** have been thought to influence the incidence of acute renal failure after contrast injection [3]. While recent studies do not definitely support their importance, the evidence is far from clear [1].

6. **High-osmolar versus low-osmolar contrast media.** Still controversial. In studies of patients with normal renal function or with Cr less than 2.0 mg/dl, there appears to be no significant decrease in the incidence of contrast-induced nephropathy when the more expensive nonionic and lower osmolality agents are used. There is evidence however that these agents may benefit patients with Cr above 2.5 mg/dl, especially if they have diabetes [5, 6, 7].

7. **Patients on dialysis.** It should be noted that once patients are already on dialysis, either peritoneal or hemodialysis, contrast-induced renal failure is no longer a consideration (see discussion regarding dialysis patients).

Evaluation

PATIENTS WITH RENAL INSUFFICIENCY, BUT NOT ON DIALYSIS

1. **Evaluation** prior to iodinated contrast administration. This evaluation does not preclude standard preangiography evaluation for all patients.
   a. **History**
      (1) Allergies, especially to contrast or topical anesthetics.
      (2) Medical illness, especially diabetes mellitus, acute or chronic renal disease, multiple myeloma, CHF.
      (3) Symptoms that might reveal or lead to volume depletion, such as diarrhea, vomiting, fluid intake.
      (4) Symptoms that might reveal fluid overload, such

as shortness of breath, edema, rapid weight gain, orthopnea.

(5) Medications that might affect renal or volume status, such as diuretics, nonsteroidal antiinflammatory agents, especially in patients with preexisting renal disease, chemotherapy with nephrotoxic agents (e.g. cisplatin, aminoglycosides).

(6) Recent prior study with iodinated contrast (< 1 month).

(7) History of prior episodes of contrast-induced renal failure.

b. Physical

(1) Check for signs of volume depletion: orthostatic BP drop (> 20 mm Hg drop in systolic or standing pressure or 10 mm Hg in diastolic pressure after dangling legs for 1 minute).

(2) Unexplained tachycardia.

(3) Poor skin turgor, dry mucous membranes.

(4) Check for signs of fluid overload—neck vein distention, rales, S3 gallop, peripheral edema.

c. Laboratory Data

(1) BUN and Cr—must be related to body size, age, and sex.

(2) The following formula closely approximates glomerular filtration rate (for women, multiply result by 0.85)

$$Cr_{Cl} = \frac{(140 - age) \times LBW\,(kg)}{72 \times S_{Cr}}$$

where Cr_{Cl} = creatinine clearance; LBW = lean body weight; S_{Cr} = serum creatinine.

(3) Urinalysis.

(4) Total protein, albumin, and globulin (if multiple myeloma is suspected).

(5) Bleeding time (for invasive procedure), if patient has Cr over 4.5 mg/dl.

2. Prophylaxis against further renal failure from contrast administration

a. Most patients with preexisting renal disease (Cr > 1.5 mg/dl) will benefit from 24 hour hospitalization prior to contrast injection to adequately assess states of hydration and give proper volume expansion. Consultation with internist or nephrologist is usually appropriate.

b. Procedures should be done only when there are specific indications and no alternative studies or procedures are available.

c. The dose of contrast should be as low as necessary to get an adequate study. A helpful formula for contrast dose is [8]:

$$\frac{5\,ml\,contrast\,/\,kg\,body\,weight}{S_{Cr}}$$

where S_{Cr} = serum creatinine.

d. Prior to the study, determine if patient has a history of CHF, or is clinically fluid overloaded. In general, patients with severe renal failure (Cr > 4.5 mg/dl) can be considered to potentially have a problem with fluid overload.

e. If there is no problem with fluid overload, hydration with 0.45% saline at a rate of 1 ml/kg/hr for 12 hours before and 12 hours after the administration of radiocontrast agents appears, at the present time, to be the most beneficial means of preventing contrast-induced nephropathy in patients with and without diabetes.

In the past, the use of mannitol and/or furosemide to induce a diuresis was thought to be protective [9]. Two recent prospective studies have cast doubt on this conventional wisdom [10, 11]. In both, mannitol was found to be of no benefit and possibly even detrimental in diabetics. The second showed no benefit of furosemide diuresis in either diabetics or nondiabetics [11]. One of the studies did show protective effects of low-dose dopamine and saline infusion, mannitol and saline infusion, and infusion of atrial natriuretic factor in saline in nondiabetic patients [10]. Since there is no consensus, only saline infusion can be recommended at this time.

f. For patients with severe renal failure, or for those who have poor urine output or are in CHF, volume should be optimized by right heart catheterization prior to any procedure involving contrast administration.

g. Future considerations may include the use of calcium antagonists as part of a pretreatment regimen [12]. Preliminary work in dogs has demonstrated that calcium antagonism with several different agents lessens the magnitude and duration of radiocontrast-mediated renal vasoconstriction. These studies suggest that calcium entry constitutes an important mediator in the vasoconstrictive phase after administration of iodinated contrast. The evidence for this is very preliminary, so we would not at this time recommend giving calcium channel blockers prior to a contrast study [13].

3. Follow-up of patients with chronic renal insufficiency after contrast administration

   a. Daily urine output and body weight measurement for 2 days after the procedure.

   b. Daily measurement of electrolytes, BUN, and Cr for 2 days.

   c. Monitor for fluid overload and hyperkalemia.

   d. If patient develops oliguria (< 500 ml/day or 20 ml/hr), nephrology evaluation is indicated.

   e. The fractional excretion of sodium ($FeNa^+$) is usually greater than 1% in patients with acute tubular necrosis. In patients with acute renal failure secondary to contrast, the $FeNa^+$ is variable, and may be less than 1%.

$$FeNa^+ = \frac{U\,Na\,/\,P\,Na}{U\,Cr\,/\,P\,Cr} \times 100$$

where U = urine and P = plasma.

1. Contrast-induced renal failure is not a consideration in these patients.
2. If possible, dialysis should be planned soon after a procedure with contrast, since iodinated contrast is dialyzable via hemodialysis or peritoneal dialysis. Iodinated contrast is highly osmotic, 5–8 times the osmolality of plasma, and will therefore increase the extracellular fluid compartment. Hemodialysis has a higher clearance of the contrast than peritoneal dialysis.
3. Dialysis patients should not receive magnesium-containing substances as preparation for procedures since clearance of magnesium is reduced in renal failure. Alternate cathartics such as 70% sorbitol, 50 ml PO q2h until clear can be used.
4. Extreme care should be taken not to put pressure on the patient's vascular access site during any procedure. No blood should be drawn from the arm with vascular access and no IV lines started. No contrast should be given into that arm unless a fistulogram or shuntogram is being performed.
5. In general, patients on peritoneal dialysis who are going for abdominal x rays should be instructed to empty the fluid before having the procedure.
6. For invasive procedures (angiography, venography) desmopressin may be considered for reducing the risk of bleeding. This can be given IV at a rate of 0.3 μg/kg in 100 ml D5W over 20 minutes prior to the procedure.
7. Radiologists and other personnel should take extreme care to follow universal precautions.

Cholesterol Emboli Versus Contrast Nephrotoxicity

Cholesterol emboli are a serious but rare complication of angiographic procedures. Atheroembolic disease has been described following angiography [14]. The mechanical manipulation of the catheter causes ulceration of the large atheromatous plaques, releasing cholesterol crystals. They are more likely to occur after a difficult procedure that involves manipulation of a catheter within a severely diseased aorta but also have been reported following uncomplicated procedures [15].

The rate of this complication is difficult to determine. In one series of percutaneous peripheral angioplasty [16], one episode of atheroemboli was noted out of approximately 1500 cases. After renal angioplasty, atheroembolism to the kidney has been described in 1.4–3% of patients [17]. The kidney is a frequent target organ when cholesterol emboli are found. Renal involvement has been found in 80% of autopsy-proven cases of atheroembolic disease. Although clinically observed only rarely, one series of autopsies done on patients within 6 months of an angiographic procedure found cholesterol emboli in 30% of patients [18].

1. **Clinical features** include acute renal failure, livedo reticularis, disseminated intravascular coagulation, abdominal pain and pancreatitis, gangrene of the lower extremities, cerebral infarction, and retinal emboli. Other organs that

can be involved include the colon, small intestine, or spinal cord. Patients may develop a "multiple cholesterol emboli syndrome" that resembles polyarteritis nodosa and is manifested by fever myalgias, eosinophilia, and penile and scrotal skin necrosis. Symptoms can begin immediately after the procedure or as late as 2–6 weeks after the procedure. One clue to the development of cholesterol emboli is peripheral gangrene in the presence of good peripheral pulses.

2. **Laboratory findings** are nonspecific. Transient eosinophilia and an elevated sedimentation rate may be present. Urine sediment is usually nondiagnostic. Serum complement may be low. These laboratory findings may be confusing and suggest a diagnosis of vasculitis.

3. **Differentiation of cholesterol emboli and contrast-induced renal failure** is very important. Contrast nephropathy usually occurs immediately after the radiologic procedure; cholesterol emboli can occur from 2–6 weeks later. Acute renal failure secondary to contrast is usually transient, with renal failure improving over a 10-day to 2-week period. Cholesterol emboli usually lead to progressive irreversible renal failure, although return of renal function to normal has been reported and renal function may stabilize if the ulcerated plaque epithelializes [19]. A transient hypertension that may be difficult to control has been reported with cholesterol emboli.

4. **Treatment.** Unfortunately, treatment for sequelae from cholesterol embolization is ineffective. Anticoagulation is considered to be detrimental because it interferes with the healing of cholesterol plaques. Patients on chronic anticoagulation therapy, who have had no procedures, have been shown to develop spontaneous cholesterol emboli. Antiplatelet agents and corticosteroids do not seem to be effective. Blood pressure should be controlled. Most patients do poorly and there is a high mortality rate in spite of dialysis, because mortality is related more to the underlying severe vascular disease than to the emboli themselves. Some patients, however, do recover renal function.

References

1. Barrett BJ, Parfrey PS. Clinical Aspects of Acute Renal Failure Following Use of Radiocontrast Agents. In K Solez, LC Racusen (eds.), *Acute Renal Failure: Diagnosis, Treatment and Prevention.* New York: Marcel Dekker, 1992. Pp. 481–500.

2. Berkseth RO, Kjellstrand CM. Radiologic contrast-induced nephropathy. *Med Clin North Am* 68:351–370, 1984.

3. Porter GA, Bennet WM. Nephrotoxin-Induced Acute Renal Failure. In JH Stein, BM Brenner (eds.), *Acute Renal Failure.* New York: Churchill Livingstone, 1980. Pp. 123–162.

4. Loggins CH, Fang LST. Acute Renal Failure Associated with Antibiotics, Anesthetic Agents and Radiographic Contrast Agents. In BM Brenner, JM Lazarus (eds.), *Acute Renal Failure.* New York: Churchill Livingstone, 1988. Pp. 295–352.

5. Parfrey PS, et al. Contrast material induced renal failure in patients with diabetes mellitus, renal insufficiency or both. *N Engl*

J Med 320:143–149, 1989.

6. Barrett BJ, et al. A comparison of nonionic, low-osmolality radio-contrast agents with ionic, high-osmolality agents during cardiac catheterization. *N Engl J Med* 326:431–436, 1992.

7. Rudnick MR, et al. Nephrotoxicity of ionic and nonionic contrast media in 1196 patients: A randomized trial. *Kidney Int* 47:254–261, 1995.

8. Cigarroa RG, et al. Dosing of contrast material to prevent contrast nephropathy in patients with renal disease. *Am J Med* 86:649–652, 1989.

9. Anto HR, et al. Infusion intravenous pylography and renal function effects of hypertonic mannitol in patients with chronic renal insufficiency. *Arch Intern Med* 141:1652–1656, 1981.

10. Weisberg LS, Kurnik PB, Kurnik BR. Risk of radiocontrast nephropathy in patients with and without diabetes mellitus. *Kidney Int* 45:259–265, 1994.

11. Solomon R, et al. Effects of saline, mannitol and furosemide on acute decreases in renal function induced by radiocontrast agents. *N Engl J Med* 331:1416–1419, 1994.

12. Loutzenhiser RD, Epstein M, Hayashi K. Renal hemodynamic effects of calcium antagonists. *Am J Cardiol* 64:41F–45F, 1989.

13. Bakris GL, Burnett JC. A role for calcium in radiocontrast-induced reductions in renal hemodynamics. *Kidney Int* 27:465–468, 1985.

14. Harrington JG, Dommers SC, Kassirer JP. Atheromatous emboli with progressive renal failure. *Ann Intern Med* 68:152–160, 1968.

15. Henderson MJ, Manhire AR. Case report. Cholesterol embolization following angiography. *Clin Radiol* 42:281–282, 1990.

16. Belli AM, et al. The complication rate of percutaneous peripheral balloon angioplasty. *Clin Radiol* 43:380–383, 1990.

17. Weitz Z, et al. Cholesterol emboli in atherosclerotic patients: Reports of four cases occurring spontaneously or complicating angioplasty and aortorenal bypass. *J Am Geriatr Soc* 35:357–359, 1987.

18. Ramirez G, et al. Cholesterol embolization, a complication of angiography. *Arch Intern Med* 138:1430–1432, 1978.

19. Colt HG, et al. Cholesterol emboli after cardiac catheterization. Eight cases and a review of the literature. *Medicine* 67:389–400, 1988.

Needles, Guidewires, Catheters, and Stents

Krishna Kandarpa
Oun J. Kwon

Needles

Needles are designed to be efficient and safe for their intended use. Numerous designs are marketed by competing manufacturers. Table 31-1 describes a few commonly used needles.

Guidewires

Guidewires are constructed of a tightly wound fine-spring steel wire and a stiff inner mandrel core wire. The outside of the guidewire is coated with Teflon to reduce friction and may be impregnated with heparin to reduce thrombogenicity. However, the heparin coating is shorter-lived and catheters should be double-flushed after each removal of the wire. The wire should be wiped before it is placed in a heparinized bath. The inner core, which provides rigidity, is often tapered to a point toward the introduction end of the guidewire and ends at a variable distance from the tip, depending on the type of wire. This allows for a flexible end, with a gradual decrease in the stiffness toward the tip. Various lengths of distal core wire are available. Some wires have movable cores so that the length of flexible tip can be changed at will. A fine inner safety wire is provided in most guidewires to prevent accidental intravascular breakage and loss of wire fragments.

Standard wires are generally used for routine percutaneous introduction of catheters through a superficial artery. Tip flexibility allows the wire to buckle and avoids dissecting the vessel. However, the tip of any wire can cause damage to the wall as it first emerges from the catheter. Heavy-duty wires with a stiff inner core, once in place, allow the catheter to be introduced through tortuous vessels without buckling. Sometimes, even a standard wire within a catheter will provide longitudinal rigidity to allow the latter to be translated without buckling. Movable core wires have a retractable nontapered inner mandrel providing the advantage of a flexible tip for maneuvering through tortuous vessels; the wire can subsequently be stiffened by advancing the mandrel so as to allow the catheter to pass easily over the wire. Specially constructed wires with extra torsional rigidity (torquable wires) allow the wires to be steered into arterial branches. Exchange wires are long and allow enough length of wire between the target site and external end so that a new catheter may be introduced without losing wire purchase internally. Specialty wires have specific uses as outlined below.

Table 31-2 describes some commonly used guidewires.

Table 31-1. Needles commonly used for intraluminal access

Needles	Diameter (gauge)	Maximum guidewire diameter (in.)	Common length	Application
Seldinger (double-wall puncture)	18 (thin wall)	0.038	2¾ in.	Widely used for arterial and venous access. Similar gauge needles made of thinner wall tubing can accommodate larger wires.
	19	0.025		
	20	0.021		
	21	0.018		
Potts	18	0.038	2¾ in.	Stylet hub has hole to show back-bleeding. For single-wall or axillary puncture.
	20	0.021		
Amplatz (5 Fr. Teflon sheath over cannula)	18	0.038	2½ in.	Femoral/axillary arterial access, grafts and dialysis access fistulas.
	20	0.021		
Butterfly venipuncture	19	0.028	Various	Venous access; plastic extension tubing to hub.
	21	0.021		
Jelco IV (with Teflon sheath)	18	0.035	Various	Venous access.
	20	0.025		

Coaxial Micropuncture Set	21	0.038	5–15 cm	21-gauge beveled needle allows 0.018-in. wire. Two coaxial sheaths serve as vessel dilators; with the inner sheath removed; the outer sheath allows the 0.038-in. wire.[a]
Syringe needles	18 20 21	0.035 0.021 0.018	Various	Injection, aspiration.
Chiba ("Skinny" needles)	22 (21,23)	0.018	15 and 20 cm	Percutaneous transhepatic cholangiography, some biopsies. Generally for deep targets, but the flexible needle may deviate from desired path.
Sheath needle (Teflon sheath with metal stylet)	16 sheath (19 stylet)	0.038	24 cm	Percutaneous transhepatic biliary drainage and nephrostomy. Drainage of other fluid collections. Stiff stylet minimizes deflection of needle from desired route.
"Blood-containment needles"	Standard	Standard	Standard	Sos Pulse-Vue Bloodless Entry Needle[b] Arrow Fischell Evan Needle[c]; both needles are designed to provide access to the blood vessel without exposing personnel to blood.

[a]Cook, Inc., Bloomington, IN.
[b]AngioDynamics, Inc., Glens Falls, NY.
[c]Arrow International, Inc., Reading, PA.

Angiographic Catheters

Catheters are designed for safe and efficient cannulation of vessel orifices. Efficient cannulation is determined by the shape of the catheter and its torquability. The ability to retain shape and torquability and to sustain injection pressures safely is in turn determined by the characteristics of the material from which the catheter is manufactured (Table 31-3). Commonly used catheters are listed in Tables 31-4 and 31-5).

DETERMINATION OF FLOW RATE AND BURSTING PRESSURE

Flow Rate
$[Q = \Delta P\,(\pi r^4)/8\,\mu(L)]$; where ΔP = pressure drop across catheter, r = radius, L = catheter length, μ = viscosity of undiluted contrast; flow rate varies with internal radius to the fourth power and is inversely proportional to the length.

Catheter Bursting Pressure
$P = T(t/r)$; where T = tensile strength of catheter material, t = wall thickness, r = internal radius. Thicker walls and smaller internal diameters make stronger catheters.

Technical Facts about Catheters and Wires

1. There is no standard color coding corresponding to a catheter French size.
2. Watch for weak points in catheter (holes, etc.)—catheters usually burst at the hub where pressure limits are exceeded first.
3. Watch for "lack of fit" (between catheters/sheaths/wire).
   a. Recommended manufacturing tolerances are ± 0.3 Fr. on diameter; ± 5% on length.
   b. Dimensional discrepancy (can exist between products from the same manufacturer).
   c. This can prolong procedures, increasing risk to patient.
4. Watch for leakage or separation or both at connections.
5. Some catheters are not radiopaque (because either size, material, or manufacturing process does not allow barium sulfate impregnation).
6. Catheters are not normally heparinized. Thrombogenicity of catheters is minimized by improving the smoothness of the catheter surface. The ability to make this surface smooth depends on the catheter material (including additives) and manufacturing process. Significant factors in thrombus formation are the relative size of the catheter outer diameter to the vessel inner diameter and the indwelling time. An occlusive catheter will almost always result in an intravascular thrombus.
7. Heparinized wires. Heparin coating is short-lived (10 minutes) in vivo. The wire should be kept in the body for no longer than 3 minutes. It must be wiped clean and kept in a heparinized saline (2500 IU/500 ml NS) bath when not in use. Catheters must be double flushed after removing the wire and single flushed q3min when in the artery

Table 31-2. Commonly used guidewires

Wire	Diameter (0.001 × in.)	Maximum length (cm)	Tip radius (mm)	Flexible-tip length (cm)	Comments
Standard fixed core					
J-GW	18, 21, 25, 28, 32, 35, 38	50, 80, 100, 125, 145	1.5, 3, 7.5, 15	5, 6, 8, 10	For catheter introduction by Seldinger technique
Straight	18, 21, 25, 28, 32, 35, 38	50, 80, 100, 125, 145	—	3	
Flexible-tip wires					
Tapered core (Newton)					
J-GW	35, 38	125, 145	3–15	LT = 10 cm LLT = 15 cm LLLT = 20 cm	Facilitate safe negotiation of tortuous or stenotic vessels
Straight	32, 35, 38	125, 145			
Bentson[a]	32, 35, 38	145	Straight	15 (taper), distal 1 cm is very flexible	Negotiates tortuous iliacs

Table 31-2. (continued)

Wire	Diameter (0.001 × in.)	Maximum length (cm)	Tip radius (mm)	Flexible-tip length (cm)	Comments
Amplatz[b]	35	145	6	15	Very flexible tip
Movable core	32, 35, 38	125, 145	1.5–15.0 and straight	Variable (5 cm)	Core movable 5 cm; for tortuous and stenotic vessels
Exchange wires					
Standard	35, 38	260	Straight	3	Extra length for exchanging catheters
Heavy-duty Standard	35, 38	145	Straight	3	Large diameter core for extra stiffness
Rosen[b]	35, 38	145, 260	1.5 and straight	2	Provides good support for advancing a catheter Moses wire[a] is similar a 38-Rosen

Lunderquist Exchange ("coathanger")[c]	35, 38	120	Straight	8	Solid stainless steel shaft for catheter support. *Not for intravascular use*
Amplatz Super-Stiff[d]	35, 38	145, 260	Straight	7	Large core for stiffness. Smooth transition to a soft tip
Torquable guidewires					
Ring[a]	35	145	A = straight, B = slight curve, C = moderate curve	—	Standard wire construction with weld every 5 cm to improve torquability. *Not for intravascular use*
Lunderquist-Ring[a]	38	125	Shapeable tip		1 : 1 torque control, shapeable tip
Hi-torque steerable (Wholley[e]/Amplatz)	35, 38	150	Straight, floppy, mod-J (90 degrees)	—	
Hydrophilic-coated Glidewire[d] Roadrunner[a] NaviGuide (formable tip)[c]	18, 25, 35, 38	150	Straight, angled	3	Elastic alloy core with a hydrophilic coating that reduces friction when wet. Regular and stiff shafts, with straight, angled, and variable-taper tips are available.
Coronary steerable[b]	14, 16, 18	175, 300 (exchange)	Straight (shapeable) and J-tip	Variable	Teflon-coated solid shaft with flexible platinum tip. Needs pin-vice handle for torquing. Also available in very flexible and **Flex-J** version

Table 31-2. (continued)

Wire	Diameter (0.001 × in.)	Maximum length (cm)	Tip radius (mm)	Flexible-tip length (cm)	Comments
Hi-torque floppy	14, 18	175, 300 (exchange)	Straight	Variable (shapeable)	Stiff shaft torquable with extremely flexible tip; needs pin-vice
Tapered tip wires TAD[e]	35 down to 18 at the tip	145, 200	Shapeable	2 cm (soft tip), 10–15 cm (taper)	Tapered attenuated diameter: excellent for crossing a stenosis, tip minimizes trauma to distal vessel; the larger diameter of shaft provides good support for advancing a balloon catheter
Platinum Plus GW[d]	18 25	150 180	Shapeable	short (ST) & long (LT)	Shorter, flexible tips require less purchase within the vessel
Specialty wires Tip-deflecting[a]	25, 28 38, 45	65, 80 100	Deflected radius: 5, 10	Wire should remain within catheter at all times	Special handle fits onto proximal wire Tip can be deflected to facilitate selective catheterization
Variable stiffness[a]	35	145	Straight	Flexible	Deflector handle is used to stiffen the wire body and facilitate catheter advancement

Hi-torque J-GW[f]	35	45 (with proximal handle) 100 (no handle)	3, 5, 10	15	Translumbar aortography (version with handle cannot be used for exchanges)
Open-ended injectable Sos-wire[b]	35, 38	145	Straight	—	Inner removable stiffening wire (0.014–0.018) is used for selecting vessels and for advancing the outer wire
Cragg FX-wire[d]	38 (0.027-in. ID)	145	Straight	12 cm	
Curry intravascular retriever set[a]	21 spring GW	300	—	Entire length	For foreign body removal
Amplatz Goose-Neck snares[g]	Loop diameter: 5–10 mm (4 Fr.) 120 15–35 mm (5 Fr.)	120	—	—	Snare wire is made of kink resistant Nitinol; used coaxially

GW = guidewire.
[a]Cook, Inc., Bloomington, IN.
[b]USCI Bard Radiology, Billerica, MA.
[c]Meadox/Surgimed, Oakland, NJ.
[d]Medi-Tech, Watertown, MA.
[e]Advanced Cardiovascular Systems, Temecula, CA.
[f]Argon Medical Corp., Athens, TX.
[g]Microvena Corp., Vadnais Heights, MN.

Table 31-3. Material characteristics of catheters

Catheters	Material characteristics
Polyurethanes (PU)	Soft unbraided tip; stainless steel braided body; provides for good torque control, but wall is thicker and internal diameter is smaller; unbraided catheters available Highest coefficient of friction between catheter surface and tissues, and catheter and guidewire
Polyethylenes (PE)	Soft and flexible but stiffer than unbraided catheters (i.e., better torsional rigidity), therefore better torque When unbraided, follows tight corners well Commonly used plastic Coefficient of friction much less than PU
Polypropylenes	Good memory: less likely to lose shape at body temperature Lower coefficient of friction than PU
Teflons	Stiff, good memory, lowest coefficient of friction; material strength allows for manufacture of thin-walled (large inner bore, small outer caliber) catheters May kink easily if bent too sharply
Nylon	Combined with PU for manufacture of high-flow 4–5 Fr. catheters
Balloon PTA catheters	
Balloon	Irradiated PE: sustains high pressure without stretching PU: dimension changes with repeated inflation; bursts easily Polyvinylchloride (PVC): tends to stretch, low dilating force but follows bends well
Catheter	PE PVC

(and on removal if needed again). *Double flush:* Use first syringe to aspirate blood from catheter and discard into waste bowl. Use a second syringe with fresh heparinized saline to aspirate a little blood and forward flush briskly to fill catheter. Shut off stopcock while still flushing forward.

8. Teflon-coated wires have smoother surfaces, reducing friction and thrombogenicity.
9. Likelihood of infection increases with the amount of time a catheter is left in the body.

Table 31-4. Commonly used catheters[a]

Application	Name	Tip shape
Aortography[b] Venacavography[b] Pulmonary arteriography (with tip deflector wire)	Pigtail	
Pulmonary arteriography	Grollman	
Iliac and antegrade femoral angiography	Straight side-hole (flush) or end-hole	
Selective catheterization of hepatic and renal veins	Multipurpose (curve)	
Inferior mesenteric artery; also for hooking contralateral iliac	IMA (Rosch visceral)	
Left gastric arteriography	LGA	
Selective arteriography (adult visceral and extremity)	Cobra C1–C3 C2 and C3 have wide primary curves Levin (distal tip is angled less acutely than a Cobra)[c] Sos-Omni (see Simons curve)[d]	
Selective renal arteriography	Renal curve (good for RA with downward course)	
Selective aortic arch (brachiocephalic) arteriography[c]	Modified headhunter (see Simons)	
Selective visceral and brachiocephalic arteriography[e] (shape must be reformed in the artery; numbers reflect increasing radius of primary curve)	Simons 1: narrow aorta (Sos-Omni Selective has smaller curve but similar shape and use) 2: normal aorta 3: wide aorta 4: elongated aorta	
Right heart pressures	Balloon wedge pressure catheter (Swan-Ganz type)[f]	

Table 31-4. (continued)

Application	Name	Tip shape

Coronary arteriography	Judkins left and right
	  coronary catheter:
	  JL4 (4-cm arm)
	  JL5 (5-cm arm)
	  JR4 and JR5	

	Amplatz left and rig
	  coronary catheter
	  AL2, AL3
	  AR1, AR2	

[a]Consult package inserts and manufacturer for available Fr. sizes (guidewire accommodation), lengths, and possible flow rates.
[b]Tennis Racket (Medi-Tech, Watertown, MA) and Halo (AngioDynamics, Gler Falls, NY) may also be used.
[c]Available through Cook, Inc., Bloomington, IN.
[d]Available through AngioDynamics, Inc., Glens Falls, NY.
[e]Berenstein (hockey-stick shape with a simple angled tip) is also extremely use
[f]Available through Arrow International, Inc., Reading, PA.

Nonvascular Catheters and Stents

Catheters and stents of various materials and designs are commercially available for nonvascular use (e.g., biliary, urinary, and gastrointestinal tracts), for purposes such as access (for feeding), drainage, or stenting. A partial list of some commonly used items is given below.

INTERNAL AND EXTERNAL BILIARY DRAINAGE CATHETERS

1. **Ring biliary duct drainage catheter** (Cook, Inc., Bloomington, IN). The original biliary drainage catheter is made of opaque polyethylene that is slightly stiff. It is available in an 8.3 Fr. size, 50 cm in length, with 32 side ports.
2. **Biliary drainage catheter** (Cook, Inc.). Made of polyurethane or Ultrathane (Cook, Inc.) (8.5, 10.2, and 14 Fr., 40 cm in length with 32 side ports with Cook-Cope [Cook, Inc.] type loop or Cook Simp-Loc [Cook, Inc.] locking loop).
3. **VTC biliary systems** (Medi-Tech, Watertown, MA). Percuflex locking pigtail catheters (8, 10, 12, and 14 Fr., 35 cm working length).

EXTERNAL BILIARY DRAINAGE CATHETERS

1. **Amplatz anchor system** (Medi-Tech). 8, 10, 12, and 14 Fr.; 30-cm-long Percuflex (Medi-Tech) catheters with small two-wing Malecot-type locking tip.
2. **Hawkins accordion catheter drainage set** (Cook, Inc.). A 6.5 Fr. × 20 cm opaque Teflon catheter with a drawstring for forming a small accordion configuration tip.

INTERNAL BILIARY STENTS (endoprostheses)

1. **Miller double mushroom biliary stent** (Cook, Inc.). 10, 12, or 14 Fr. size, and 2.5, 5, or 7.5 cm length stents of

Table 31-5. Commonly used infusion catheters[a]

Application	Name	Comment
Pulse-spray and slow infusion (side holes)	PRO-pressure responsive side slits[b]	4 or 5 Fr.; 90 or 135 cm long; 10 or 20 cm infusion length; 0.035-in. tip-occluder wire for pulse-spray. Slow infusion without wire.
	Mewissen[c] infusion catheter	5 Fr.; 35, 65, or 100 cm long; 5, 10, or 15 cm infusion length.
	Katzen infusion wire[c]	Can be used with Katzen wire. 0.035-in. OD; 145 cm, removable hub; 3, 6, 9, or 12 cm infusion length with side holes. Teflon coated.
	Multi-sideport infusion catheter[d]	5 Fr.; 65 or 100 cm long; 0.035 or 0.038-in. GW; 4, 7, 11, 15 cm infusion lengths.
	McNamara[d] coaxial catheter infusion set	Outer 5.5 Fr. catheter with coaxial inner 3 Fr. multi-sidehole catheter. Can be used for pulse-spray. Advantage: infusion length can be adjusted to match the thrombus length without catheter exchanges.
	EDM[e] catheter	4.7 Fr.; 90 or 135 cm long, five-lumen, four-sidehole catheter, 0.018-in. inner wire; 4, 5, 6, 9, 12, 15, 18, 30, 35, 40 cm infusion lengths
	Micro-Soft Stream[f] T3 : Teflon[c,d]	3 Fr. small vessel catheter with distal marker. 3 Fr. end-hole slow infusion catheters, 80, 100, 120, 135, or 150 cm long.
Slow infusion (end-hole only)		May be used for microembolization.

Table 31-5. (continued)

Application	Name	Comment
Slow infusion (end-hole only)	Sos-wire[g]	0.035 or 0.038-in. OD, end-hole Teflon catheter; 0.018 or 0.021-in. inner wire for coaxial introduction.
	Cragg convertible wire[c]	0.038-in. OD (accommodates inner 0.025-in. wire), 145 or 170 cm long, removable hub. Teflon jacket, 12 cm distal floppy tip. Cragg FX[c] (fixed hub) also for microembolization.
	Fast-Tracker[f]	3 Fr. end-hole catheter with clear radiopaque distal marker. These small catheters are designed to track easily through small tortuous arteries; excellent for microembolization.
	Hieshima microcatheter[h]	3 Fr. tapering to 2 Fr. (or 2.3 Fr.) distally. Tip lengths 5, 10, 15 cm. Overall lengths 40, 60, 100, 150 cm. Need 0.016 in. or 0.018 in. guidewires.
Percutaneous central venous access and infusion	PICC[d,i]	3 Fr. to 5 Fr. percutaneously and peripherally inserted catheters for intermediate-term venous parenteral nutrition, infusion of antibiotics and certain chemotherapeutic agents. Single and double lumen catheters are available.

OD = outer diameter; GW = guidewire diameter

[a]Consult package inserts and manufacturer for available French sizes (guidewire accommodation), lengths, and possible flow rates.
[b]AngioDynamics, Glens Falls, NY.
[c]Medi-Tech, Watertown, MA.
[d]Cook, Inc., Bloomington, IN.
[e]Advanced Cardiovascular Systems, Temecula, CA.
[f]Target Therapeutics, Freemont, CA.
[g]USCI Bard, Billerica, MA.
[h]Microvena, White Bear Lake, MN.
[i]Pharmacia-Deltec, St. Paul, MN.

radiopaque polyethylene. Stents have double (proximal and distal) mushroom (Malecot-type) tips, which help to maintain their position. The set contains a peel-away sheath and a positioner.

2. **Carey-Coons soft stent biliary endoprosthesis** (Medi-Tech). 12 Fr. and 14 Fr., 20 cm long Percuflex stents designed to be placed across the ampulla. The stent's distal 5 cm is bent to lie into the duodenum. A button with a string attaching it to the stent is placed subcutaneously to prevent distal migration (optional).

3. **Wallstent biliary endoprosthesis** (Schneider [Pfizer], Minneapolis, MN). The only metallic self-expanding permanent flexible stent approved for endobiliary use. The new "Unistep" delivery system has simplified its deployment. The stent is mounted on a 7 Fr. delivery catheter. The deployed stent provides a large unrestricted lumen favoring it over smaller caliber plastic stents—especially across malignant strictures and occlusions. The stent retracts from both ends following deployment; proper initial positioning is important. The stent may be dilated with a balloon to expand it to its maximum unconstrained diameter. Available sizes (UD = unconstrained diameter; UL = unconstrained length): 8 mm UD × 20, 40, 60, and 80 mm UL; 10 mm UD × 20, 42, 68, and 94 mm UL; and 12 mm UD × 40, 60, and 90 mm UL. These stents are also widely used for transjugular intrahepatic portosystemic shunting (TIPS). (See Chap. 16.)

PERCUTANEOUS CHOLECYSTOSTOMY CATHETERS

1. **McGahan percutaneous multipurpose drainage catheter needles** (Cook, Inc.). This moderately stiff catheter has multiple side holes in its pigtail tip and is mounted on an 18- or 19-gauge trocar needle. Used with either single-stick trocar or a needle-guidewire technique. Available in 6.7 Fr. or 8.3 Fr. size, and 17 cm length.

2. **vanSonnenberg gallbladder catheter** (Medi-Tech). Catheter is less stiff than the one above. One size of 7 Fr. with a 30 cm length.

NEPHROSTOMY CATHETERS

The most common catheter for external drainage of urine from the renal pelvis has multiple distal side holes and a distal pigtail-tip for securing it internally. This is a versatile and simple design that can be used for other types of drainage as well. A less commonly used design provides a Malecot-type (mushroom) securing tip.

1. **Polyurethane or Ultrathane nephrostomy catheters** (Cook, Inc.). 6.5, 8.5, 10.2, 12, or 14 Fr. size, with a 25 cm length. Cook-Cope (Cook, Inc.) type loop catheters or Sim-Loc (Cook, Inc.) locking loop catheters allow external urine drainage from the renal pelvis.

2. **VTC nephrostomy catheter systems** (Medi-Tech). 8, 10, 12, or 14 Fr., with a 30 cm length.

3. **BUD drainage catheters** (Medi-Tech). 6 Fr., with a 15 cm length; 8.3 Fr. and 10.3 Fr., with a 30 cm length. There is no locking mechanism for its distal pigtail.

4. **Malecot nephrostomy catheter** (Medi-Tech). 14, 16, 20, or 24 Fr., with a 35 cm length. Percuflex (Medi-Tech) catheters with multiwing Malecot design for securing catheter and maximizing available space for drainage.

NEPHROURETEROSTOMY STENT

In addition to the distal pigtail tip that is positioned in the bladder, the stent has a proximal loop that is formed in the renal pelvis. These catheters are used for internal drainage from the renal pelvis to the bladder while maintaining external access to the stent. Several lengths (22, 24, 26, 28 cm) between the pigtails are available.

1. **Ultrathane Cope nephroureterostomy stents** (Cook, Inc.). Type A (for diversion) and B (for drainage) in 8.5 Fr. and 10.2 Fr.
2. **Nephroureteral stent systems** (Medi-Tech). 8 Fr. and 10 Fr.
3. **Internal ureteral stents.** Double pigtail stents made of Ultrathane (Cook, Inc.) (Amplatz ureteral stents) or Percuflex (Medi-Tech) are more easily advanced than the much softer stents made of Silastic. Available in several lengths (between pigtails) of 20, 22, 24, 26, and 28 cm.
4. **Ultrathane Amplatz ureteral stents** (Cook, Inc.). 8.5 Fr. and 10.2 Fr.
5. **Medi-Tech ureteral stent systems** (Medi-Tech). 8 Fr. and 10 Fr.
6. **TempTip** (Medi-Tech). Drainage catheter, internal ureteral stents, and nephroureteral stents are available with this short temporary tip made of material that dissolves away once it is placed in the body. The "TempTip" tapers to the diameter of a standard wire (0.038 in.) to facilitate insertion of the catheter/stent, but when it dissolves a large unrestricted distal opening is created (internal diameter of main catheter).

GASTROSTOMY TUBES

In addition to specific products commercially available for percutaneous placement, Foley catheters or loop nephrostomy catheters of a large size may also be used for feeding and/or suction drainage.
Multipurpose drainage catheters (Cook, Inc.). Ultrathane drainage catheters, 8.5, 10, 12, and 14 Fr., with six side ports. Available with Cook-Cope type or Simp-loc locking loops.

GASTROJEJUNOSTOMY AND JEJUNOSTOMY CATHETERS

1. **Dawson-Mueller gastrojejunostomy** (Cook, Inc.). A 14 Fr. single-lumen Ultrathane catheter in 30 cm and 53 cm lengths. A peel-away introducer is provided for transgastric jejunal feeding tube placement. Does not have gastric ports for suction.
2. **Carey-Alzate-Cooks gastrojejunostomy set** (Cook, Inc.). 16.5 Fr. × 80 cm length radiopaque polyurethane catheter with friction-lock Malecot tip; available with or without a double lumen.

3. **MIC gastro-enteric tube** (Medical Innovations Co., Milpitas, CA). Dual-lumen design allows gastric and jejunal access. Available in 16–30 Fr. with 28-cc securing balloon for adult use and 16 or 18 Fr. with 5-cc balloon for pediatric use.
4. **MIC jejunal tubes** (Medical Innovations). 14–24 Fr. (even sizes) with a 28-cc balloon; for surgical placement or replacement of surgically placed jejunal tubes.

ABSCESS DRAINAGE CATHETERS

Specifically designed sump drainage catheters are available for abscess or fluid drainage. In addition, single-lumen catheters with a straight, J-curved, pigtail, Malecot, or accordion tip are also available.

1. **Ring-Mclean sump drainage sets** (Cook, Inc.). 14 Fr., 30 cm length Ultrathane or 12, 16, and 24 Fr., 30 cm length polyvinylchloride catheters mounted on a trochar needle.
2. **vanSonnenberg sump catheters** (Schneider [Pfizer]). 12, 14, or 16 Fr., with 30 cm or 35 cm length, J tip or pigtail tip, Percuflex catheters.
3. **vanSonnenberg chest drain set** (Schneider [Pfizer]). 12 Fr. Percuflex catheter with "TempTip" (see above) and locking pigtail, mounted on a trochar needle.

Selected Readings

FOR PRACTICAL TECHNICAL HINTS

Gerlock AJ, Mirfakhraee M. *Essentials of Diagnostic and Interventional Techniques.* Philadelphia: Saunders, 1985.
Johnsrude IS, Jackson DC, Dunnick NR. *A Practical Approach to Angiography* (2nd ed.). Boston: Little, Brown, 1987.
Ring EJ, McClean GK. *Interventional Radiology.* Boston: Little, Brown, 1981.
Kadir S. *Diagnostic Angiography.* Philadelphia: Saunders, 1986.
Kadir S. *Current Practice of Interventional Radiology.* Philadelphia: B.C. Decker, 1991.

FOR CLINICAL INFORMATION ON ANGIOGRAPHY
AND INTERVENTIONAL RADIOLOGY

Abrams HL (ed.). *Abrams' Angiography: Vascular and Interventional Radiology* (3rd ed.). Boston: Little, Brown, 1983.
Athanasoulis CA, et al. *Interventional Radiology.* Philadelphia: Saunders, 1982.
Ring EJ, McClean GK. *Interventional Radiology.* Boston: Little, Brown, 1981.
Reuter SR, Redman HC, Cho KJ. *Gastrointestinal Angiography* (4th ed.). Philadelphia: Saunders, 1986.
Kadir S. *Diagnostic Angiography.* Philadelphia: Saunders, 1986.
Kadir S. *Current Practice of Interventional Radiology.* Philadelphia: B.C. Decker, 1991.

Equipment and Techniques for Angiography

Basics of Angiographic Equipment

Maria M. Damiano

Krishna Kandarpa

Equipment should be tailored to the specific needs of the angiography suite. A brief review of the major components found in an angiographic suite today is presented below.

1. **Generators.** A generator provides electrical power for the x-ray tube. A generator with a stable constant output and precise control systems is indispensable. A state-of-the-art generator for angiographic applications will be a constant potential generator, a high-frequency generator or a three-phase (12-pulse) unit, with a power rating of 85–100 kilowatts (kW) at 100 kilovolts (kV). With such ratings, short exposure times are possible—eliminating motion artifact and allowing rapid filming.

   A constant potential generator is intrinsically immune to line fluctuations and is more likely to provide accurate output and greater reproducibility. The high-frequency generators available on modern machines are well suited for fast image acquistion and are able to provide self-compensation of line fluctuations. The generator is an expensive component, but cost should be a secondary consideration, while it is inappropriate to couple an inadequate generator with sophisticated secondary image-processing equipment. On the other hand, it is also a needless expense to purchase an excessively high-powered generator if it is to be put to limited use.

   Ideally, the control panel should allow stepless kV adjustment and selection of exact exposure times. A technologist should be able to use the lowest possible exposure times at the highest possible current (mA). The voltage (kV) employed should be low enough to maximize radiographic contrast but high enough to adequately penetrate the part being examined and reduce potential radiation exposure. Exposure factors (for radiographic technique and automatic brightness control for fluoroscopy) are set during installation within a preestablished range and should follow the highest current/lowest exposure time guideline.

2. **X-ray tubes.** Consist of a tungsten filament cathode that provides the incident beam of electrons that hit the anode (target) and generate x rays. The focal spot is the area on the tungsten anode that is bombarded by electrons from the cathode.

   a. The choice of **focal spot size** should be determined by the specific application. A small focal spot produces better resolution but may reduce the field size. In angiography, small focal spots are desired. For most nonmagnification radiography, a 0.6-mm focal spot size is recommended. This will produce sharper vessel borders than the usual 1.0- or 1.2-mm focal spot size used for a plain film of the abdomen. However, a 1.0- or 1.2-mm focal spot size will allow higher tube loading for studies such as lateral abdominal aortograms. For magnification angiography, a 0.3-mm focal spot size is required. When performing greater than 2 : 1 magnification, such as in neuroangiography, a 0.1- or 0.2-mm focal spot size is used. Multiple focal spot x-ray tubes are now available (with as many as six possible sizes) to accommodate various tube loading needs for angiographic (including digital subtraction angiography [DSA]) and interventional procedures.

   b. Anode angle. Angiographic x-ray tubes have high-speed rotating anodes with higher heating capacity. The angle between the anode surface and incident electron beam from the cathode is the anode angle (usually 10 or 12 degrees for angiography). A smaller anode angle will have a higher tube loading capability but also a smaller apparent focal spot, and therefore a small field size. As an alternative to calculating anode heat units, heat monitoring devices are available that display percentage of target capacity and also have an audible signal or alarm when target approaches maximum thermal capacity.

3. Image intensifier. Converts the x-ray image to a brighter but smaller light image. Image intensifiers are available in many different sizes, ranging from 4–16 in. and are built in single-, double-, or triple-field size modes. A smaller field-of-view size (magnification mode) is ideal for interventional procedures when panning is limited. A large field-of-view size is an important feature in a dedicated digital imaging suite, if a rapid serial film changer has not been installed. A video or cine camera can be coupled to the image intensifier. This image can also be digitized for later image processing. A digital spot film device with single and/or rapid acquisition is useful in imaging during (nonvascular) interventional procedures.

4. Fluoroscopy. Modern angiography units allow adjustments in fluoroscopic quality by selecting settings on the generator control system. Low-dose fluoroscopy is possible during catheter placement and high-dose fluoroscopy is available for critical positioning of wires and catheters during interventional procedures which require sharper high-resolution images. Pulsed-fluoroscopy tries to optimize the image quality while minimizing exposure to radiation. Digital fluoroscopy technology provides further flexibility during the procedure.

5. Television monitors. The standard resolution of a TV monitor is 525 lines/frame. However, most monitors used in angiography suites today have higher resolution screens (1024 lines/frame). High-resolution TV systems are necessary if the TV chain is being used for image recording (e.g., DSA). In discussing high-resolution images, a distinction should be made between the acquisition resolution and the display resolution (on the TV monitor). Standard fluoroscopic acquisition is at 525 lines/frame. High-line fluoroscopic acquisition is at 1024 lines/frame. High-resolution acquisition and display results in a high-quality, high-contrast image. "Upscaning" is a postacquisition processing maneuver that displays the image at twice the acquisition resolution, giving the perception of a "smoother" fluoroscopic image. An image acquired at 1024 lines/frame can be displayed as an upscanned image on a modern monitor with a 2000 lines/frame screen resolution.

6. **Patient tables.** The tables should be made of a low-absorption material with minimal beam attenuation. Lower-extremity angiography is performed on tables that are programmed to shift (step) with the bolus of contrast. The table should provide enough range of panning during fluoroscopy in order to facilitate the study. Table height is usually adjustable and some tables pivot around the base. The option of a tilting table top for interventional procedures is desirable but may not be available with a "floating" top table.

7. **Cut-film film changers.** Some film changers have film supply magazines and receivers that can be used for both anteroposterior and lateral filming. Other magazines can only be used in one projection. Size and weight of magazines can affect their ease of use. Newer magazines are smaller in size and weight and allow film to be rolled into the receiver (versus flat film storage). Loading of magazines is easier in newer models as interleaving between sheets of film during loading is no longer necessary. Newer film changers have a keyboard-operated alpha-numeric film-marking labeling system instead of removable flash cards. Other available options are: the number of films per magazine, maximum filming rate, and the ability to fluoroscope through the changer in order to check the position or projection before filming.

8. **Gantry stands.** Designs include a C-arm, a U-arm, or a parallelogram on which the filming and/or digital acquisition system is integrated. A well-designed system should allow easy access to the patient. The arm should be easily cleared away from the patient in case of an emergency, and the organ of interest should stay at isocenter with angulation. Some machines step the gantry rather than the table for vascular runoff studies. This option is desirable if there are space limitations. There are many **advantages** to using these systems over the previously discussed ceiling-suspended x-ray tube and stationary film changer.

   a. Oblique views can be obtained without ever moving the patient.

   b. Compound angles can be used (however, this can result in increased exposure due to scattered radiation to the angiographers).

   c. Rapid switching from frontal to lateral fluoroscopy is possible. This can aid in depth determination and is very convenient in tube placements and biopsies.

   d. Automatic centering with rapid interchange of image intensifier and film changer are possible.

9. **Contrast injectors.** The contrast injector arm can be ceiling-suspended or placed on the table near the patient where it will move with the table during panning or stepping. The injector control unit can either be rack-mounted or placed in a remote location. Injection volume, peak injection rate, and acceleration to peak rate are adjustable. A mechanical stop on the volume injected is a good safety feature. Programming options allow the injector, film changer, and table motion to be synchronized.

10. **DSA** is a computer-based digital image-processing technique by which an initial noncontrast mask is electronically subtracted from subsequent serial images of an angiogram. Modern DSA systems are capable of acquiring true (high-resolution) 1024×1024 pixels per image frame or more. DSA systems have many useful features. **Density reversal** provides the option of viewing an image black-on-white or vice versa. **Masking** features allow any image within a series to be selected or used as a mask. **Remasking** allows the use of different images to be used as masks within a single series. **Pixel shifting** can be used to adjust a mask to save an image marred by motion. **Landmarking** provides localizing anatomic reference points on the images. **Window and level adjustments** may be made during postprocessing. Image annotation and identifying marks can be included. Other features such as edge enhancement and electronic magnification are also available. Special software programs provide the ability to measure volumes, degree of vessel stenosis, and size of a lesion. Digital subtraction "road-mapping" provides a stored image of the area of interest (e.g., a stenosis to be dilated) over which a live fluoroscopic image may be superimposed, providing image guidance for placement of wires and catheters during interventional procedures.

    While DSA has not yet completely replaced cut-film imaging, it does have many **advantages.**

    a. Less contrast is required per study; dilute contrast can be used because DSA systems are sensitive to very small differences in density.

    b. There is a considerable savings on the cost of film, since only selected images need to be processed and printed.

    c. Postprocessing of images may resolve questions without the need to repeat a study.

    d. Exquisitely processed hard-copy reproductions of the acquired images are possible with modern laser printing technology.

    e. Digital angiography/radiography may be employed without utilizing subtraction capability. Angiographic images (single exposure "spot films" or rapid sequence acquisition) are obtained and printed "digitally" instead of with standard analog cut-film radiography. This is a step toward the "filmless" angiography/interventional suite.

    f. Other features that contribute to ease of operation and efficiency are remote control review of images in the procedure room and remote selection and dispatching of images directly to the printer during a procedure (without the need for the technologist to leave the suite).

g. To enhance the flexibility of this expensive equipment multitasking features are available (e.g., dual-room digital interfaces or simultaneous acquistion, review, and printing capability). In the future, digital archiving, retrieval, and display will become more universal.

Selecting Optimal Radiographic Technique

Maria M. Damiano
Krishna Kandarpa

General Principles

1. **Kilovoltage** (kV). Generally determines contrast on image.

   a. 70 kV is ideal for cerebral, thoracic, and abdominal arteriography. It is high enough to provide adequate penetration in most projections, while low enough to maintain an optimal scale of radiographic contrast and latitude.

   b. Lower kV may be employed for peripheral arteriography (e.g., 50–65 kV).

   c. For abdominal aortography in the lateral projection, kV should be increased (e.g., 85 kV) to ensure adequate penetration to the thicker part and to reduce scattered radiation.

2. **Milliamperes/Seconds** (mAs). Determines overall density of image. Once the mAs has been selected, the shortest exposure time (milliseconds) and highest current (mA) value should be employed.

   a. Highest mA will maximize number of photons and will prevent excessive image noise due to quantum mottle.

   b. Shortest possible exposure time will minimize vessel motion artifact. The maximum exposure time for arteriography should not exceed $1/10$ second (or 100 mAs) (Some x-ray generators will automatically select lowest exposure time for a given mAs).

3. **Focal spot.** Determines image resolution.

   a. The smaller the focal spot size, the less the x-ray output but the sharper the vessel borders. In magnification studies, vessel unsharpness (or penumbra) will occur unless even smaller focal spot sizes are employed.

   b. For nonmagnification arteriography

      (1) Size 0.6 mm.

      (2) 1.0 or 1.2 mm for lateral aortography.

   c. For magnification arteriography

      (1) 0.2 or 0.3 mm for 2 × magnification.

      (2) 0.1 mm for greater than 2 × magnification.

4. **Film-screen combination**

   a. A slower speed system provides better resolution but may require higher kV (resulting in less radiographic contrast) and longer exposure time (resulting in blurring of vessels due to arterial motion).

b. Selection of a film-screen combination depends on the type of exam most commonly performed (we employ 800 speed system).

5. Digitally acquired images may be photographed using laser printers.

Injection Rates and Image-Acquisition Programs

Maria M. Damiano

Injection rates and image-acquisition programs should be tailored for the patient when indicated. However, for the vast majority of studies, routine programs are useful. The following programs may be used for cut-film or digital acquisitions. Digital acquisition protocols may be adapted to closely emulate the sequences suggested below (Tables 32-1, 32-2, 32-3, 32-4).

Table 32-1. Visceral and peripheral angiography

Study and injection site	Total volume and rate[a]	Image-acquisition program[b]
Abdominal aortogram (above celiac axis)	50 ml @ 25/sec	3/sec × 2 sec 1/sec × 2 sec two delays
Thoracic aortogram (ascending aorta)	70 ml @ 35/sec	3/sec × 3 sec 1/sec × 2 sec
Bilateral lower extremity runoff (distal aorta)	60–80 ml @ 6–8/sec	0 for 4 sec, then 1/sec × 3 sec = pelvis 1/sec × 2 sec = thigh 1/sec × 4 sec = knee four delays = calf
Standing pelvic arteriogram (distal aorta)	30 ml @ 15/sec	2/sec × 3 sec 1/sec × 3 sec
Unilateral lower extremity runoff (ipsilateral common iliac artery)	25 ml @ 8/sec	1/sec × 2 sec = pelvis 1/sec × 2 sec = thigh 1/sec × 3 sec = knee four delays = calf
Renal transplant (iliac fossa; ipsilateral common iliac artery)	20 ml @ 8/sec	3/sec × 2 sec 2/sec × 2 sec two delays

Table 32-1. (continued)

Study and injection site	Total volume and rate[a]	Image-acquisition program[b]
Renal transplant (iliac fossa; selective ipsilateral hypogastric artery)	14 ml @ 7/sec	3/sec × 2 sec 2/sec × 2 sec two delays
Unilateral renal arteriogram (proximal ipsilateral renal artery)	12 ml @ 6–8/sec	3/sec × 2 sec 1/sec × 2 sec two delays (for donors only—five delays)
Selective renal postepinephrine	12 ml @ 3/sec	1/sec × 4 sec four delays
Celiac arteriogram (selective)	60 ml @ 8–10/sec	2/sec × 2 sec 1/sec × 6 sec six delays
Hepatic arteriogram (selective)	30 ml @ 6–8/sec	2/sec × 2 sec 1/sec × 4 sec two delays
Gastroduodenal arteriogram (selective)	15 ml @ 4/sec	2/sec × 2 sec 1/sec × 3 sec three delays
Splenic arteriogram (selective)	40–50 ml @ 6–8/sec	1/sec × 4 sec seven delays
Left gastric arteriogram (selective)	20 ml @ 4/sec	1/sec × 6 sec three delays
Dorsal pancreatic arteriogram (selective)	10 ml @ 3/sec	1/sec × 6 sec three delays
Superior mesenteric arteriogram (selective)	50–60 ml @ 6–8/sec	1/sec × 9 sec six delays
Inferior mesenteric arteriogram (selective)	15 ml @ 3/sec	2/sec × 2 sec 1/sec × 3 sec four delays
Lumbar arteriogram (selective)	6 ml hand	1/sec × 8 sec
Inferior phrenic arteriogram (selective)	12 ml @ 3/sec	1/sec × 8 sec

Table 32-1. (continued)

Study and injection site	Total volume and rate[a]	Image-acquisition program[b]
Middle or inferior adrenal arteriogram (selective)	8 ml hand	1/sec × 8 sec
Subclavian arteriogram (distal to cephalic arteries)	20–25 ml @ 6–8/sec	*shoulder* 2/sec × 3 sec 1/sec × 3 sec *arm* 0 × 1 sec 1/sec × 6 sec four delays *hand* 0 × 3 sec 1/sec × 10 sec three delays
Hand arteriogram (mid-brachial artery)	16 ml @ 4/sec	0 × 2 sec 1/sec × 8 sec two delays

[a]Based on Hypaque 76.
[b]Delay = one film every other second.

Table 32-2. Peripheral venous angiography

Study and injection site	Total volume and rate	Image-acquisition program*
Inferior venacavogram (iliac vein or IVC)	50 ml @ 20/sec	2/sec × 4 sec
Common femoral vein (selective)	25 ml @ 8/sec	2/sec × 4 sec
Renal venogram (selective ipsilateral renal vein)	25 ml @ 10/sec after injecting epinephrine into renal artery	2/sec × 4 sec 1/sec × 2 sec
Adrenal venogram (selective)	*left:* 8 ml by hand *right:* 5 ml by hand	2/sec × 4 sec 1/sec × 2 sec
Superior venacavogram (unilateral or bilateral antecubital vein)	30 ml @ 6/sec	0 × 3 sec 1/sec × 12 sec
Lower extremity venogram (foot vein)	80–200 ml Conray 43 hand infusion with fluoroscopic monitoring	AP and lateral calf AP thigh AP pelvis
Wedge hepatic venogram (superselective hepatic vein)	12 ml @ 3/sec	2/sec × 3 sec 1/sec × 3 sec

AP = anteroposterior.
*Delay = one film every other second.

Table 32-3. Coronary and pulmonary angiography

Study and injection site	Total volume and rate	Image-acquisition program*
Coronary arteriogram (selective)	*left:* 6–9 ml hand *right:* 4–6 ml hand	Cine or spot films @ 4/sec
Left ventriculogram (intracavitary)	35–50 ml @ 12–15/sec	Cine
Unilateral pulmonary arteriogram (selective)	40–50 ml @ 20–25/sec	3/sec × 3 sec 2/sec × 1 sec 1/sec × 3 sec
Lobar pulmonary arteriogram (superselective lobar artery)	25 ml @ 15/sec	3/sec × 3 sec 2/sec × 1 sec 1/sec × 3 sec
Right ventriculogram (intracavitary)	50 ml @ 15/sec	Cine
Right atriogram (intracavitary)	50 ml @ 25/sec	Cine

Table 32-4. Useful obliquities for peripheral angiography

Carotid bifurcation	Lateral and AP (with head turned to opposite extreme)
Siphon	Lateral
Circle of Willis	Transfacial with head turned 10 degrees to either side
Aortic arch (to open arch)	AP and steep (70 degrees) RPO
Aortic arch (for brachiocephalic vessels)	Body at 45-degrees RPO with head true lateral, chin raised, shoulders dropped down
Selective pulmonary artery	AP and lateral *or* left 45–60-degrees RPO; right 45–60-degrees LPO Opposite obliques if necessary
Origins of mesenteric vessels	Lateral aorta
Hepatic artery branches	*left:* LPO 30–45 degrees *right:* RPO 30–45 degrees
Origin of renal arteries	*left:* 15-degrees RPO *right:* 15-degrees LPO
Common iliac bifurcation	Ipsilateral posterior oblique 45 degrees (side of interest down)
Common femoral bifurcation	Contralateral posterior oblique 45 degrees (side of interest up)

AP = anteroposterior; RPO = right posterior oblique; LPO = left

Selected Readings

Abrams, HL. *Abrams' Angiography: Vascular and Interventional Radiology* (4th ed.). Boston: Little, Brown, 1994.

Curry TS, Dowdey JE, Murry RC. *Christensen's Introduction to Physics of Diagnostic Radiology* (3rd ed.). Philadelphia: Lea & Febiger, 1984.

Moore RJ. *Imaging Principles of Cardiac Angiography.* Rockland, MD: Aspen, 1990.

Thompson, TT. *A Practical Approach to Modern Imaging Equipment* (2nd ed.) Boston: Little, Brown, 1985.

Radiation Safety

Stuart J. Singer

Primary Safety Caveats [1–4]

1. **Scatter radiation.** This main source of exposure to the operator (Tables 33-1, 33-2) decreases exponentially as the fluoroscopic field size is decreased from 30 × 30 cm². The scatter radiation plateaus at field sizes greater than 30 × 30 cm² [3].
2. **Distance from primary beam.** The scatter exposure falls off as the inverse square of the distance from the primary beam. The scatter radiation intensity is 1/1000 of the primary beam 1 meter from the skin entrance site with a 20 × 20 cm field size [3,4].
3. **X-ray tube position.** There is at least a twofold increase in scatter radiation exposure to the primary operator with an overhead C-arm x-ray tube when compared to an under-patient x-ray tube [1,2].
4. **Cineangiography.** Scatter exposure to the primary operator during cineangiography accounts for about 50% of the total scatter exposure to the primary operator during cardiac catheterization [2].
5. **Video recording.** Incorporation of a single-frame video recording device in the fluoroscopy system will decrease fluoroscopy time as will judicious use of fluoroscopy.
6. Judicious use of **fluoroscopy** will protect both personnel and patient (Table 33-3).

Protective Equipment

1. **Lead protective clothing.** 0.50-mm lead equivalent protection is required.
   a. Thyroid shields are highly recommended because thyroid exposure is 1.7 times that recorded by the collar radiation badge [1,4,5].
   b. A commercially available maternity lead apron has 1.0-mm lead equivalent protection from the xiphoid to the pubic bone. The remainder of the apron has 0.50-mm lead equivalent. This apron decreases maternal exposure by a factor of 5 over a 0.50-mm lead equivalent apron. This reduces the theoretical maximum occupational gestational fetal exposure from 500 to 100 mrem. The maternal apron weighs 14 lb; a standard frontal apron weighs 9.5 lb [6].
   c. Scheduled fluoroscopic evaluation for cracks or tears in the lead apron is necessary [7].
2. **Leaded eyeglasses.** There is a 20-mrem absorption by the lens during a cardiac catheterization. The primary operator would be limited to 5 cases/week if lens exposure is not to exceed 5 rem/year. Cataract formation is estimated to have a single dose threshold of 200 rem, with a 20-year latency period. Leaded eyeglasses absorb at least 70% of scatter exposure. Side shields are mandatory since

Table 33-1. Radiation doses to radiologist and personnel

References	Procedure	Fluoroscopy time (min): mean (range)	Dose (mrem) to radiologist: mean (range)		Dose (mrem) to assisting nurse: mean (range)
			Forehead/neck	Hand/finger	
a	Percutaneous transhepatic portography	35 (8–84)	(1–21)	(30–800)	(1–6)
a	Percutaneous transhepatic cholangiography	13 (8–18)	(5–9)	(30–600)	(1–4)
b	Percutaneous transhepatic cholangiography	14 (3–57)	—	478	—
c	Abdominal angiography	29 (3–57)	<2	18 (2–112)	5 (2–11)
d	Cardiac catheterization	—	28 (19–46)	26 (2–69)	—
e	Cardiac catheterization + cineradiography	16[h] (2–40)	4 (0–34)	5 (2–16)	—
f	Cardiac catheterization	12 (2–33)	8	35	4
g	Percutaneous renal calculus removal	18 (4–65)	10 (2–32)	27 (10–200)	4 (1–11)

Note: Doses are given in millirems for simplicity; 1 rem = 10^{-2} Sv.

[a]Gustafsson M, Lunderquist A. Personnel exposure to radiation at some angiographic procedures. *Radiology* 140:807–811, 1981.

[b]Cruikshank JG, Fraser GM, Law J. Finger doses received by radiologists during Chiba needle percutaneous cholangiography. *Br J Radiol* 53:584–585, 1980.

[c]Kaude J, Svahn G. Absorbed, gonad, and integral doses to the patient and personnel from angiographic procedures. *Acta Radiol [Diag]* 15:454–464, 1974.

[d]Wold GJ, Scheel RV, Agarwal SK. Evaluation of physician exposure during cardiac catheterization. *Radiology* 99:188–190, 1971.

[e]Ardran GM, Fursdon PS: Radiation exposure to personnel during cardiac catheterization. *Radiology* 106:517–518, 1973.

[f]Stacey AJ, Davis R, Kerr IH: Personnel protection during cardiac catheterization with a comparison of the hazard of undercouch and overcouch x-ray tube mountings. *Br J Radiol* 47:16–23, 1974.

[g]Bush WH, Jones D. Brannen GE. Radiation dose to personnel during percutaneous renal calculus removal. *AJR* 145:1261–1264, 1985.

[h]Plus 35 sec for cineradiography.

Source: Modified from Bush WH, Jones D, Brannen GE. Radiation dose to personnel during percutaneous renal calculus removal. *AJR* 145:1261–1264, 1985.

Table 33-2. Maximum permissible radiation dose for occupationally exposed personnel

Area	Annual (rem)	Quarterly
Whole body (gonads, lens, bone marrow) = about 100 mrem/week	5	3
Hands	75	25
Forearms	30	10
Thyroid	15	5
Fetus (entire gestation)	0.5	

Source: TS Curry, JE Dowdey, RC Murray. *Christensen's Introduction to the Physics of Diagnostic Radiology.* Philadelphia: Lea & Febiger, 1984.

Table 33-3. Patient doses (in mrad) from angiography

Abdominal angiography	
Maximum skin	37,000
Testes	900
Ovaries	7000
Red bone marrow	2800
Thyroid	<1
Uterus	7000
Cerebral angiography	
Maximum skin	17,000
Testes	<1
Ovaries	<1
Red bone marrow	500
Thyroid	4000
Uterus	<1
Coronary angiography	
Maximum skin	28,000
Testes	20
Ovaries	30
Red bone marrow	1800
Thyroid	1800
Uterus	30
Superior mesenteric angiography	
Maximum skin	11,000
Testes	10
Ovaries	100
Red bone marrow	2000
Thyroid	50
Uterus	100

Source: PF Judy, RE Zimmerman. Dose to critical organs. In BJ McNeil, HL Abrams (eds.), *Brigham and Women's Hospital Handbook of Diagnostic Imaging.* Boston: 1986. Pp. 318–324. Published by Little, Brown and Company.

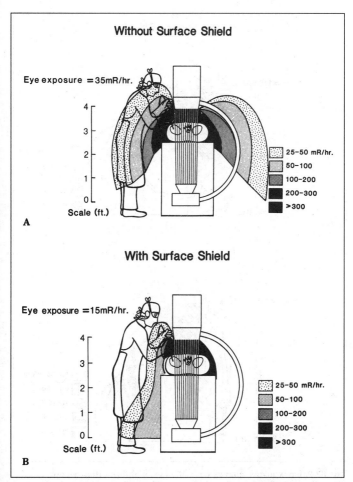

Fig. 33-1. Isoexposure curves with vertical fluoroscopy (A) without surface shield and (B) with 25- × 15-cm surface shield (0.75-mm lead equivalent) in place. (From AT Young et al. Surface shield: Device to reduce personnel radiation exposure. *Radiology* 159:801–803, 1986.)

the primary beam and scatter source are at an angle to the fluoroscopy monitor [8]. Eye exposure is twice the scatter exposure measured by the collar radiation badge [2].

3. **Lead shields.** They must not hinder table and image intensifier activity.
   a. Ceiling suspended facial shields absorb about 95% of scatter exposure to the head and neck. They also force the primary operator to move away from the primary beam. The shields should be covered with sterile clear plastic [1].

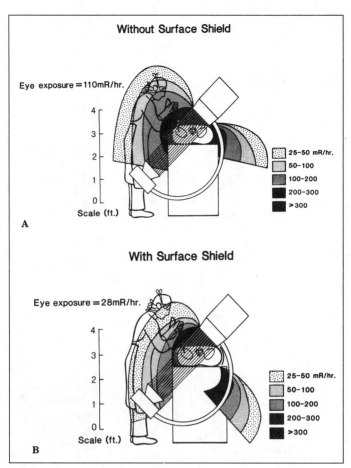

Fig. 33-2. Isoexposure curves with 45-degree oblique fluoroscopy (A) without surface shield and (B) with 25- × 15-cm surface shield (0.75-mm lead equivalent) in place. (From AT Young et al. Surface shield: Device to reduce personnel radiation exposure. *Radiology* **159:801–803, 1986.)**

    b. Leaded leaves suspended from the image intensifier absorb 25–70% of scatter exposure. They are most effective when the primary beam is angled toward the primary operator [1].

    c. Leaded curtains at the side of the fluoroscopy table absorb about 85% of scatter exposure to the legs of the primary operator [1].

    d. Leaded surface shields with 0.75-mm lead equivalent can be secured to the patient's flank with up to 75% reduction in scatter radiation during interventional uroradiology. The surface shield (20 × 25 cm) can have a central hole to permit biliary interventions. The surface shield does limit fluoroscopy to 20 degrees obliquity (Figs. 33-1, 33-2) [9].

4. Leaded gloves. Sterile "radiation resistant" gloves give 0.38-mm lead equivalent protection but are somewhat cumbersome to use. They attenuate 22% of the scatter at 80 kV(p) and 16% at 100 kV(p). They are advisable when the hands are close to the primary beam as in percutaneous nephrolithotomy [5].

References

1. Kosnik IT. Personnel exposure in the cardiac catheterization laboratory. *Health Phys* 50:144–147, 1986.
2. Rueter FG. Physician and patient exposure during cardiac catheterization. *Circulation* 58:134–139, 1978.
3. Curry TS, Dowdey JE, Murray RC. *Christensen's Introduction to the Physics of Diagnostic Radiology.* Philadelphia: Lea & Febiger, 1984.
4. Boone JM, Levin DC. Radiation exposure to angiographers under different fluoroscopic imaging conditions. *Radiology* 180:861–865, 1991.
5. Bush WH, Jones D, Brannen GE. Radiation dose to personnel during percutaneous renal calculus removal. *Am J Radiol* 145:1261–1264, 1985.
6. Witrak B, Sprawls P. Maternity lead apron. *Radiology* 150:597, 1984.
7. Glaze S, LeBlanc AD, Bushong SC. Defects in new protective aprons. *Radiology* 152:217–218, 1984.
8. Richman AH, Chan B, Katz M. Effectiveness of lead lenses in reducing radiation exposure. *Radiology* 121:357–359, 1976.
9. Young AT, et al. Surface shield: Device to reduce personnel radiation exposure. *Radiology* 159:801–803, 1986.

Infection Control

Julie M. Sniffen

The first infection control measure was as simple as washing hands between contact with patients. While this still remains the basis for infection control, many more practices have become important. The most recent, referred to as "universal blood and body fluid precautions" or simply "universal precautions," was developed to protect health-care workers from exposure to blood-borne pathogens, primarily hepatitis B virus (HBV) and human immunodeficiency virus (HIV).

Introduced in August 1987 by the Centers for Disease Control (CDC) and updated in June 1988 [1,2], these guidelines have become the standards for infection control. Guidelines for the prevention of occupational exposures, published in 1989 by the CDC, reviewed methods of HBV and HIV transmission in the workplace and outlined infection control recommendations [3].

The U.S. Department of Labor Occupational Safety and Health Administration (OSHA) published their standards and enforcement procedures in 1991 [4]. This standard took effect March 6, 1992, and has mandated infection control and occupational safety standards in health-care settings. Surveys by OSHA are conducted to assess compliance.

In angiography, because most procedures involve intravascular manipulation and contact with blood, and needles or sharp instruments ("sharps"), strict adherence to hospital infection control policies is essential for maintaining a safe work environment.

This chapter outlines some basic guidelines.

Universal Precautions

1. Blood and body fluid precautions must be used in the care of all patients (i.e., treat blood and other body fluids from all patients as potentially infective).
2. Persons performing procedures, and anyone within the sterile field during a procedure, are required to wear eye and face protection (protective eyewear or face shield and a mask) in addition to sterile gloves and impervious sterile gowns.
3. Persons assisting in procedures, not within the sterile field, must have face protection available to them.
4. All sharps must be disposed of in labeled, puncture-resistant containers located at the site of use.
5. Needles and sharps must never be manually recapped.
6. Specifically designed sterile needle and blade holders, safety needles, and needleless IV administration systems should be evaluated and employed whenever possible. Closed flushing systems may help reduce the risk of splashing.
7. All blood-soaked trash must be disposed of in labeled, impervious containers. (Disposal is according to hospital policy and state regulations).

Personnel Policies

1. All personnel whose job may expose them to blood or body fluids must
   a. Receive in-service training regarding OSHA infection control policies at the time of employment and at least annually,
   b. Be offered hepatitis B vaccination, *and*
   c. Be informed of and have access to the hospital exposure control plan (OSHA).
2. All departments must have infection control guidelines. These must be reviewed and updated every 2 years (according to JCAHO, Joint Commission for the Accreditation of Healthcare Organizations).
3. All procedures or tasks performed by a department must be assessed for risk of exposure to blood and body fluids (OSHA).
   Example:

Task	Exposure risk	Minimum protective equipment
Percutaneous procedures (angiography, venography, angioplasty, visceral puncture, drainages)	Hand contact Splash Puncture	Gloves Eye and face protection Impervious gowns

4. Job categories must be assessed for risk of contact and exposure to blood and body fluids (OSHA).

Cleaning

1. Blood spills must be cleaned promptly using an absorbent material and/or hospital-approved disinfectant (e.g., tuberculocidal quaternary ammonia, phenol, bleach diluted 1 : 10 with water).
2. Horizontal surfaces (tables, counter tops, floors) should be cleaned on a regular basis, and when soiling occurs.
3. Vertical surfaces (e.g., walls, curtains, blinds) need be cleaned only when visibly soiled.
4. Persons who clean equipment must wear appropriate personal protective equipment (i.e., heavy-duty utility gloves and face protection with impervious gown when the risk of splashing is present).
5. Manufacturer and/or hospital guidelines must be followed for the cleaning of and disinfection and sterilization of equipment.

Other Issues

1. The presence of certain bacteria such as methicillin-resistant *Staphylococcus aureus* (MRSA), vancomycin-resistant enterococcus (VRE), and some multiple-drug-resistant Gram-negative rods, may require the use of contact pre-

cautions in addition to universal precautions. Persons having contact with these patients should wear a gown and gloves. All equipment that was in contact with the patient should be cleaned before being used on another patient.

2. Precautions for patients with known or suspected pulmonary or laryngeal tuberculosis (TB) are currently being addressed by the CDC. Special masks (dust mist or equivalent), as opposed to surgical masks, should be worn by persons in contact with patients with TB. In addition, these patients should be in rooms at negative air pressure and vented outside of the institution.

References

1. Centers for Disease Control. Recommendations for prevention of HIV transmission in health care settings. *MMWR* 36(suppl):2S–18S, 1987.
2. Centers for Disease Control. Update: Universal precautions for prevention of transmission of human immunodeficiency virus, hepatitis B virus, and other bloodborne pathogens in health-care settings. *MMWR* 37:377–388, 1988.
3. Centers for Disease Control. Guidelines for prevention of transmission of human immunodeficiency virus and hepatitis B virus to health-care and public safety workers. *MMWR* 38(suppl 6):1–37, 1989.
4. Department of Labor. Occupational Safety and Health Administration. (29 CFR Part 1910.1030). Occupational exposure to bloodborne pathogens; final rule. *Federal Register*. December 6, 1991.

Risk Management

Albert L. Bundy

The Concept of Risk Management [1,2]

The concept of risk management evolved as the response of health-care professionals to the malpractice crisis. Health professionals realize that they must play an active role in identifying risks that could lead to negligence or malpractice litigation. Once identified, these risks should be prevented or minimized. Malpractice underwriting companies and administrative agencies require hospitals and physicians to establish formal risk-management programs. Some states, such as Massachusetts, require that a physician earn a certain number of continuing medical education (CME) credits in risk management annually to maintain a current license.

The Medical Malpractice Crisis [1,3–5]

Medical malpractice litigation was relatively rare prior to 1960. Claims were few and outcomes generally favored the defendant physicians. Fortunately, the latter is still generally true today [4]. However, the 1970s saw a dramatic increase in medical negligence litigation. This came to be known as the medical malpractice crisis. Legislation enacted to do away with the immunity of both government and charitable hospitals exposed these institutions to potential liability from negligent acts of their employees. The situation was further complicated with the introduction of Medicare and Medicaid into the health-care system.

Other important factors were also contributed to this crisis. The personalization of medicine was declining and the physician-patient relationship was being eroded. Patients who are upset about their clinical outcome ("unrealized expectations") find it easier to sue physicians they do not know or with whom they have had little contact—often, the radiologist. Most early litigation involving radiologists resulted from injuries related to radiation therapy. Today the crisis has spread to all of radiology. Although, invasive procedures account for about 20% of lawsuits brought against radiologists, they account for about 70% of radiology-related payments [5].

The Law of Medical Negligence [3]

The legal concept of negligence is "conduct which falls below the standard established by law for the protection of others against unreasonable risk of harm."

1. For most medical practice cases, negligence is the primary theory of liability. **An act of negligence has four basic elements:** duty, breach, proximate causation, and damages. The plaintiff (the one bringing the suit) has the burden of establishing

    a. That the defendant physician owed him a **duty of care**;

    b. That the defendant violated the applicable standard of care resulting in the **breach**;

    c. That the defendant's alleged **negligence proximately caused the injury**; and

    d. That identifiable **damages** resulted.

2. Negligence law is based on a uniform standard of behavior on which to judge the actions of the defendant. The legal standard on which the courts rely is known as the **"reasonable man standard."** This means that the interventional radiologist is expected to behave like a reasonable interventional radiologist under like circumstances (e.g., community radiologists, whose practice generally defines and establishes the local standard). Since the judge and jurors are usually laypersons regarding medical matters, expert testimony often is necessary to establish the applicable standard of care.

Four Steps of a Risk Management Program

A risk management program should be based on providing "good patient care, communication, documentation, quality assurance, and follow-up" [4]. The four basic steps are

1. **Identify all potential risks**

   This step should ideally result in recognition of areas of risk before legal action. Often, however, risky situations may only come to attention after litigation has begun.

2. Develop methods to **measure the potential impact** of each risk

   a. More frequently occurring risks can be predicted fairly accurately. More severe, less frequent, risks are more difficult to predict.

   b. The interventional radiologist should be aware of the frequency of minor contrast media reactions, infiltrations of contrast media into the skin, groin or axillary hematomas after arterial punctures, and infections caused by needle puncture.

   c. The interventional radiologist should be able to assign a frequency to severe risk such as death, paralysis, stroke, or other catastrophes resulting in organ damage.

3. Develop a program to **manage** situations with potential risk

   a. Without a comprehensive program, the frequency of observed risks will not be altered.

   b. Establish reasonable means and methods for obtaining **informed consent** prior to performing invasive procedures.

   c. Other approaches include

       (1) Adequate preprocedure patient evaluation, competence in procedural skills, postprocedure follow-up, and documentation of outcomes.

       (2) Periodic analyses of data obtained for an ongoing program to deal with a particular risk, with corrective action as required.

       (3) In-service training for personnel on equipment

and methods, including emergency situations (e.g., training in cardiopulmonary resuscitation or advanced life support, fire evacuation drills).

(4) Physical inspection of work areas to identify potential hazards and establish equipment maintenance programs.

4. Establish a system to **monitor and control** improvements obtained as a result of implementing the above steps.

   a. The motivating force for this step is the anticipated reduction of the frequency and severity of claims.

   b. Reducing claims protects the assets of the insurers, which should result in premium savings for the insured.

   c. A malpractice insurance policy should not substitute for a good risk-management program. Malpractice litigation has encouraged many physicians to practice "defensive medicine." This type of practice neither leads to better patient care nor averts lawsuits but is one of the factors responsible for rising medical care costs.

The Concept of Informed Consent [3,4,6]

1. The rationale behind informed consent is to strengthen communication between the physician and the patient. Verbal communications must be documented in writing.

   a. The **physician-oriented standard** of disclosure requires a physician to disclose only information that other reasonable physicians would disclose under the same or similar circumstances.

   b. The **patient-oriented standard** of disclosure requires physicians to disclose all information that a reasonable patient should want to know under the same or similar circumstances (i.e., any information that could influence the patient's ultimate decision).

   c. When in doubt, it is prudent to err on the side of disclosure. The interventional radiologist must be aware of the standard used in his or her jurisdiction.

2. Verbal discussion with the patient about the procedure, its risks, and its alternatives is of special importance to the interventional radiologist. The patient must be given an opportunity to ask any and all questions related to the proposed procedure, and honest answers must be provided. These discussions must be documented.

3. **SIGNED INFORMED CONSENT IS REQUIRED BY LAW.** The signature on the consent form should only be obtained after the above discussion with the patient by the physician who will perform the procedure (and not by the referring physician). A signature obtained while the patient is on medications that may alter mentation may not be legally valid. There are four major exceptions to the requirement of informed consent:

   a. Emergency situations (permission to proceed may be granted by the hospital's legal officer on-call if immediate family or legal guardian is unavailable).

b. Patient's mental incompetence (legally documented).
c. Patient's desire not to be informed; this must be documented.
d. If such information may aggravate the patient's condition (usually psychiatric patients).

References

1. Bundy AL. Risk management concept and application. *Radiol Report* 2:108–110, 1989.
2. Hirsh HL, Gibbs RF. Medical Liability, Risk Management. In *Legal Medicine, Legal Dynamics of Medical Encounters.* St. Louis: Mosby–Year Book, 1988. Pp. 468–479.
3. Bundy AL. *Radiology and the Law.* Rockville, MD: Aspen, 1988. Pp. 1–28, 109–120.
4. vanSonnenberg E, Barton JB, Wittich GR. Radiology and the law, with an emphasis on interventional radiology. *Radiology* 187:297–303, 1993.
5. Bowyer EA. High radiology losses related to invasive procedures. *Risk Manag Found Forum* 6:1–8, 1985.
6. Andrews LB. Informed consent statutes and decision making process. *J Leg Med* 5:163–217, 1984.

Nursing Management

Nursing Management During Angiography and Interventional Procedures

Eileen M. Bozadjian

Preprocedure Patient Assessment

For patients who will undergo procedures as outpatients or on the same day of admission, a preprocedure patient assessment is best accomplished a minimum of 48 hours in advance. This provides sufficient time for patient workup and preparation, which should include a complete medical history, review of pertinent laboratory values and tests, physical examination, nursing assessment and care plan, informed consent, patient teaching, and the development of a sedation and analgesia plan.

Establishing preprocedure/admitting protocols and communication between the referring physician's office and radiology scheduling can coordinate and streamline patient workup (e.g., laboratory visits, office visits, radiology clinic visits) to occur on a single day with minimal patient inconvenience.

FUNCTIONAL HEALTH PATTERN ASSESSMENT—
A PATIENT-COMPLETED QUESTIONNAIRE

1. **Current concerns and health history**
   a. What health problem(s) bring the patient here?
   b. What are the patient's expectations regarding this procedure?
   c. List date(s) and reasons for any previous hospitalization(s).
   d. List date(s) and reasons for any previous angiographic or interventional procedure(s).
2. **Nutrition**
   a. Does the patient follow a special diet?
   b. Does the patient have food allergies?
   c. Has the patient been having any problems with nausea or vomiting?
   d. What are the patient's eating habits?
3. **Integumentary**
   a. Does the patient have any conditions of the skin and mucous membranes?
   b. Are there any broken areas, ulcers, sores, or rashes?
4. **Elimination**
   a. Does the patient have any difficulty urinating?
   b. Does the patient have any difficulty with bowel movement?
5. **Sleep/rest**
   a. Does the patient have any difficulty lying flat?
   b. Does the patient have any problems with the back, knees, hips, shoulders, elbows, or neck?
6. **Exercise**
   a. To what extent does the patient exercise?

    b. Is there discomfort with exercise? (For example, leg or buttock cramps, shortness of breath, chest pain.)

7. Cognitive/sensory
    a. Does the patient have vision impairment or wear glasses?
    b. Does the patient have hearing loss or use a hearing aid?
    c. Is the patient intellectually impaired; are there cognitive deficits (e.g., memory loss or problems integrating information)?
    d. Does the patient have any psychomotor deficits?

8. Activities of daily living: role and responsibilities
    a. Is the patient dependent on others for all or part of his/her care?
    b. Is the patient ambulatory; dependent, on crutches, cane, or walker?
    c. Does the patient usually take care of someone or something (e.g., pet) at home?
    d. For outpatient procedures, is there someone who will be able to drive the patient home and care for the patient in the immediate postprocedure period?
    e. Does the patient anticipate any problems going home from the hospital?

9. Coping and adaptation
    a. How concerned are the patient and family about this illness?
    b. How concerned are the patient and family about this procedure?
    c. What are the patient's primary support structures?
    d. How do the patient and family usually respond to stress?

10. Behavior and habits
    a. Alcohol and drug use: addiction, dependence, abuse.
    b. Smoking history: packs per day, years.
    c. Emotional or stress-related problems?

NURSE'S REVIEW OF MEDICAL HISTORY

1. Hypertension: severity; treated with medications?
2. Diabetes: insulin-dependent, oral hypoglycemics, diet control.
3. Angina: stable/unstable (date of last episode and precipitating factors).
4. Previous myocardial infarction: with or without angina.
5. Congestive heart failure.
6. Cardiac valvular disease.
7. Neurologic diseases: seizures, myasthenia gravis, intracranial hypertension.
8. Stroke/transient ischemic attack.
9. Endocrinologic: hypo-/hyper- thyroidism/parathyroidism, Addison's disease, etc.
10. Musculoskeletal: rheumatism or arthritis, unstable fractures with or without open reductions, joint replacements, contractures, muscle disease, or bone disease.
11. Lung disease: chronic obstructive pulmonary disease (COPD), arthritis, pulmonary hypertension, asthma, cystic fibrosis, bronchitis.

12. Hepatic disease: cirrhosis, hepatitis, cholangitis, cholecystitis, biliary or cystic stones.
13. Renal disease: dialysis, transplant, nephrectomy, kidney stones or obstruction, hematuria, renal failure.
14. Hematologic/oncologic: carcinoma(s), metastasis and treatment, pheochromocytoma, lymphoma, myeloma, leukemia, polycythemia vera, sickle cell disease, brain or spinal tumors, coagulopathies, hypo- or hypercoagulopathies.
15. Glaucoma.
16. Benign prosthetic hypertrophy.
17. Naso-oropharangeal disease.
18. Fevers, infections, communicable diseases.
19. Previous surgeries.
20. Reproductive history; currently pregnant.
21. Recent barium exams or cholecystogram.

CURRENT MEDICATIONS

1. List all patient medications, dosage routes, and frequency.
2. List all current allergies to food, drugs, and environment. Has the patient had IV contrast in the past? Was there an adverse response to contrast?

LABORATORY TESTS TO BE CONDUCTED
(tailor to specific procedure)

1. Coagulation: PT, PTT, platelets.
2. Hematology: Hct and Hgb.
3. Chemistry: BUN, Cr, electrolytes.
4. ECG for all patients with cardiac disease and those undergoing cardiopulmonary procedures.
5. Review results of all pertinent prior studies: noninvasive studies, CT, MRI/MRA, nuclear medicine, etc.
6. Will there be requirements for blood or blood product transfusion? If so, screen for blood type.

PHYSICAL EXAMINATION

1. Prepare patient for physical examination and assist radiologist who is evaluating the patient.
2. Extremity exam, skin condition and color (rashes, dermatitis) ulcers, capillary refill, peripheral pulses: palpation, segmental Doppler pressures, sensation and motion.
3. Baseline vital signs, BP in both arms (if possible).
4. Assessment of airway patency, naso-oropharangeal abnormalities, breath sounds.
5. Chest and cardiac exam, current ECG.
6. Actual weight and height.
7. Examination of planned percutaneous access site(s). Note any skin abrasions, infections, wounds, or inguinal scars.
8. Neuromotor deficits, baseline Glasgow Coma Scale.

ANALGESIA AND SEDATION RATIONALE

1. Risk assessment: American Society of Anesthesiologists (ASA) Physical Status Category score.
2. Capacity of patient to adapt to:
    a. Comorbidity associated with the procedure.
    b. Duration of the procedure.

     c. Physical positioning required by procedure.

     d. Discomfort associated with the procedure.

3. Pain assessment. Specify location, duration, and frequency

     a. Local anesthetic.

     b. Type of pain anticipated (e.g., ischemic, biliary or renal colic, pressure).

     c. Baseline pain assessment: scale of 0–10, 0 = no pain and 10 = worst possible.

4. Level of patient anxiety.

Nursing Care Plan: Preprocedure Preparation and Patient Education

The plan for nursing care prescribes nursing interventions aimed at achieving established goals for actual or potential patient problems noted in the nursing diagnosis.*

1. Preprocedure teaching. Verbal review of written instructions should be done during preprocedure or preadmission patient assessment.

     a. Medication adjustments. For example, discontinue warfarin sodium (Coumadin), split morning insulin dose. Outpatients should bring their regular daily medications in their labeled containers to be taken during postprocedure recovery period.

     b. Contrast allergies. Careful review of pretreatment with steroids/antihistamines should be made with patient and family. Provide patient with unit doses or prescriptions and ensure they have written instructions.

     c. Diet. NPO after midnight except for sips of clear liquids with regular medications. Encourage patients to hydrate orally and avoid alcoholic beverages the day before the exam. A late dinner or bedtime snack will help allay morning hunger.

     d. Encourage patients to report onset of cold, flu, or fever.

     e. Outpatients must arrange for someone to drive them home and stay with them the evening following the procedure.

     f. Advise patient of required restriction of physical activity after the procedure.

     g. Describe procedure process, environment, and expected activities of special procedure staff.

     h. Orient the patient to the use of the pain scale.

2. Patient identification. Outpatient or same-day patients should provide a valid identification. Patient should be given a hospital wrist band on admission to the department if one has not been previously issued.

3. Verify that there is a completed and signed procedure consent form.

---

*Standards of Care established by the American Radiologic Nurses Association. The American Radiological Nurses Association (ARNA, 2021 Spring Road, Suite 600, Oak Brook, IL 60521) develops and approves standards of practice and care. Further information may be obtained directly from this organization.

4. Review preadmission nursing assessment, medical history, results of labs and tests, physical exam, and the rationale for sedation and analgesia.
5. Verify that all elements of preprocedural patient preparation have been completed: pretreatments or premedications, NPO and time of last meal, medications brought in from home, outpatient discharge arrangements completed.
6. Verify the appropriateness of the procedural environment
   a. **Procedure room fully stocked.** Suction equipment and catheters, bite blocks, intubation kit, airways and masks, self-inflating positive pressure oxygen supply system capable of delivering 90% oxygen at 15 liter/minute flow rate.
   b. **Monitoring equipment.** Cardiac monitor, automated BP unit and sphygmomanometer with multiple cuff sizes, stethoscope, pulse oximeter, capnometer.
   c. **Stock medications.** In-room stock medication should be checked monthly for expiration. Medication should include routine procedure, drugs for contrast reactions, medications for emergency reversal of sedatives and analgesics, first-line emergency care drugs.
   d. **Emergency cart and resuscitation equipment.** Emergency code cart properly checked daily and restocked weekly per protocol. Cardiac defibrillator should be configured for battery operation and include quick look: anteroposterior defibrillation and cardioversion and external cardiac pacing features.
7. Check for functional IV line (18- or 20-gauge angiocath). If not, place before procedure.
8. Institute cardiac and oxygen-saturation monitor, document baseline heart rate, rhythm, and oxygen saturation.
9. Assess and document baseline vital signs, Glasgow Coma Scale score, pain scale.
10. Will a Foley catheter be required? If so, place one before draping for the procedure.
11. Will intravascular pressure measurement be made? If so, prepare equipment.
12. Are there special patient positioning requirements for the planned procedure? Discuss with radiologist and technologist.
13. Review sedation and analgesia plan. Document patient response, e.g., Glasgow Coma Scale, pain scale, vital signs, oxygen saturation, presence of protective reflexes, adequacy of respiration.

Intraprocedural Nursing Interventions

1. **Document vital signs** q15min, after each contrast injection, and prior to the administration of medications. With changes in the patient's condition, document q5min.
   a. Continuous cardiac monitoring. Note rate, rhythm, conduction abnormalities, and presence of ischemic changes. This is especially important if cardiac chambers are being traversed. Inform operating physician immediately of all changes.
   b. Intravascular pressure monitoring as needed for conti-

nuity of care, and for the management of hypo- and hypertensive events.

c. Thermometer, skin, or axillary temperature preprocedure and predischarge.

2. Maintain fluid balance

a. Hourly documentation of intake and output.

b. Hourly calculation of IV contrast load per kg of body weight. Observe for intolerance to contrast (e.g., hyperosmolar effects, tachycardia, tremors, shortness of breath, pulmonary edema).

c. Administration of IV fluids to maintain normal fluid and electrolyte balance. Where not contraindicated, normal saline or Ringer's lactate are preferable for procedures in which IV ionic contrast media are used.

3. **Continuous surveillance of respiratory status**

a. Check position of head to ensure patency of airway.

b. Skin color, nail beds, and mucosa should be visually monitored and recorded q15min.

c. Respiratory rate and rhythm should be assessed with a stethoscope q15min and recorded to ensure the adequacy of rate and tidal volume.

d. Continuous pulse oximetry. Supplemental oxygen therapy for all patients receiving conscious sedation.

e. Capnography. Recommended for all patients receiving high-dose conscious sedation who are at risk for carbon dioxide retention (e.g., obese patients supine or prone, known carbon dioxide retainers, elderly patients, and those with multisystem organ failure, compromised cardiac output, abdominal/thoracic trauma or surgery, and shock.

4. **Prevention and early detection of spasm, thrombosis, embolism, hemorrhage, and dissection.**

a. Assess and document condition of distal extremity used for intravascular access and document color, sensation, and motion temperature and capillary refill, q15min.

b. Assess vascular access distal extremity pulses q15min.

c. **Continuous** surveillance of the distal extremity (subjected to intervention as in **a** and **b** above).

d. Monitor for signs of bleeding. Hematoma formation, hypotension and reflexive tachycardia, cold clammy skin, pale mucous membranes, alterations in consciousness. Confirm as necessary with laboratory assessment and verify that the patient has blood-type screening on current file in blood bank.

5. **Physical support**

a. Proper anatomic positioning. Support all joints and place all extremities in a nondependent position; lumbar support; position thorax and abdomen to maximize airway and maintain maximal tidal volume with respiration. Minimize pressure points (e.g., heels, knees, shoulders, elbows with additional padding).

b. Protect patient from exposure to cold. Minimize fluid saturation of drapes and bedding; layering of blankets is better than one heavy blanket. Keep the patient covered as much as possible while preparing and draping. Place absorbent underpads while patient uses bed pan or urinal.

c. Offer bed pan or urinal frequently.

d. Assist patient to move unrestricted extremities as frequently as possible.

e. Moisten lips and mouth prn.

6. Psychosocial support

a. Explain all procedures and activities.

b. Provide consistent reinforcement and elicit patient's cooperation.

c. Utilize diversional techniques, progressive muscle relaxation, and modeling to assist patient to cope with rigors of the procedure.

d. Provide patient (and when possible, family) with frequent progress reports.

e. Keep the noise level in the procedure room to a minimum. Avoid inadvertent arousal of patients who are sleeping following sedation.

f. The patient's need for dignity, privacy, and emotional support should be met continuously throughout the duration of his or her stay in the department.

7. Sedation and analgesia. 1992 JCAHO (Joint Commission for the Accreditation of Healthcare Organizations) standards mandate that "in the interest of assuring patient and staff safety, training programs, policies and procedures, and monitoring systems should be in place wherever anesthesia is used within the hospital." Therefore, guidelines for intravenous conscious sedation by nonanesthetists for diagnostic and interventional procedures should be developed in cooperation with the anesthesia department.

a. Institute sedation and analgesia plan as ordered by the radiologist.

b. Explain the goals of the plan to the patient. Contract with the patient regarding what to expect and how to participate in pain management. Use a pain scale and a sedation scale as a guide for nurse-patient collaboration in the assessment of the efficacy of treatment plan.

c. Institute patient monitoring and documentation as described previously and per your approved hospital and departmental standards.

d. Verify that outpatients have written home-care instructions (including precautions that should be taken following sedation) and a responsible adult who can take them home.

e. All sedated patients must remain monitored until they return to their preprocedure state or are transferred to a properly monitored level of care.

Postprocedure Evaluation and Follow-up

Reassessment of the patient is conducted as follows: (1) reconsideration of the nursing diagnosis, (2) revision of goals, and (3) modification and implementation of the follow-up nursing care plan. Patient and family participation is included in the development of the nursing care plan.

1. Provisions for short- and long-term follow-up are identified. Outpatient discharge plans are written and reviewed with patient and family.
2. Continuity of patient care is ensured via the immediate implementation and documentation of the postprocedure orders, verbal and written nursing reports, and transfer note.
3. Conduct a 24-hour postprocedure outpatient follow-up telephone interview. During this follow-up, assess and document the condition of the vascular (or nonvascular) access site, extremity involved in the procedure, the patient's temperature, and ability to eat and void. Identify any problems or signs of complications. Assess and document the patient's general response to the care given and the adequacy of preparation for discharge and home care.

Communications with Floor Nurses

1. Special procedure record is sent to the patient unit or floor with the medical record.
2. Following the completion of the special procedure, the nurse should communicate directly with the floor nurse who will be responsible for the follow-up care of the patient and relay information on the patient's status.

Selected Readings

AORN. Recommended practices: Monitoring the patient receiving IV conscious sedation. *AORN J* 57:978–983, 1993.

Beyer JD, Aradine CR. Patterns of pediatric pain intensity: A methodological investigation of a self-report scale. *Clin J Pain* 3:120–141, 1987.

JCAHO Manual of Accreditation of Hospitals, 1992. Pp. 165–166.

Lind LJ, Mushlin PS. Sedation, analgesia and anesthesia for radiologic procedures. *Cardiovasc Intervent Radiol* 10:247–253, 1987.

Merrick P. Nursing care for the patient undergoing intravenous conscious sedation for imaging studies. *Images* 112:1–4, 1993.

Outpatient Drainage-Catheter Care

Kathleen Reagan

Outpatient Nephrostomy Catheter Care

As with the biliary catheters, nephrostomy catheters are not sutured to the skin but affixed with an adhesive disk. Therefore, gentle handling of the tube is important.

Home Tube Care

1. Emptying the drainage bag (usually a leg bag) should be done several times a day, using a clean technique. At night, conversion to a larger gravity drainage bag to eliminate the need for emptying the smaller bag frequently is recommended.
2. A clean dressing should be applied daily over the tube site and adhesive disk.
3. Tub baths are not permitted. The patient may shower if the skin entry site is adequately protected from getting wet. Washcloth body baths are acceptable.
4. The majority of nephrostomy tubes do not require flushing.

Problems

Patients are instructed to call the interventional radiology service in the event of

1. Discharge or breakdown of skin around the catheter.
2. Leakage of large amounts of urine around the catheter; dressings soaked with urine.
3. Fever or chills, flank pain, diminished nephrostomy tube drainage.
4. Catheter position changed or pulled out.

Long-Term Follow-up

See Table 37-1.

Outpatient Biliary Catheter Care

After biliary tract decompression has been achieved with a drainage catheter (usually to external drainage), tube care is important in maintaining the patency of the catheter. During the first 24–48 hours following catheter placement, it is not unusual to have some discomfort at the tube insertion site or slightly blood-tinged biliary drainage. The catheter is not sutured to the skin but secured with an adhesive disk; patient cooperation, therefore, is needed in handling the tube gently.

Table 37-1. Long-term outpatient tube follow-up[a]

	Nephrostomy tube	Biliary drainage tube
Phone follow-up	q3–4weeks	q3–4weeks
Tube check	q6–8weeks	q6weeks
Tube change[b]	q3–4months	q3months

[a]If problems arise between scheduled tube checks and changes, the patient should be evaluated as soon as possible. Adjustments or tube changes can be handled on an elective basis if necessary.
[b]Internal ureteral stents are changed cytoscopically q3months.

Home Tube Care

1. The properly functioning biliary catheter should be forward flushed once daily with 10 ml of normal saline, using clean technique.
2. The biliary drainage bag may be emptied as necessary. This should be done with clean technique as well.
3. A fresh dressing should be applied daily over the tube insertion site and adhesive disk.
4. Because the tube is secured to the skin with only an adhesive disk, tub baths are not permitted. Showers are permitted if the patient can protect the skin entry site from getting wet. Similarly washcloth "baths" are acceptable.

Problems

Patients are instructed to call the cardiovascular and interventional service for

1. Leakage of large amounts of bile around the catheter.
2. Fever of 101°F lasting several hours without other obvious cause (such as sore throat, flu, etc.).
3. Diminished bile drainage, which may be associated with right upper quadrant pressure or pain.
4. Catheter pulled out or back.

Long-Term Follow-up

See Table 37-1.

Drugs and Dosages

Drug Administration

Krishna Kandarpa
Eileen M. Bozadjian

Guidelines for Premedication

1. Do not premedicate hypovolemic patients or those with severe chronic obstructive pulmonary disease (COPD) (carbon dioxide retention) or increased intracranial pressure [1–4].
2. Premedication should be provided cautiously in patients who are elderly or obtunded, and those with severe hepatic or renal disease, COPD, cardiovascular compromise, or intracranial lesions [1–4].
3. Premedication orders should never be routine but must be individualized considering patient's age, weight, medical and physical condition, anxiety level, allergy history, previous drug reactions, tolerance or abuse of drugs, and duration and type of procedure [1–4].

Guidelines for Drug Administration in Angiography Suite

Prior to the administration of any medication, the following steps should be taken.

1. Each patient has a qualified nurse assigned to him or her for individualized care and monitoring during the entire time that the patient is in the special procedures area. When the patient arrives, the nurse obtains and documents baseline vital signs, oxygen saturation, acetylsalicylic acid status, age, weight, height, pertinent past medical history including allergies and contrast reactions, premedications given, level of anxiety or discomfort, and level of consciousness. Oral intake and hydration status is rechecked. Body temperature is assessed on admission to and discharge from the area.
2. All patients are reevaluated by a radiologist prior to the beginning of the procedure. The completed chart of the patient is reviewed: a brief physical examination is conducted, current laboratory data, ECG, and pertinent radiographic studies are reviewed. Assistance from the anesthesiologist will be required in selected cases (see Chap. 39), but this is usually prearranged on the day before.
3. Informed consent (see Chap. 35) is obtained for the specific procedure by the radiologist who will be performing it.
4. All patients must have a patent functional large-bore IV line (e.g., 20-gauge, capable of delivering 80 ml/min) free of signs of infiltration, phlebitis, or thrombosis.
5. Continuous cardiac monitoring and pulse oximetry must be started on all patients who are candidates for conscious sedation. BP, heart rate and rhythm, respiratory rate, blood-oxygen saturation (and capnography as needed) are documented q15min throughout the procedure and during the recovery period. Frequency of documentation is in-

creased to q5min if there is a deterioration in the patient's condition. Intravascular (arterial) hemodynamic monitoring is instituted in selected procedures when indicated.

6. All patients undergoing conscious sedation receive supplemental oxygen unless contraindicated. The need for supplemental oxygen is reassessed periodically during the procedure and recovery period. Patients who have undergone conscious IV sedation continue to receive oxygen and remain under continuous observation for a minimum of 30 minutes, or until they have returned to admission baseline status. Adequate protective reflexes must have been regained for at least 30 minutes. Cardiac and respiratory resuscitative equipment must be readily available.

7. Medications are to be administered by an R.N. or M.D., under specific direction of the attending radiologist, after continuous BP and ECG monitoring have been instituted. Drug doses are titrated following the patient's subjective and physiologic response, which are monitored q15min. Specific attention must be addressed to vital signs, airway patency, oxygen saturation, presence of protective reflexes (especially, gag reflex and ability to swallow), and level of pain control and sedation.

8. All medications are recorded on a Special Procedure Record, which should include any untoward patient responses. Outpatients are given written discharge orders and on-call contact telephone numbers. A telephone follow-up is conducted at 24 hours in order to evaluate and correct late sequelae of the procedure or medication.

Dosage Calculations

Abbreviations		**Equivalents**	
microgram	μg	1000 micrograms	= 1 mg
milligram	mg	1000 milligrams	= 1 gm
gram	gm	1000 grams	= 1 kg
kilogram	kg	1 kilogram	= 2.2 lb
microdrop	μgtt	60 microdrops	= 1 ml
milliliter	ml	1000 milliliters	= 1 liter

UNITS

1. Body weight is measured in kilograms (kg)
2. Drug concentration in micrograms/milliliter (μ/ml)
3. Dosage in micrograms/kilogram (of body weight) per minute (μ/kg/min).
4. Drop factor = 60 microdrops/milliliter.

Calculating Drug Concentrations

$$\text{Concentration } (\mu g/ml) = \frac{\text{weight of drug } (\mu g)}{\text{volume of solution } (ml)}$$

$$\text{Weight of drug per microdrop} = \frac{\text{concentration } (\mu g/ml)}{\text{microdrops/milliliter}}$$

$$= \frac{\text{concentration } (\mu g/ml)}{60 \ (\mu gtt/ml)}$$

$$= \text{concentration } (\mu g/\mu gtt)$$

EXAMPLE

$$3000 \ \mu g/ml = \frac{3000 \ \mu g/ml}{60 \ \mu gtt/ml} = 50 \ \mu g/\mu gtt$$

Calculating Infusion Doses

Dose in $\mu g/min$ = dosage ($\mu g/kg/min$) $\times$ body weight (kg)
Dose in ml/min = dose ($\mu g/min$)/concentration ($\mu g/ml$)
Dose in $\mu gtt/min$ = dose (ml/min) $\times$ drop factor ($60 \ \mu gtt/ml$)

References

1. *Physicians' Desk Reference* (49th ed.). Oradell, NJ: Medical Economics Company; 1995.
2. Gilman AG, et al. *The Pharmacological Basis of Therapeutics* (8th ed.). New York: Macmillan, 1990.
3. Lind LJ, Mushlin PS. Sedation, analgesia, and anesthesia for radiologic procedures. *Cardiovasc Intervent Radiol* 10:247–253, 1987.
4. Hulbert BJ, Landers DF. Sedation and analgesia for interventional radiologic procedures in adults. *Semin Intervent Radiol* 4:151–160, 1987.

Selected Reading

Dison N. *Simplified Drugs and Solutions for Nurses* (5th ed.). St. Louis: Mosby, 1972.

Sedation, Analgesia, and Anesthesia

Leonard J. Lind
Paul M. Chetham

The practice of cardiovascular and interventional radiology often requires the use of medication to relieve anxiety, provide sedation, and minimize discomfort. Unfortunately, administration of local anesthetics, sedatives, and opioids can impose an additional element of risk to patients, mandating care in patient preparation, monitoring, and discharge from the radiology suite [1].

Available Options for Analgesia and Anesthesia

1. **Local anesthesia**
   a. Infiltration of skin and underlying tissues.
   b. Peripheral nerve block (e.g., intercostal nerve block).
2. **Local anesthesia with sedation**
   a. Provision of care by radiology team.
   b. Provision of sedation by anesthesia team.
3. **Regional anesthesia.** Induction of segmental anesthesia and muscle relaxation with local anesthetics (e.g., spinal or epidural anesthesia).
4. **General anesthesia.** Induction and maintenance of a controlled state of unconsciousness characterized by a loss of protective airway reflexes, absence of response to painful stimuli, and inability to recall procedural events.

Indications for Specific Analgesia and Anesthesia Techniques

1. **Local anesthesia.** Brief diagnostic procedures in adult patients who are cooperative and tolerate the initial local anesthetic infiltration at the puncture site.
2. **Local anesthesia with sedation provided by radiology care team**
   a. Appropriate for most patients undergoing diagnostic and interventional procedures.
   b. May require consultation with an anesthesiologist concerning choice of medication and appropriate dosage. Choice of medication is particularly important in patients during the first trimester of pregnancy.
3. **Local anesthesia with sedation provided by anesthesia care team**
   a. With poor-risk, critically ill, or difficult patients. Often, difficult patients have a history of poor tolerance for invasive procedures, usually resulting from inadequate analgesia and sedation.
   b. When intense analgesia or deep levels of sedation are required.
   c. When procedure or positioning may compromise the airway.

4. Regional anesthesia
   a. When intense analgesia for the procedure and the post-procedural period is required without the use of excessive opioid medication.
   b. When muscle relaxation is desirable or required.
5. General anesthesia
   a. Appropriate for the uncooperative patient or the patient who refuses local or regional anesthesia.
   b. When there is potential for airway obstruction as a result of the procedure or when airway patency or protection may be severely compromised by sedative medication.

Patient Evaluation

1. History and physical examination
   a. Age. Advanced age alters dose requirements and elimination of many medications. For sedatives and analgesics, the elderly patient usually requires smaller increments and less frequent dosing intervals, compared to young adults. A dosage reduction of 30–50% is recommended. Metabolism and drug elimination are both slowed in the elderly, which can result in excessive postprocedure sedation and delayed recovery [2,3].
   b. Cardiovascular disease. A myocardial infarction within the last 6 months, congestive heart failure (CHF), ectopic beats, or a nonsinus rhythm are important findings that are associated with increased risk of postoperative cardiac complications [4]. Well-controlled hypertension does not present an increased risk [5].
   c. Pulmonary disease. Smoking is a cause of increased perioperative morbidity and mortality. Prior to a procedure, cessation of smoking should be encouraged. This will result in a decrease in carboxyhemoglobin levels (12–24 hours), minimize the sympathetic stimulation from nicotine (12–24 hours), and reduce sputum volume (1–2 weeks) [6].
   d. Hepatic disease. Reduced hepatic mass is associated with a decreased production of coagulation and drug-binding proteins (e.g., albumin). Initial doses of sedative and analgesic medications should be reduced, since altered drug-protein binding can allow excessive "free" (i.e., unbound) drug to enter the CNS. In addition, drug metabolism can be markedly slowed resulting in prolonged postprocedural sedation [3].
   e. Renal disease. Impairment of renal function will slow the ultimate elimination of many drugs. Initial and maintenance doses may not require reduction; however, dosing intervals should be lengthened. Caution should be exercised with administration of meperidine (Demerol), since noremeperidine (a primary metabolite) can accumulate in patients with renal dysfunction, leading to CNS stimulation, excitement, and seizures [7].

   f. Medication history. Assessment of **drug usage patterns** and **adverse reactions** to medications are essential to the provision of safe patient care. Often, a drug effect or side effect (e.g., nausea) is described as an allergy. True allergic reactions to amide local anesthetics (lidocaine and bupivacaine) or benzodiazepines (diazepam and midazolam) are rare.

   (1) Maintenance **cardiovascular medication** (e.g., antianginal and antihypertensive medications) should be continued prior to the procedure. These can be given with sips of water, while maintaining the patient in an otherwise fasted state.

   (2) The **insulin-dependent diabetic patient** requires special consideration. Elective studies in these patients should be scheduled for early in the day. Often, one-half the usual morning dose of insulin is given and an infusion of 5% dextrose is begun on the day of the procedure. For lengthy procedures, frequent blood sugar determinations should be performed, and an insulin infusion (1–3 units/hour) should be considered [8].

2. Laboratory testing

   a. Overview. Preprocedural and preoperative laboratory screening is expensive and often contributes little to patient care. When tests are ordered by protocol without specific indications, few significant abnormalities are found, and many of these determinations could be eliminated [9].

   b. Indications

   (1) Risk assessment for **cardiovascular morbidity** (e.g., ECG).

   (2) Risk assessment for **hemorrhagic complications.**

   (3) Evaluation of **hepatic and renal function.**

   (4) Guide for preprocedural medical therapy (e.g., transfusion, electrolyte repletion, additional medical consultation).

   c. Basic laboratory screening

Age < 40	Hct/Hgb
	Coagulation profile
Age 40–60	Hct/Hgb
	Coagulation profile
	ECG
	Blood glucose
	BUN/Cr
Age > 60	Hct/Hgb
	Coagulation profile
	ECG
	Glucose
	BUN/Cr
	Electrolytes
	LFTs

Recommended Monitoring

1. **Standards.** Most anesthesia-related morbidity or mortality is believed to be preventable with meticulous cardiovascular and respiratory monitoring [10,11]. In an effort to improve patient saftey during anesthesia, minimum standards for monitoring have been outlined and implemented in many institutions [10].
2. **Designated monitoring personnel.** An individual (R.N. or M.D.) must be designated to be responsible for monitoring vital signs, administering medication, and record keeping. This person should be in attendance throughout the procedure and have no other significant responsibilities during the monitoring period.
3. **Recommendations.** For radiologic procedures, minimum monitoring standards should be adopted (Table 39-1).

Required Resuscitation Equipment

1. **In procedure room**
   a. Oxygen source.
   b. Face masks and nasal prongs for oxygen delivery.
   c. Oral and nasal airways.
   d. Suction.
   e. Functional bag and mask device (e.g., Ambu bag).
   f. IV supplies (e.g., catheters, tubing, infusion pumps).
   g. Naloxone (Narcan).
   h. Epinephrine.
2. **In radiology suite**
   a. Intubation equipment (e.g., laryngoscopes, tracheal tubes).
   b. Defibrillator.
   c. Advanced life-support medications (e.g., epinephrine, lidocaine, sodium bicarbonate, dopamine).

Table 39-1. Recommended monitoring parameters for various forms of anesthesia

Parameter	Monitor	Local	Local with sedation	Regional	General
Circulation	BP	X	X	X	X
Cardiac rhythm	ECG	X	X	X	X
Oxygenation	Pulse oximeter		X	X	X
Respiratory depression	Respiration rate		X	X	X
Ventilation	ETCO$_2$				X
Extent of block	Sensory level			X	

ETCO$_2$ = endotracheal carbon dioxide.

Medication Prior to Procedure

See Chap. 40.

1. **Goals of premedication**
   a. Decrease apprehension.
   b. Sedation.
   c. Induce amnesia.
   d. Analgesia.
   e. Prevent nausea and vomiting.
   f. Prophylaxis against contrast media reaction.
2. **Guidelines** (see also Chaps. 36, 38, 40). The adminis-tration of medication prior to a procedure should never be routine. The choice of agent, dosage, and route of administration must be individualized, especially in the elderly patient. After oral and intramuscular adminis-tration, sufficient time (30–60 min) must be allowed for drug absorption to obtain desired effects. If continuous patient observation cannot be provided after an IM in-jection, intravenous administration of medication just prior to the procedure (with patient monitoring) is recom-mended.
3. Summary of frequently used drugs (for a more detailed discussion see Chap. 40).
   a. Diazepam (Valium)
      (1) Indications: decrease in apprehension, induction of sedation and amnesia.
      (2) Dose/route of administration: 5–10 mg PO or 1–5 mg IV; avoid IM injections (painful, erratic ab-sorption).
      (3) Adverse effects: prolonged sedation in elderly, pain on injection, postinjection thrombophlebitis.
      (4) Contraindication: first trimester of pregnancy.
   b. Midazolam (Versed)
      (1) Indications: decrease in apprehension, induction of sedation and amnesia.
      (2) Dose/route of administration: 2–7 mg IM or 1–3 mg IV.
      (3) Adverse effects: profound sedation in patients over 70 years old. In patients 60–69 years, midazolam, 2–3 mg IM is usually quite effective [12].
      (4) Contraindication: first trimester of pregnancy.
   c. Droperidol (Inapsine)
      (1) Indications: prevention of nausea and vomiting.
      (2) Dose/route of administration: 2.5–5.0 mg IM or 0.625–1.250 mg IV.
      (3) Adverse effects: prolonged sedation with IM ad-ministration, hypotension, extrapyramidal symp-toms and exacerbation of Parkinson's disease.
   d. Hydroxyzine (Vistaril)
      (1) Indications: prevention of nausea and vomiting, sedation, decrease in apprehension.
      (2) Dose/route of administration: 25–100 mg IM.
      (3) Adverse effects: excessive sedation, dry mouth.
   e. Diphenhydramine (Benadryl)
      (1) Indications: sedation, prophylaxis against con-trast reaction.

      (2) Dose/route of administration: 25–50 mg PO or 25–50 mg IM or 12.5–25.0 mg IV.

      (3) Adverse effects: excessive sedation, dizziness, dry mouth, difficult urination, thickening of bronchial secretions.

f. Morphine sulfate (Duramorph)

      (1) Indications: analgesia, sedation.

      (2) Dose/route of administration: 2–10 mg IM or 1–3 mg IV.

      (3) Adverse effects: respiratory depression, hypotension, nausea, vomiting, itching, biliary spasm.

g. Meperidine hydrochloride (Demerol)

      (1) Indications: analgesia, sedation.

      (2) Dose/route of administration: 25–100 mg IM or 12.5–25.0 mg IV.

      (3) Adverse effects: respiratory depression, hypotension, nausea, vomiting, biliary spasm.

      (4) Contraindication: patients on monoamine oxidase (MAO) inhibitors.

h. Fentanyl citrate (Sublimaze)

      (1) Indications: analgesia.

      (2) Dose/route of administration: 25–50 μg IV.

      (3) Adverse effects: respiratory depression, bradycardia, nausea, vomiting, muscle rigidity, biliary spasm.

i. Butorphanol tartrate (Stadol)

      (1) Indications: sedation, analgesia.

      (2) Dose/route of administration: 1–2 mg IM or 0.5–1.0 mg IV.

      (3) Adverse effects: excessive sedation, limited analgesia, dysphoria. Concomitant administration of butorphanol and other opioids (e.g. fentanyl, morphine, and meperidine) may result in ineffective analgesia.

      (4) Biliary tract: less elevation of biliary pressure compared to morphine, meperidine, and fentanyl [13].

j. Nalbuphine hydrochloride (Nubain)

      (1) Indication: analgesia, sedation.

      (2) Dose/route of administration: 5–10 mg IM or 1–3 mg IV.

      (3) Adverse effects: excessive sedation, nausea, vomiting, dizziness, limited analgesia, restlessness, reversal of analgesia produced by other opioids.

      (4) Biliary tract: less elevation of biliary pressure than fentanyl and butorphanol [14].

k. Ketorolac (Toradol)

      (1) Indication: analgesia without respiratory depression; can be used in combination with opioids [15].

      (2) Dose/route of administration: 30–60 mg IM.

      (3) Adverse effects: reversible platelet dysfunction (24–48 hours after drug discontinuation), gastritis, peptic ulceration, and inhibition of renal autoregulation.

      (4) Not approved for use in obstetric or pediatric patients.

    l. Prednisone
- **(1)** Indication: prophylaxis against contrast reaction.
- **(2)** Dose/route of administration: 50–75 mg PO the evening before and 1–2 hours prior to the examination.
- **(3)** Adverse effects: hyperglycemia, hypertension, fluid retention.

    m. Methylprednisolone (Solu-Medrol [IV/IM], Medrol [PO])
- **(1)** Indication: prophylaxis against contrast reaction [16].
- **(2)** Dose/route of administration: 32 mg PO the evening before and 1–2 hours prior to the examination.
- **(3)** Adverse effects: hyperglycemia, hypertension, fluid retention.

Techniques of Sedation, Analgesia, and Anesthesia During the Procedure

LOCAL ANESTHESIA

1. **Indications:** analgesia at puncture site.
2. **Drug classification**
   - **a. Amides:** lidocaine (Xylocaine), mepivacaine (Carbocaine), bupivacaine (Marcaine, Sensoracaine).
   - **b.** Esters: chloroprocaine (Nesacaine), procaine (Novocaine).
3. **Choice of drug.** Most commonly used agents are amide local anesthetics. These local anesthetics are preferred over the esters because of increased potency, prolonged duration, and far fewer documented allergic reactions. For radiologic procedures, lidocaine (1–1.5%) is the most frequently used amide local anesthetic since it has a rapid onset of action and a duration of 1.0–1.5 hours. However, both mepivacaine (1.0–1.5%) and bupivacaine (0.5%) provide longer durations of action (1.5–4.0 hours).
4. **Alkalinization of local anesthetics.** Subcutaneous and intradermal infiltration of local anesthetics can be painful. However, alkalinization of local anesthetics (with the addition of sodium bicarbonate) can lessen the discomfort associated with skin and subcutaneous infiltration [17]. For lidocaine, 1 mEq of sodium bicarbonate is added to 10 ml of anesthetic. Alkalinization of bupivacaine is not recommended since even small amounts of sodium bicarbonate may result in precipitation of the local anesthetic.
5. **Injection technique and dosage.** Careful needle placement, aspiration prior to injection and after each 3–5 ml, and frequent patient observation during infiltration are required to avoid intravascular injections of local anesthetic. Rapid IV injection of 100–200 mg can cause toxic manifestations (see Chap. 40). The total dose of lidocaine should not exceed 4–5 mg/kg (healthy adult), while bupivacaine doses should not exceed 3 mg/kg. A dose reduction of 30–50% is recommended in elderly patients, and those with hepatic dysfunction and CHF. Excessive local anes-

thetic doses, resulting in high serum concentrations, can result in prolonged lethargy following cardiac catheterization [18].

LOCAL ANESTHESIA WITH SEDATION/ANALGESIA

1. **Indications**
   a. Anxious patient.
   b. Procedures that produce discomfort distant from puncture site.
2. **Anesthesia consultation**
   a. Extremes of age.
   b. Unstable patient.
   c. Severe cardiovascular or pulmonary disease.
   d. Multiple maintenance medications (especially MAO inhibitors).
   e. Pregnancy.
3. **Anesthesia attendance**
   a. Critically ill patients.
   b. Procedures that require intense analgesia or deep levels of sedation (e.g., difficult percutaneous biliary drainage or nephrostomy).
   c. Procedures or positioning that may comprise the airway.
4. **Sedatives**
   a. Diazepam: 1–3 mg IV q1–2h.
   b. Midazolam: 0.5–2.0 mg IV q30–60min.
   c. Diphenhydramine: 12.5–25.0 mg IV q1–2h.
5. **Opioid analgesics**
   a. Fentanyl: 25–75 μg IV q15–60 min.
   b. Morphine: 1–5 mg IV q30–60min.
   c. Meperidine: 12.5–25.0 mg IV q30–60min.
   d. Butorphanol: 0.5–1.0 mg IV q30–60min.
   e. Nalbuphine: 1–5 mg IV q30–60min.
6. **Biliary procedures.** There may be an advantage to use of butorphanol or nalbuphine during procedures involving the biliary tree. These "agonist-antagonist" opioids appear to provide analgesia without marked elevations in biliary duct pressures and resistance to bile flow [13,14]. Intramuscular ketolorac can provide additional pain relief, when used in combination with the agonist-antagonist opioids, and can improve patient comfort during these procedures.
7. **Coadministration of benzodiazepines and opioids.** Extreme care must be exercised when administering these medications in combination. Hypoxemia, apnea, and marked elevations in PCO_2 (partial pressure of carbon dioxide in blood) may occur. Supplemental oxygen must be given to these patients, and personnel skilled in airway management must be available to attend these procedures [19].

REGIONAL ANESTHESIA (Table 39-2)

1. **Indications**
   a. Intense analgesia without excessive opioid medication.
   b. Muscle relaxation.
   c. Postprocedure pain management.

Table 39-2. Types of regional anesthesia: indications and complications

Block	Procedural indication	Complications
Cervical plexus	Carotid puncture Carotid angiogram*	Bleeding Pneumothorax Intravascular injection
Intercostal	Lung biopsy Rib biopsy Biliary drainage and stents Subphrenic drainage	Pneumothorax Bleeding Intravascular injection
Axillary/interscalene	Brachial catheterization (especially with cutdown) Hand angiograms*	Bleeding Intravascular injection Pneumothorax (interscalene)
Epidural/spinal	Femoral catheterization Lower extremity angiogram* Nephrostomy drainage and stents Embolization of kidney	Motor blockade Hypotension Urinary retention Postdural puncture headache Intravascular injection (epidural)

*Consider low-ionic, low-osmolar contrast to decrease discomfort.
Source: Reprinted from LJ Lind, PS Mushlin. Sedation, analgesia and anesthesia for radiologic procedures. *Cardiovasc Interv Radiol* 10:247–253, 1987.

GENERAL ANESTHESIA

1. **Indications**
   a. If procedure may compromise the patient's airway.
   b. Highly anxious patients who refuse local anesthesia with sedation or regional anesthesia.
   c. Patients who are unable to cooperate, and potentially combative due to a mental disability.
2. **Disadvantages**
   a. Risks of inherent to general anesthesia.
   b. Need to arrange anesthesia coverage and transport of anesthesia equipment to the radiology suite.
   c. Increased patient care costs.

Considerations Following the Procedure

1. **Monitoring.** Patient's vital signs should be monitored in a recovery area and observed for complications following

interventional procedures performed with sedative/opioid medication, regional or general anesthesia.

2. Discharge criteria for outpatients
- **a.** Vital signs returning to preprocedural values and stable for 1 hour.
- **b.** Must be sufficiently recovered from sedative/hypnotic medications to allow ambulation with assistance.
- **c.** Should be oriented.
- **d.** Able to void and to tolerate oral fluids.

3. Discharge instructions for outpatients
- **a.** Should be written and given to the responsible companion.
- **b.** Expected problems should be listed.
- **c.** Should have a telephone or beeper number to call for questions or complications.

4. Discharge criteria for inpatients
- **a.** Vital signs should be stable.
- **b.** Adequate analgesia.
- **c.** If regional or general anesthesia has been employed, the patient should be sufficiently recovered from the anesthetic. Standards for adequate recovery should be adapted from your institutional Postanesthesia Care Unit (PACU) standards.

5. Follow-up
- **a. Inpatient.** All patients should be visited after an interventional procedure. A chart note documenting the effectiveness of sedation or anesthetic technique employed and any complications of the procedure is recommended. These comments can be invaluable in planning future interventional radiologic and surgical procedures.
- **b. Outpatient.** Outpatient follow-up is also important and can be accomplished via a telephone call or mailed patient questionnaire [20].

References

1. Lind LJ, Mushlin PS. Sedation, analgesia and anesthesia for radiologic procedures. *Cardiovasc Intervent Radiol* 10:247–253, 1987.
2. Greenblatt DJ, Sellers EM, Shader RI. Drug disposition in old age. *N Engl J Med* 306:1081–1088, 1982.
3. Cheng EY, Cheng RM. Impact of aging on preoperative evaluation. *J Clin Anesth* 3:324–343, 1991.
4. Goldman L, et al. Multifactorial index of cardiac risk in noncardiac surgical procedures. *N Engl J Med* 297:845–850, 1977.
5. Goldman L, Caldera DL. Risks of general anesthesia and elective operation on the hypertensive patient. *Anesthesiology* 50:285–292, 1979.
6. Pearce AC, Jones RM. Smoking and anesthesia: Preoperative abstinence and perioperative morbidity. *Anesthesiology* 61:576–584, 1984.
7. Kaiko RF, et al. Central nervous system excitatory effects of meperidine in cancer patients. *Ann Neurol* 13:180–185, 1983.

8. Alberti KG, Thomas DJ. The management of diabetes during surgery. *Br J Anaesth* 51:693–710, 1979.

9. Kaplan EB, et al. The usefulness of preoperative laboratory screening. *JAMA* 253:3576–3581, 1985.

10. Eichhorn JH, et al. Standards for patient monitoring during anesthesia at Harvard Medical School. *JAMA* 256:1017–1020, 1986.

11. Tobin, MJ. Respiratory monitoring, *JAMA* 264:244–251, 1990.

12. Wong HY, Fragen RJ, Dunn K. Dose-finding study of intramuscular midazolam preanesthetic medication in the elderly. *Anesthesiology* 74:675–679, 1991.

13. Radnay PA, et al. Common bile duct pressure changes after fentanyl, morphine, meperidine, butorphanol and naloxone. *Anesth Analg* 63:441–444, 1984.

14. McCammon RL, Stoelting RK, Madura JA. Effects of butorphanol, nalbuphine and fentanyl on intrabiliary tract dynamics. *Anesth Analg* 63:139–142, 1984.

15. Dahl JB, Kehlet H. Non-steroidal anti-inflammatory drugs: Rationale for use in severe postoperative pain. *Br J Anaesth* 66:703–712, 1991.

16. Lasser EC, et al. Pretreatment with corticosteroids to alleviate contrast reactions to intravenous contrast material. *N Engl J Med* 317:845–849, 1987.

17. Ferrante FM, et al. 1% lidocaine with and without sodium bicarbonate for attenuation of pain of skin infiltration and intravenous catheterization. *Anesthesiology* 75:A736, 1991.

18. Palmisano JM, et al. Lidocaine toxicity after subcutaneous infiltration in children undergoing cardiac catheterization. *Am J Cardiol* 67:647–648, 1991.

19. Bailey PL, et al. Frequent hypoxemia and apnea after sedation with midazolam and fentanyl. *Anesthesiology* 73:826–830, 1990.

20. Lind LJ, Mushlin PS, Schnitman PA. Monitored anesthesia care for dental implant surgery: Analysis of effectiveness and complications. *J Oral Implant* 16:106–113, 1990.

Commonly Used Medications

Krishna Kandarpa

Sedatives

Diazepam (Valium)

MODE OF ACTION

A commonly used benzodiazepine that probably increases the responsiveness of brain receptors to the inhibitory neurotransmitter gamma-aminobutyric acid.

INDICATIONS

1. Sedation.
2. Induction of anterograde amnesia.
3. Treatment of seizures.

CONTRAINDICATIONS

1. Known hypersensitivity to the drug.
2. Acute narrow-angle glaucoma.
3. Untreated open-angle glaucoma.

ADVERSE REACTIONS

1. Drowsiness, fatigue, ataxia. Watch for mental status changes, especially in the elderly.
2. Respiratory depression may occur with large IV doses, especially in patients with chronic obstructive pulmonary disease (COPD).
3. Has additive effect with other CNS depressants (especially opioids).
4. Venous thrombosis at injection site.
5. Pain on injection.

PREPARATION

Available in 10-ml vials, 2-ml ampules, 2-ml disposable syringes; also 2-mg, 5-mg, and 10-mg tablets.

DOSAGE AND METHOD

Premedication: 5–10 mg PO. Premedication of elderly patients prior to arrival at the angiography suite is not recommended. 2–3 mg IV/dose over 1 minute (maintenance 2–3 mg IV q20–30min monitoring vital signs; maximum recommended dose, 10 mg/hour for a 2-hour study). Use lower doses for elderly patients. 10 mg IV for **toxic convulsions.**

KINETICS

1. Onset of action is within 2–3 minutes after IV injection (up to 1 hour after oral dose).
2. Duration up to 6–10 hours.
3. Sedative effects are long-lived but amnestic effects are not (1–30 minutes).
4. Distribution half-life: 1–2 hours.

5. Elimination half-life: 24–48 hours.
6. Liver dysfunction and aging retard metabolization. Metabolites are excreted through the kidney.

REVERSAL

1. General supportive measures; monitor vital signs.
2. Maintain intravenous fluids and airway.
3. Hypotension may be treated with norepinephrine bitartrate (Levophed) or metaraminol (Aramine).
4. Physostigmine (Antilirium) 1 mg IV slowly or aminophylline 1–2 mg/kg IV can reverse the CNS depression.
5. Flumazenil is a specific benzodiazepine antagonist that has undergone extensive clinical trials. 1–10 mg will reverse the CNS and respiratory depressant effects of benzodiazepines. Additional doses may be required 1–2 hours later.

Midazolam (Versed)

MODE OF ACTION

A short-acting benzodiazepine CNS depressant. Midazolam has anxiolytic, hypnotic, muscle relaxant, antegrade amnestic, and anticonvulsant properties. The potency is approximately 3–4 times that of diazepam (Valium).

INDICATIONS

Induction of conscious sedation and amnesia during angiographic or interventional procedures.

ABSOLUTE CONTRAINDICATIONS

1. Known hypersensitivity to the drug.
2. Acute narrow-angle glaucoma (benzodiazepines in general); however, treated open-angle glaucoma is not a contraindication.
3. Acute alcohol or drug intoxication and shock.

RELATIVE CONTRAINDICATIONS

1. Pregnancy—potential hazard to the fetus and neonatal CNS depression (midazolam is not recommended for obstetric use, especially in the first trimester).
2. Nursing mother.

ADVERSE REACTIONS

1. Fluctuations in vital signs including serious cardiopulmonary events. Apnea is more likely to occur with higher dose and speed of injection.
2. During conscious IV sedation, hypotension can occur with concomitant narcotic premedication (e.g., meperidine).
3. With IV administration, a greater than 1% incidence of the following has been reported: hiccups, nausea, vomiting, coughing, oversedation, headache, drowsiness.
4. Patients with COPD are extremely sensitive to the respiratory depressant effect of this drug.
5. Profound and prolonged amnesia can occur.

PREPARATION

1. Available in 1-, 2-, 5-, and 10-ml vials at 5-mg midazolam/ml. Also 2-ml Tel-E-Ject (Roche Laboratories, Nutley, NJ) disposable syringe (5 mg/ml).
2. Midazolam can be diluted in D5W, NS, or Ringer's lactate solution to 2–5 times the original volume for titration of the dose.

DOSAGE AND METHOD

Administer only if continuous cardiac and respiratory monitoring are available. **For intravenous conscious sedation** (incidence of venous irritation and thrombophlebitis is significantly less than for diazepam).

1. Initial titration dose given immediately prior to procedure
   a. **Average healthy adult:** 1.0–2.0 mg (0.035 mg/kg) given over 2–3 minutes.
   b. **Debilitated or elderly adult:** 0.5–1.5 mg given over 2–3 minutes.
   c. With the above doses, cardiovascular depression and clinical evidence of respiratory depression are usually minimal. End point of titration should be slurred speech.
2. If further sedation is needed, wait 2 minutes and, if the vital signs are stable, the dosage may be titrated in small increments (25%) of the initial dose.
3. Dose to maintain sedation is 25% of the initial dose required to obtain that level of sedation.
4. **Total** recommended dose for an average healthy adult: 0.10–0.15 mg/kg.
5. Narcotic medication (e.g., fentanyl, meperidine, morphine sulfate) is often concomitantly administered. If this is done, the dosage of midazolam should be lowered by 25–30%. In patients who are debilitated or older than 60 years, dosage should be cut by 50% and rate and frequency of administration should be slower. Drug effect is prolonged in the elderly.
6. For obese patients, single IV dose may be determined by true body weight, but continuous infusion and maintenance should be based on ideal body weight.
7. If used for **outpatient procedures**
   a. The patient should be instructed not to operate vehicles or machinery until the next day.
   b. Postprocedure instructions should be written or given to accompanying responsible adult.

KINETICS

1. Onset of action is rapid (1–2 minutes) and duration of action is short (30 minutes) following an IV (5 mg) dose.
2. Plasma elimination half-life: 2–4 hours (normal healthy patients). Elimination half-life is about 10-fold less than diazepam. About 45–57% of the dose is excreted in urine as a major (conjugated) metabolite. The elimination half-life is increased 1.5–2.0 times in patients with chronic renal failure and 2–3 times with congestive heart failure.

Hepatic dysfunction does not appear to affect the elimination half-life when small IV doses (5 mg) are administered.

REVERSAL

1. Manifestations of overdosage: sedation, somnolence, confusion, diminished reflexes, etc. (similar to other benzodiazepines).
2. Monitor vital signs—especially early signs of apnea (this can result in hypoxic cardiac arrest).
3. Oxygen and equipment to maintain airway patency should be immediately available.
4. General supportive measures including patent IV access.
5. Hypotension is treated with IV fluid infusion, Trendelenburg position, vasopressors.
6. Midazolam-induced sedation may be reversed with physostigmine 1 mg IV administered over 2 minutes (for adults). Atropine sulfate is an antagonist for physostigmine.
7. Respiratory depressant effects of midazolam **cannot** be reversed by naloxone (Narcan).

Diphenhydramine (Benadryl)

MODE OF ACTION

Blocks histamine$_1$ receptors.

INDICATIONS

1. Sedation.
2. Treatment of contrast-induced pruritus or urticaria.
3. Antiemetic.
4. Precontrast prophylaxis in high-risk patients (controversial).
5. Anticholinergic (decreased secretions and bronchodilation).

CONTRAINDICATIONS

1. Hypersensitivity to drug or chemically similar antihistamines.
2. Should **not** be used to treat lower respiratory tract symptoms including asthma, in conjunction with MAO inhibitors, or in nursing mothers.

ADVERSE REACTIONS

1. Sedation, sleepiness, dizziness, distorted coordination.
2. Epigastric distress.
3. Thickening of bronchial secretions.
4. Urinary retention.
5. Urticaria, drug rash, chills, dry mouth.

PREPARATION

50 mg in 1-ml disposable syringe.

DOSAGE AND METHOD

25–50 mg PO (also available IV/IM). Maximum dose during 2 hours study should be limited to 100 mg.

KINETICS

Onset of action after oral dose: 30–60 minutes. Duration of activity (average PO dose): 4–6 hours. Metabolites formed in the liver are excreted within 24 hours.

REVERSAL

1. General supportive measures: monitor vital signs, fluid intake, and output.
2. If drug is administered orally, induce vomiting or consider gastric lavage.
3. Maintain intravenous line.
4. Vasopressors for hypotension.
5. Do not use stimulants.

Analgesics

Morphine Sulfate (Duramorph)

MODE OF ACTION

Phenanthrene narcotic analgesic.

INDICATIONS

1. Analgesia.
2. Sedation.

CONTRAINDICATIONS

1. Allergy to morphine or other opiates.
2. Acute bronchial asthma.
3. Upper airway obstruction.
4. Biliary obstruction.
5. Hepatic insufficiency. Results in poor metabolization and prolonged duration of drug effect.
6. Nursing mothers.

ADVERSE REACTIONS

1. Respiratory depression (reduces brainstem response to carbon dioxide).
2. Convulsions (high IV dose).
3. Nausea and vomiting.
4. Causes rise in common bile duct pressure, decrease in gastric emptying, bronchoconstriction, and urinary retention.
5. Orthostatic hypotension without significant change in cardiac rate, rhythm, or output.

PREPARATION

10 mg/10-ml (1 mg/ml) disposable syringe.

DOSAGE AND METHOD

   a. 2–3 mg IV/dose slowly over 1 minute (titer monitoring vital signs; maximum dose, 10 mg/hour for a 70-kg patient **OR** not to exceed total dose of 0.2 mg/kg).
   b. Hold maintenance dose if there is any change in BP or heart rate greater than 20%, or if respiration rate is less than 10/minute.

    c. As premedication: 1 mg/10 kg IM. Administer with extreme caution in elderly or debilitated patients.

KINETICS

1. Immediate onset of action (5–7 minutes) with peak analgesia about 20 minutes after IV injection.
2. Analgesia and respiratory depression last several hours depending on dose (3–4 hours).
3. Elimination half-life: 1.5–2.0 hours. Major metabolic pathway is via conjugation with glucuronic acid in the liver. Ninety percent of intravenously administered morphine is eliminated via urine in 24 hours. About 10% of the administered dose is eliminated in the feces.

REVERSAL

1. Maintain adequate airway.
2. General supportive measures: monitor vital signs, fluid input/output.
3. Naloxone hydrochloride (Narcan) 0.1–0.2 mg/dose over 2–3 minutes titered to desired effect (adequate ventilation, alertness without undue pain). Duration of effect is 30–45 minutes, therefore patient must be monitored for 1–2 hours.

Meperidine Hydrochloride (Demerol)

MODE OF ACTION

A synthetic analgesic.

INDICATIONS

1. Analgesia.
2. Sedation.

CONTRAINDICATIONS

1. Hypersensitivity to drug.
2. Concomitant MAO-inhibitor therapy (potential life-threatening hypertension and hyperthermia can occur) or other narcotic therapy.
3. Use with extreme caution in patients with asthma or other respiratory conditions.

ADVERSE REACTIONS

1. Tachycardia following IV injection (anticholinergic effect).
2. Respiratory depression (effect equal to morphine sulfate).
3. May lower seizure threshold.
4. Lightheadedness, dizziness, sedation, nausea, vomiting, and sweating less than morphine sulfate.
5. Orthostatic hypotension, similar to morphine sulfate.
6. Lesser rise in biliary pressure than morphine sulfate.
7. Urinary retention (rare).
8. Urticaria, drug rash (rare).

PREPARATION

100-mg injectable cartridge needle.

DOSAGE AND METHOD

1. Titrate up to 0.5–1.0 mg/kg. During the procedure, fractional doses (10 mg) may be repeated q30min to 1 hour as needed by the patient. Meperidine has a shorter duration and one-tenth the analgesic potency of morphine sulfate.
2. 50–100 mg IM (if used as premedication 30–45 minutes before procedure).

KINETICS

Onset of action (3–5 minutes after IV injection) is slightly more rapid than morphine sulfate and duration is slightly shorter (2–4 hours). Redistribution half-life is about 7 minutes; elimination half-life is about 4 hours. Metabolized by the liver.

REVERSAL

1. Maintain adequate airway.
2. General supportive therapy.
3. Naloxone, (0.1–0.2 mg/dose over 2–3 minutes titered to desired effect (adequate ventilation, alertness).
4. Oxygen, IV fluids, vasopressors as needed.

Butorphanol Tartrate (Stadol)

MODE OF ACTION

A potent synthetic opioid agonist-antagonist analgesic. (Its antagonist activity is $1/40$ that of naloxone.)

INDICATIONS

1. Sedation and analgesia with a notably milder respiratory response than opioids.
2. Produces less elevation in biliary tract pressures and reduces smooth muscle tone, providing potential advantages in gastrointestinal procedures.

CONTRAINDICATIONS

1. Hypersensitivity to drug.
2. Butorphanol should be avoided in individuals who are dependent on narcotics because symptoms of withdrawal may occur.
3. Once butorphanol has been administered, the effects on an opioid agonist (e.g., morphine) are unpredictable due to its weak antagonistic effect at the supraspinal narcotic receptors.

ADVERSE REACTIONS

1. Sedation (40% patients), nausea (6%), sweating (6%).
2. Respiratory depression (2-mg butorphanol = 10-mg morphine); however, the magnitude of respiratory depression does not increase beyond a dose of 4 mg.
3. Increases load on heart and therefore should be avoided, if possible, in patients with acute myocardial infarctions and patients with ventricular or coronary insufficiency.

PREPARATION

2 mg/ml, 1-ml disposable syringe.

DOSAGE AND METHOD

1. Premedication may be given on floor: 1–2 mg butorphanol IM with 25–50-mg hydroxyzine pamoate (Vistaril) IM.
2. Titration to desired effect in angiography suite, administer 0.5 mg IV slowly and q15min (while assessing patient's response) up to a dose of 2 mg.
3. After adequate analgesia has been established, additional 0.5-mg increments of butorphanol may be given q30min up to a total of 6 mg, depending on the patient's size, age, and level of debilitation.
4. It is difficult to "catch up" with pain, thus adequate medication is the key.

KINETICS

Rapid onset of action (10 minutes) and peak analgesia (30 minutes) following IV administration. Duration of action is 3–4 hours.

REVERSAL

1. Naloxone (Narcan) 0.1–0.2 mg/dose over 2–3 minutes; titrate to desired effect (adequate ventilation, alertness).
2. General supportive therapy, including oxygen, IV fluids, vasopressors as necessary.

Fentanyl Citrate (Sublimaze)

MODE OF ACTION

Short-acting synthetic opioid.

INDICATIONS

1. Analgesia 50–100 times the analgesic potency of morphine with generally acceptable cardiovascular effects.
2. Sedation (not effective alone).

CONTRAINDICATIONS

1. Known intolerance to the drug.
2. Avoid in patients using MAO inhibitors.
3. Use with caution in patients with respiratory problems.

ADVERSE REACTIONS

1. Respiratory depression (peaks at 5–15 minutes).
2. Bradycardia (depends on dose and rate of injection; prophylactic atropine prevents bradycardia).
3. Nausea.
4. Dizziness.
5. Laryngospasm.
6. Muscle rigidity causing stiff-chest syndrome: occurs with rapid injection, especially in elderly patients. Muscle relaxants are useful for treatment.

PREPARATION

2-ml and 5-ml ampules (50 μg/ml).

DOSAGE AND METHOD

1. Load: 25–50 μg IV over 1–2 minutes.
2. Maintenance: 25–50 μg q30min.
3. Maximum dose: 3 μg/kg/hour.
4. 100 μg fentanyl = 10 mg morphine = 100 mg meperidine.
5. Monitor for vital signs. Hold maintenance if any *change* in BP or heart rate greater than 20% or respiratory rate less than 10/minute.
6. Adjust dosage appropriately for elderly and debilitated patients.

KINETICS

When administered intravenously, onset of action is immediate (2–5 minutes), but maximum analgesia and respiratory depression take several minutes (about 15 minutes). Duration of action for single IV dose of 100 μg is 30–60 minutes.

REVERSAL

1. Respiratory support.
2. General supportive care.
3. Naloxone (Narcan): 0.1–0.2 mg/dose over 2–3 minutes, titered to desired effect (adequate ventilation, alertness without significant pain or discomfort).

Lidocaine Hydrochloride (Xylocaine)

MODE OF ACTION

Stabilizes neuronal membrane preventing initiation and conduction of nerve impulses.

INDICATIONS

1. Local anesthetic at skin puncture site prior to catheterization; peripheral nerve block.
2. Additive to contrast to reduce pain during intraarterial contrast injection.

CONTRAINDICATIONS

1. Known history of hypersensitivity to amide-type local anesthetics or components of the injectable formulation. Consider infiltration with procaine-type local anesthetic or with sterile normal saline alone.
2. Use with caution if there is inflammation or sepsis, or both, at proposed site of injection.

ADVERSE REACTIONS

1. Drowsiness is an early sign of high blood level of lidocaine due to inadvertent intravascular administration or rapid absorption of the drug.
2. Nervousness, dizziness, blurred vision, tremors, seizures (usually of short duration), and possibly respiratory arrest.
3. Hypotension, bradycardia, cardiovascular depression are dangerous late signs.

PREPARATION

1. For local subcutaneous infiltration 0.5% solution = 5 mg/ml.
2. Mix 10 ml of 2% lidocaine (without epinephrine) in 100-ml contrast, 2 mg/ml (2% solution = 20 mg/ml).

DOSAGE AND METHOD

1. Percutaneous infiltration. Start with small subcutaneous skin wheal, then deep infiltration with aspiration prior to each injection to avoid intravascular injection—maximum dose 0.5% lidocaine (without epinephrine). Should not exceed about 4 mg/kg in a healthy adult.
2. As additive to contrast: see **2.** in Preparation.

KINETICS

Metabolized by the liver and excreted by the kidney. Local anesthetic effect and duration depends on volume and concentration infiltrated. Plasma half-life is approximately 2 hours.

REVERSAL

Treatment of toxic manifestations. Maintain patent airway and ventilation. Support circulatory system with IV fluids and vasopressors as required. Treat convulsions as necessary.

Nalbuphine Hydrochloride (Nubain)

MODE OF ACTION

Potent synthetic narcotic agonist-antagonist analgesic.

INDICATION

Analgesia and sedation (with less elevation of biliary pressure than fentanyl and butorphanol).

CONTRAINDICATIONS

1. Known hypersensitivity.
2. Contains metabisulfite and may cause allergic-type reaction in patients with sulfite sensitivity and in asthmatics.

ADVERSE REACTIONS

1. Excessive sedation.
2. Nausea and vomiting.
3. Dizziness.
4. Restlessness.
5. Limited analgesia.
6. Reversal of analgesia produced by other opioids.
7. In nondependent patients, may show additive effect with other narcotics; reduce dose of drugs.
8. Respiratory depression. Use in low doses and cautiously in patients with respiratory problems.
9. Bradycardia.

PREPARATION

10 mg/ml in 1-ml ampules.

DOSAGE AND METHOD

1. 5–10 mg IM, or
2. 1–3 mg IV.
3. Maximum recommended for pain refief is 10 mg for a 70 kg adult. May be repeated every 3–6 hours.

KINETICS

Onset of action is within 5 minutes of IV injecction, and 15 minutes of IM or SQ injection. Plasma half-life: 5 hours. Duration of analgesia: 3–6 hours. Metabolized in the liver, excreted by the kidneys.

REVERSAL

1. Naloxone.
2. Resuscitative equipment must be available.
3. Oxygen and supportive measures.

Vasodilators

Nifedipine (Procardia)

MODE OF ACTION

Calcium (slow) channel blocker. Relaxes and prevents arterial spasm (decreases peripheral vascular resistance and increases flow to distal bed).

INDICATION

As a vasodilator during angioplasty to prevent or treat vasospasm caused by catheter or wire manipulation.

CONTRAINDICATIONS

Known hypersensitivity.

ADVERSE REACTIONS

Watch for hypotension. Generally there are few problems with a one-time 10-mg dose.

PREPARATION

Supplied as 10-mg capsule.

DOSAGE AND METHOD

During peripheral angioplasty; 10 mg PO or sublingual (puncture hole in capsule and squeeze contents sublingually; then ask patient to swallow capsule).

KINETICS

Plasma half-life: 2 hours. Approximately 80% of this drug and its metabolites are excreted by the kidney. Clearance may be prolonged with impaired renal function.

REVERSAL

Cardiovascular support. Monitor vital signs, elevate extremities, monitor fluid input and output, and adjust as necessary. Vasoconstrictors may be beneficial.

Nitroglycerin (Nitro-Bid IV)

MODE OF ACTION

Relaxes vascular smooth muscle; a short-acting vasodilator.

INDICATIONS

1. Vasodilator during percutaneous transluminal angioplasty to prevent or treat vasospasm caused by catheter or wire manipulation.
2. To treat angina pectoris.

CONTRAINDICATIONS

1. Known hypersensitivity to nitroglycerin or known idiosyncratic reaction to organic nitrates.
2. Hypotension.
3. Increased intracranial pressure due to trauma or hemorrhage.
4. Constrictive pericarditis or pericardial tamponade.

ADVERSE REACTIONS

1. Headache (2% of patients).
2. Tachycardia, nausea, vomiting, retrosternal discomfort, palpitation (< 1%).

PREPARATION

15 mg in 150 ml of D5W (100 µg/ml). Prepare, store, and administer in glass containers. Protect from light until use.

DOSAGE AND METHOD

1. **During angioplasty.** 100–200 µg (bolus directly into artery that is to undergo angioplasty).
2. **For angina pectoris.** 0.3 mg sublingual as needed.

KINETICS

Rapid onset of action and short duration of effect. Plasma half-life: 1–4 minutes.

REVERSAL

Cardiovascular support. Monitor vital signs, elevate extremities, monitor fluid input and output, and adjust as necessary.

Tolazoline Hydrochloride (Priscoline)

MODE OF ACTION

Direct peripheral vasodilator (alpha blocker) decreases peripheral resistance and increases venous capacitance.

INDICATIONS

1. Useful during peripheral arteriography to elicit hyperemic pressure gradients.
2. To better visualize the portal venous system (in noncirrhotics) during visceral arteriography or peripheral vessels in extremity arteriography.

CONTRAINDICATIONS

1. Hypersensitivity to the drug.
2. Patients with mitral stenosis, coronary artery disease, and arrhythmias.

ADVERSE REACTIONS

1. Systemic hypotension.
2. Tachycardia.
3. Nausea and vomiting.
4. Skin flushing.
5. Oliguria.

PREPARATION

Ampules—4 ml (25 mg/ml).

DOSAGE AND METHOD

25 mg IA (diluted) prior to contrast injection given over 2 minutes.

KINETICS

Rapid onset of action and peak activity.

REVERSAL

1. Trendelenburg position.
2. Intravenous fluids.
3. General supportive measures monitor vital signs and fluid intake and output.
4. Do **not** use epinephrine or norepinephrine to reverse hypotension due to tolazoline overdosage—further reduction in BP and subsequent exaggerated rebound may occur.

Vasoconstrictors

Epinephrine (1 : 1000) for Pharmacoangiography

MODE OF ACTION

The relative composition of alpha- and beta-adrenergic receptors in a vascular bed determines its overall response to epinephrine. In the visceral and renal arteries, it is a vasoconstrictor. As a vasoconstrictor, epinephrine increases heart rate, BP, ventricular contractility, myocardial oxygen consumption, and systemic vascular resistance.

INDICATIONS

1. To differentiate normally vasoconstricting vessels from abnormal ones whose response is variable.
2. For renal arteriography and venography.
3. Visceral arteriography (rare application).

CONTRAINDICATIONS

1. Individuals with organic brain damage.
2. Narrow-angle glaucoma.
3. Use with caution in patients with cardiovascular disease, hypertension, and diabetes.

ADVERSE REACTIONS

1. Palpitations.
2. Respiratory difficulty.
3. Dizziness.
4. Headache.
5. Anxiety.
6. Ventricular arrhythmias.

PREPARATION

Mix 1 ml of 1 : 1000 in 500 ml D5W or NS (2 μg/ml).

DOSAGE AND METHOD

1. **Renal arteriography.** 3–6 μg/10 ml NS IA (follow with 5–10-ml saline flush) 30 seconds prior to contrast injection for demonstrating neoplastic vessels (decrease contrast injection rate by 30%).
2. **Renal venography.** 10–12 μg IA (follow with saline flush).
3. **Celiac and mesenteric arteriography.** 10–12 μg IA (follow with saline flush).

KINETICS

Rapid onset (within a few minutes) and short duration (within a few minutes) when administered parenterally. When administered subcutaneously, onset is rapid but action may be prolonged (hours).

REVERSAL

1. Because epinephrine is rapidly inactivated, treatment of acute toxicity (increase in arterial and venous blood pressure may cause cerebrovascular hemorrhage) is mainly supportive.
2. If necessary, a rapidly acting alpha-adrenergic blocking agent such as phentolamine may be used to counteract the pressor effect.
3. If necessary, a rapidly acting beta-blocker (e.g., Esmolol) can decrease the bradycardia.

Vasopressin (Pitressin)

MODE OF ACTION

Causes smooth-muscle contraction in the gastrointestinal tract and vascular bed (capillaries, small arterioles, vessels). Short-acting, rapid response.

INDICATIONS

Intraarterial infusion for the control of gastrointestinal bleeding. Decreases flow in mesenteric, gastric, and splenic arteries, but increases flow in hepatic arteries.

CONTRAINDICATIONS

1. Anaphylaxis or hypersensitivity to the drug.
2. Chronic nephritis with elevated BUN.
3. Angina pectoris.

ADVERSE REACTIONS

1. When using it, watch for hypertension, angina, and CNS symptoms.
2. It has an antidiuretic hormone (ADH) effect due to increased water resorption by the renal tubules.
3. Local or systemic allergic reactions: anaphylaxis, cardiac arrest or shock, or a combination of these.
4. Abdominal cramps, nausea and vomiting, diaphoresis, urticaria, bronchial constriction, vertigo, and "pounding" head.

PREPARATION

Prepare vasopressin solution as follows: vasopressin is supplied in ampules of 10 or 20 units/0.5 or 1.0 ml. Mix 100 units of vasopressin in 500 ml of NS or D5W (0.2 units/ml), or in a more concentrated form of 200 units/500 ml of solution (0.4 units/ml).

DOSAGE AND METHOD

Infuse with a constant arterial infusion pump at an initial rate of 60 ml/hour (0.2 units/minute). Protocol for gastrointestinal bleeding—see Chap. 12.

KINETICS

Rapid onset of action (20–40 minutes) is noted when used to stop gastrointestinal bleeds. Duration of action is in the order of minutes unless continuous infusion is given.

REVERSAL

Spontaneous recovery from side effects such as blanching of skin, abdominal cramps, and nausea within minutes after the infusion is stopped.

Thrombolytic Agents

Urokinase (Abbokinase)

MODE OF ACTION

Urokinase (UK) is an enzyme that directly converts plasminogen to plasmin. Plasmin is a fibrinolytic enzyme that degrades fibrinogen and fibrin.

INDICATION

Thrombolysis.

ABSOLUTE CONTRAINDICATIONS

1. Active internal bleeding.
2. Recent (2 months) cerebrovascular accident, intracranial or intraspinal surgery.
3. Intracranial neoplasm. (See Chap. 5 for relative contraindications.)

ADVERSE REACTIONS

1. Bleeding.

2. Mild bronchospasm or skin rash (serious allergic reactions are rare).
3. Fever (2–3% of patients receiving UK; treat fever with acetaminophen, not aspirin).

PREPARATION

Reconstitute UK with *nonbacteriostatic sterile H₂O;* standard preparation is *750 K IU of UK in 250 ml / D5W or NS* (concentration = 3000 IU/ml). Supplied in vials of 250 K IU containing 25 mg mannitol and 45-mg sodium chloride.

DOSAGE AND METHOD (For peripheral arterial thrombolysis)

1. Bolus (into thrombus): 30–60 K IU.
2. Infuse: 4000 IU/minute × 2 hours (80 ml/hour)
     2000 IU/minute × 2 hours (40 ml/hour)
     1000 IU/minute × 8 hours (20 ml/hour)
   Continue at this rate with periodic angiographic monitoring (see Chap. 5).
3. Systemically heparinize patient to prevent clot formation around catheter (maintain PTT at 40–50 seconds).

KINETICS

Serum half-life of 20 minutes or less (cleared by liver); but may also decrease plasma, plasminogen, and fibrinogen levels for 12–24 hours.

REVERSAL

Fresh-frozen plasma.

Streptokinase (Streptase)

MODE OF ACTION

Streptokinase first forms a complex with plasminogen. This complex then converts unbound plasminogen to plasmin. Plasmin is an enzyme that degrades fibrinogen and fibrin.

INDICATION

Thrombolysis.

CONTRAINDICATIONS

Same as urokinase.

ADVERSE REACTIONS

1. Bleeding.
2. Allergic reactions
   a. Minor: itching, urticaria, flushing, nausea, headache, musculoskeletal pain, breathing difficulty.
   b. Major: bronchospasm, periorbital swelling, angioneurotic edema.
   c. Mild and moderate allergic reactions are treated with antihistamines or corticosteroids, or both. With severe allergic reactions, discontinue streptokinase and treat with IV adrenergics, antihistamines, and corticosteroids as clinically indicated.

PREPARATION

750 K IU/500 ml NS or D5W (150 K IU/100 ml).

DOSAGE AND METHOD (FOR PERIPHERAL ARTERIAL THROMBOLYSIS)

1. Bolus (into thrombus): 50,000 IU.
2. Infuse: 5000 IU/hour × 12 hours; then 2500 IU/hour for duration of therapy.
3. Systemically heparinize patient to prevent clot formation around catheter (maintain PTT at 40–50 seconds).

KINETICS

Two to six hours in serum. Plasminogen and fibrinogen levels may be decreased for longer.

REVERSAL

Fresh-frozen plasma.

Tissue Plasminogen Activator (Activase)

MODE OF ACTION

Causes fibrin-enhanced conversion of plasminogen to plasmin.

INDICATION

Fibrinolysis (approved for use in management of acute myocardial infarction and massive pulmonary embolism in adults).

CONTRAINDICATIONS

Same as for urokinase, and other thrombolytic drugs.

ADVERSE REACTIONS

1. Bleeding.
2. Mild hypersensitivity reactions.
3. Fever.

PREPARATION

Tissue plasminogen activator is available as a sterile, lyophilized powder in 20-mg and 50-mg vacuum vials. The solution must be prepared immediately before use. When reconstituted with supplied sterile water (no preservatives, nonbacteriostatic), a solution at a concentration of 1 mg/ml (pH of 7.3) is obtained. Mix by gentle swirling. Large bubbles (from foaming) are dissipated when the solution is left to stand for a few minutes. The solution may be kept for approximately 8 hours at room temperature. The concentration may be reduced by adding the appropriate volume of normal saline or 5% dextrose solution.

DOSAGE AND METHOD

1. Recombinant tissue plasminogen activator is not FDA approved for IA use in the peripheral arteries. No optimal dosing regimen exists.
2. Initial intrathrombic bolus doses of 5 mg to 10 mg have been reported. Continuous infusion doses of 0.05 mg/kg/hour to 0.1 mg/kg/hr have been reported. The maximum recommended IV dose for both acute myocardial infarction

(given over 3 hours) and pulmonary embolism (given over two hours) is 100 mg. Doses in excess of 150 mg should not be used because there is an increased incidence of intracranial bleeding.

KINETICS

Tissue plasminogen activator is cleared rapidly (50% within 5 minutes) from the plasma, primarily by the liver.

REVERSAL

1. Stop infusion of tissue plasminogen activator and heparin (if used).
2. Fresh-frozen plasma.

Anticoagulants

Heparin (Tubex Heparin Sodium Injection)

MODE OF ACTION

Combines with antithrombin III to inactivate thrombin, a coagulation protein preventing conversion of fibrinogen to fibrin; does not directly lyse existing clot.

INDICATION

Anticoagulation (if facilities to monitor blood coagulation parameters are available).

CONTRAINDICATIONS

1. Hypersensitivity to heparin (derived from porcine intestinal mucosa).
2. Uncontrollable bleeding.
3. Thrombocytopenia (with prolonged therapy, > 25 days).
4. Hemophilia.
5. Bacterial endocarditis.
6. Excessive ethanol intake.

ADVERSE REACTIONS

1. Hemorrhage (3–8% of patients).
2. Acute thrombocytopenia.
3. Hypersensitivity, chills, fever, urticaria (2–5% of patients).
4. Vasospastic reactions.
5. Anaphylactic shock (rare).

PREPARATION

Mix 50,000 units of heparin in 500 ml of NS or D5W (= 100 IU/ml).

DOSAGE AND METHOD (CONTINUOUS IV INFUSION)

1. Bolus: 5000 units IV (2500–5000 units IV, if < 70 kg).
2. Infuse: 800–1000 units/hour (reduce rates for older patients, especially females).
3. Maintain PTT at 1.5–2.5 times normal. Check PTT at 4 hours; then q2–4h until therapeutic, then qd.

KINETICS

1. Onset: immediate (30 minutes to maximum activity).
2. Duration: 90 minutes in normal people (cleared by reticulo-endothelial cells of the liver).

REVERSAL

To reverse heparin effect (i.e., to decrease PTT), stop 6 hours prior to procedure, or administer IV protamine sulfate 10 mg/1000 units of heparin given during the procedure (drip slowly; use cautiously in diabetics taking NPH insulin).

Warfarin Sodium (Coumadin)

MODE OF ACTION

Inhibits hepatic synthesis of clotting factors II, VII, IX, and X, thereby preventing clot formation or extension of formed clot. Does not directly lyse existing clot.

INDICATION

For long-term anticoagulation (oral administration).

ABSOLUTE CONTRAINDICATIONS

1. High risk for serious hemorrhage.
2. Patient who abuses alcohol or drugs who is at risk of hemorrhage from serious trauma.
3. Pregnancy (crosses placenta, potential teratogen).
4. Lactating mother who breast-feeds infant.

RELATIVE CONTRAINDICATION

Noncompliant patient.

ADVERSE EFFECTS

1. Hemorrhage (3% of cases).
2. Hypersensitivity (rare).

PREPARATION

Available for oral administration: 2, 2.5, 5, 7.5, 10 mg. Dose is individually titered to therapeutic PT (1.5–2.5 times normal control). Concomitant administration of heparin will affect PT.

KINETICS

1. Onset of action after loading dose: 2–7 days for effective anticoagulation.
2. Duration: 4–5 days.
3. Half-life: 2.5 days. Metabolites are primarily excreted through urine.

REVERSAL

1. If an intravascular procedure is contemplated, it is best to discontinue warfarin several days before the procedure. If necessary, intravenous heparin may be given instead of warfarin until 4–6 hours prior to the procedure. Acceptable PT for intravascular procedures is 15 seconds or less.
2. Alternatively, fresh-frozen plasma may be given to normalize PT. The onset is fast and duration is short-lived.

3. Another option is to administer vitamin K, 25–50 mg IM, 4 hours prior to the procedure. Both onset of action and duration are prolonged. Unfortunately, it may take 1–3 weeks to reestablish acceptable anticoagulation with warfarin after vitamin K reversal.

Antibiotics

Published doses for antibiotic prophylaxis in interventional procedures are listed in Table 40-1.

Antiemetics

Droperidol (Inapsine)

MODE OF ACTION

A neuroleptic (tranquilizer) agent.

INDICATIONS

1. Prevention of nausea and vomiting.
2. Sedation and marked tranquilization.

CONTRAINDICATION

Known hypersensitivity.

ADVERSE REACTIONS

1. Prolonged sedation with IM injection.
2. Mild to moderate hypotension with tachycardia (via peripheral vascular dilatation).
3. Potentiates other CNS depressants; adjust other drug doses accordingly.
4. Reduces the pressor effect of epinephrine (choose other pressor agents to treat hypotension).
5. Blood pressure elevation may be noted if used in combination with fentanyl citrate.
6. Decreases pulmonary arterial pressures (especially if high). This should be taken into consideration when the procedure requires PA pressure measurement.
7. Extrapyramidal symptoms.
8. Exacerbation of Parkinson's disease.

PREPARATION

1-, 2-, 5-, and 10-ml ampules at 2.5 mg/ml of sterile, nonpyrogenic aqueous solution for IV or IM injection.

DOSAGE AND METHOD

1. 2.5–5.0 mg IM, 30–60 minutes preprocedure, or
2. 0.625–1.250 mg IV, 30–60 minutes preprocedure; similar IV doses may be used cautiously if maintenance is required.
3. Decrease the dose in elderly and debilitated patients.

KINETICS

1. Onset of action following single IV or IM injection in 3–10 minutes. Peak activity is at about 30 minutes.
2. Duration of activity 2–4 hours; altered alertness up to 12 hours.
3. Hepatic and renal metabolism and excretion.

REVERSAL

1. Supportive measures.
2. Fluids and measures to counter hypotension must be readily available.

Hydroxyzine (Vistaril)

MODE OF ACTION

Acts on subcortical CNS.

INDICATIONS

1. Prevention of nausa and vomiting.
2. Sedation.
3. Decreasing apprehension.

CONTRAINDICATIONS

1. Known hypersensitivity.
2. Pregnancy.

ADVERSE REACTIONS

1. Excessive sedation.
2. Dry mouth.
3. Potentiates CNS depressants (narcotics, barbiturates, alcohol). It is prudent to avoid concomitant CNS depressants (e.g., meperidine). If absolutely necessary, reduce their dose by 50% and use with extreme caution.
4. Counteracts pressor effect of epinephrine.

PREPARATION

Intramuscular solution. Unit dose vials of: 50 mg/ml (1 ml vial) and 100 mg/2 ml (2 ml vial).

DOSAGE AND METHOD

25–100 mg IM, must be injected deep within the body of a large muscle (e.g., upper outer quadrant of the buttock or mid-lateral thigh). Subcutaneous injection will cause tissue damage. Avoid inadvertent IV and intraarterial injection.

KINETICS

Rapidly absorbed following IM injection.

REVERSAL

1. Supportive.
2. No specific antidote.

Table 40-1. Recommended antibiotic prophylaxis in interventional radiologic procedures

Procedure	Suspected organism(s)	Recommended drug	Adult dosage and duration[a]
Vascular system			
Diagnostic angiography	None	None	—
Interventional (angioplasty, certain embolizations, infusion, etc.)	None	None	—
Biliary tract			
No clinical infection suspected	Enterobacteriaceae, (includes *Escherichia coli, Klebsiella, Enterobacter*), enterococcus, *Pseudomonas, Clostridium*	Cefazolin *or* Cefoperazone	1 gm IV/IM before and q8h for 48 h 2 gm IV/IM before and q12h for 48 h
Clinical infection suspected	Same as above	Cefoperazone (or other third-generation cephalosporin) *or* Ampicillin plus Gentamicin	2 gm IV/IM before and q12h (based on results of Gram stain and culture)[b] 2 gm IV before and q6h (based on results of Gram stain and culture)[b] 1.5 mg/kg IV before and q8h[b,c]
Outpatient procedure	Same as above	Ceftriaxone	1 gm IV/IM (single dose)

	Organism	Antibiotic	Dosing
Genitourinary system[c]			
No clinical infection suspected	None	Cefazolin *or* Cefoperazone	1 gm IV/IM before and q8h for 48 h 2 gm IV/IM before and q12h for 48 h
Clinical infection suspected	Enterobacteriaceae (includes *Escherichia coli, Klebsiella, Proteus, Enterobacter*), enterococcus, *Pseudomonas aeruginosa*	Ampicillin plus	2 gm IV before and q6h (based on results of Gram stain and culture)[b]
		Gentamicin *or* Ticarcillin or other ureidopenicillin	1.5 mg/kg IV before and q8h[b,c] Consult product insert
Drainage of fluid collection			
Tap of "clear" fluid collection (renal or hepatic cyst, lymphocele)	None	None	—

Table 40-1. (continued)

Procedure	Suspected organism(s)	Recommended drug	Adult dosage and duration[a]
Known or suspected abscess	Enteric gram-negative bacteria, enterococcus, *Bacteriaceae fragilis*, other anaerobes	Cefoxitin	2 gm IV before and q6h (based on results of Gram stain and culture)[b]
		or Cefotetan	1 gm IV before and q12h[b]
		or Gentamicin plus metronidazole	1.5 mg/kg IV before and q8h[b,c] 500 mg IV before and q6h[b]
		or Gentamicin plus clindamycin	1.5 mg/kg IV before and q8h[b,c] 900 mg IV before and q8h[b]

Endocarditis prophylaxis[d] Biliary, genitourinary, or gastrointestinal procedures that are not considered "clean"	Enterococcus	Ampicillin[e] plus *gentamicin	2 gm IV before and q8h in for 48 h 1.5 mg/kg IV before and q8h for 48 h[c]

[a]IV = intravenously, IM = intramuscularly.

[b]These drugs recommended as prophylaxis. Specific therapy should be instituted when clinically indicated and when results of cultures are available, in consultation with referring clinical staff.

[c]Dose may require modification in the presence of renal insufficiency. Consult product insert.

[d]Endocarditis prophylaxis recommended for the following cardiac conditions: prosthetic cardiac valves (including biosynthetic valves), most congenital cardiac malformations, surgically constructed systemic-pulmonary shunts, rheumatic or other valvular dysfunction, idiopathic hypertrophic subaortic stenosis (IHSS), previous history of bacterial endocarditis, mitral valve prolapse with insufficiency.

[e]When patient has penicillin allergy, substitute vancomycin, 1 gm IV before and q12h for 48 h.

Source: Modified from JB Spies, RJ Rosen, AS Lebowitz. Antibiotic prophylaxis in vascular and interventional radiology: A rational approach. *Radiology* 166:381–387, 1988.

Antiinflammatories

Ketorolac Tromethamine (Toradol)

MODE OF ACTION

A nonsteroidal antiinflammatory drug (NSAID) with analgesic and antipyretic effects. Inhibits synthesis of prostaglandins.

INDICATION

Short-term management of pain. Analgesia without respiratory depression; can be used with opioids (meperidine and morphine).

CONTRAINDICATIONS

1. Not approved for use in obstetric or pediatric patients.
2. Known hypersensitivity or prior reaction to aspirin and other NSAIDs.

ADVERSE REACTIONS

1. Reversible platelet dysfunction (24–48 hours after drug is discontinued) and may prolong bleeding time.
2. Side effects additive with other NSAIDs.
3. With long-term use
   a. Gastritis and peptic ulceration.
   b. Inhibition of renal autoregulation (use with caution in patients with renal impairment).

PREPARATION

15 mg/ml and 30 mg/ml in 1-ml syringe, or 30 mg/ml in 2-ml syringe.

DOSAGE AND METHOD (short-term use)

1. 30–60 mg IM, loading dose; followed by half of loading dose (15–30 mg) q6h as needed.
2. Ketorolac 10 mg IM gives equivalent pain relief of meperidine 50 mg or morphine 6 mg, generally with less drowsiness, nausea, and vomiting than morphine.

KINETICS

Onset of pain inhibition in about 10 minutes. Time to peak plasma level (proportional to dosage) is at about 30–60 minutes, and peak analgesia occurs about 45–90 minutes later. Primarily renal excretion.

REVERSAL

Supportive measures.

Methylprednisolone (Medrol)

MODE OF ACTION

A potent steroid antiinflammatory drug.

INDICATIONS

Prophylaxis against contrast and drug hypersensitivity reactions. (Multiple other indications are not listed here.)

CONTRAINDICATIONS

1. Hypersensitivity to compounding components (e.g., tartrazine sensitivity, which may occur in patients with aspirin hypersensitivity).
2. Systemic fungal infections, active tuberculosis.

ADVERSE REACTIONS (Depend on dosage and duration of treatment.)

1. Hyperglycemia.
2. Hypertension.
3. Fluid and sodium retention.
4. Allergic, anaphylactic, and hypersensitivity reactions have been reported following oral as well as parenteral therapy.

PREPARATION

Available in 2-, 4-, 8-, 16-, 24-, and 32-mg tablets. Solu-Medrol is available in powder form for IV and IM use.

DOSAGE AND METHOD

32 mg PO the evening before and 1–2 hours prior to contrast infusion.

KINETICS

Readily absorbed through the gastrointestinal tract and metabolized by naturally occurring steroid metabolism pathways.

REVERSAL

1. Supportive measures.
2. Long-term therapy should be gradually tapered.

Miscellaneous

Atropine

MODE OF ACTION

A muscarinic cholinergic blocking agent.

INDICATIONS

1. During vasovagal reaction for bradycardia (pulse < 60 beats per minute and systolic BP > 90 mm Hg) in an otherwise normotensive patient.
2. Given for severe bradycardia and AV block other than complete heart block (increases sinus rate and AV conduction).
3. Decreases gastrointestinal muscle tone, potential benefit during transhepatic biliary drainage procedures.

CONTRAINDICATIONS

1. Narrow-angle glaucoma.

2. Adhesions between iris and lens.
3. Severe heart disease.
4. Prostatism.

ADVERSE REACTIONS

1. Dry mouth.
2. Diminished respiratory secretions; relaxes bronchial smooth muscle.
3. Urinary retention.
4. Blurred vision.
5. Aggravation of glaucoma.
6. Sedation and confusion.

PREPARATION

Atropine sulfate injection, USP: 10-ml prefilled syringe (0.1 mg/ml) for IV, IM, or SC use.

DOSAGE AND METHOD

1. 0.5–1.0 mg q5min up to 2 mg or pulse greater than or equal to 60.
2. 0.4 mg IV may be used to prophylactically counteract bradycardia during intracoronary contrast injection.

KINETICS

Plasma half-life: about 2.5 hours; most is excreted in the urine within 12 hours.

REVERSAL

Large doses are not indicated for the purposes outlined above. However, should delirium or coma result from inadvertent administration of a large dose, physostigmine may be administered via slow IV injection (1–4 mg in adults, 0.5 mg in children).

Acetylsalicylic Acid (Aspirin)*

MODE OF ACTION

1. Low dose (e.g., 80 mg qod). Blocks cyclooxygenase, preventing formation of thromboxane A_2, a platelet-derived, platelet-aggregating agent and vasoconstrictor.
2. High dose (e.g., 1000 mg qd). Inhibits formation of endothelial prostacyclin, a platelet antiaggregant and vasodilator.

INDICATION

Platelet inhibition during and after PTA.

ABSOLUTE CONTRAINDICATIONS

1. Active bleeding (aspirin prolongs bleeding time).
2. Known aspirin hypersensitivity.

*Information provided here is pertinent only for the use of aspirin during percutaneous transluminal angioplasty (PTA).

RELATIVE CONTRAINDICATIONS

1. Hepatic or renal insufficiency.
2. Hypoprothrombinemia or other bleeding disorder.

ADVERSE REACTIONS

1. Bleeding (< 7% of patients).
2. Gastrointestinal distress (20% of patients).
3. Disturbed acid-base balance (toxic doses).

PREPARATION

Available as tablets and various other formulations.

DOSAGE AND METHOD

Prior to PTA, 80 mg PO the night before and on the morning of the procedure.

KINETICS

Aspirin is cleared from the body within a few hours (mainly through the kidney), but its effect on platelets is irreversible and lasts for the lifetime of the platelet (several days). Plasma half-life is 15 minutes but is dose-dependent and depends on urine pH as well.

REVERSAL

Discontinue drug and treat according to severity of symptoms.

Glucagon

MODE OF ACTION

1. Relaxation of smooth muscles of stomach, duodenum, small bowel, and colon.
2. Stimulates the conversion of liver glycogen to glucose.

INDICATION

Used to decrease bowel peristaltic activity during digital subtraction arteriography.

CONTRAINDICATIONS

1. Hypersensitivity to the drug.
2. Use with caution in patients with diabetes, insulinomas (can cause hypoglycemia), or pheochromocytomas (can cause severe hypertension).

ADVERSE REACTIONS

1. Nausea and vomiting.
2. Possible hypokalemia.

PREPARATION

Dissolve lyophilized glucagon in diluting solution provided.

DOSAGE AND METHOD

0.5–1.0 mg IV given a few minutes prior to study.

KINETICS

When administered intravenously, the time of onset of action for a 0.5-mg dose is 1 minute and the duration of effect is 9–17 minutes. Plasma half-life: 3–6 minutes.

REVERSAL

1. Hypoglycemia should be treated with oral or intravenous glucose and other supportive measures.
2. Hypertension (in patients with pheochromocytomas) may require 5–10 mg IV of phentolamine mesylate.

Naloxone Hydrochloride (Narcan)

MODE OF ACTION

Naloxone antagonizes the opioid effects of the drugs below under "Indication" by competing for the same receptor sites.

INDICATION

Reversal of narcotic overdosage from morphine sulfate (Duramorph), meperidine (Demerol), butorphanol (Stadol), fentanyl (Sublimaze).

CONTRAINDICATIONS

1. Known sensitivity to the drug.
2. Use with care in the very old and very young.

ADVERSE REACTIONS

Abrupt reversal of narcotic depression resulting in nausea, vomiting, diaphoresis, tachycardia, ventricular arrythmias, elevated BP, and tremulousness.

PREPARATION

1 ampule (or disposable prefilled syringe) = 1 ml = 0.4 mg/ml.

DOSAGE AND METHOD

1. Postprocedural narcotic depression: 0.1–0.2 mg IV over 2 minutes, at 2–3 minute intervals until desired degree of reversal—adequate ventilation and alertness without undue pain—is achieved. Since the duration of reversal is about 45 minutes, the patient must be monitored closely for 1–2 hours and given repeat doses of naloxone as indicated.
2. Narcotic overdosage: 0.4–2.0 mg IV, repeat at 2–3-minute intervals, up to 10 mg total dose. (If no response, question narcotic overdosage as cause of problem.)

KINETICS

1. Onset of action 1–2 minutes after IV administration.
2. Duration varies with dose (45 minutes at 0.4 mg/70 kg).
3. Serum half-life in adults is approximately 1 hour. Naloxone is metabolized in the liver by glucuronide conjugation and is excreted in the urine.

REVERSAL

There is no clinical experience with naloxone overdosage in humans.

Selected Reading

Physician's Desk Reference (49th ed). Montrale, NJ: Medical Economics, 1995.

Appendixes

Anatomy

Krishna Kandarpa

Coronary Arteries

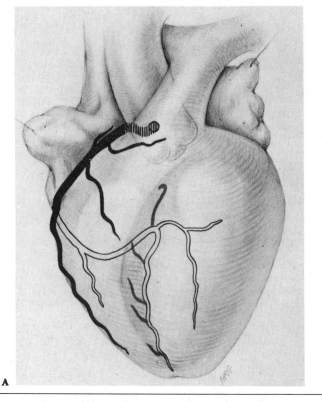

A

Fig. A-1. Right coronary artery (RCA) in left anterior oblique (A) and right anterior oblique (B) views. The proximal RCA is dashed. Vessels on near side are black (counterclockwise: conus, SA nodal, acute marginals). Those on far sides are outlined (counterclockwise: inferior right ventricular, posterior descending artery [PDA] with four shaded septal branches, and posterior left ventricular arteries.) The AV nodal artery (shaded) rises vertically from the distal RCA shown just proximal to the PDA. The vessels in the interventricular septal level are shaded. (From HL Abrams [ed.]. *Coronary Arteriography: A Practical Approach.* Boston, 1983. Published by Little, Brown and Company.)

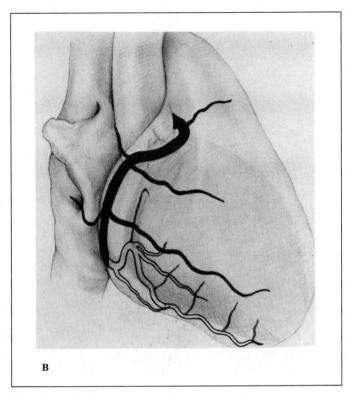

B

Fig. A-1 (continued)

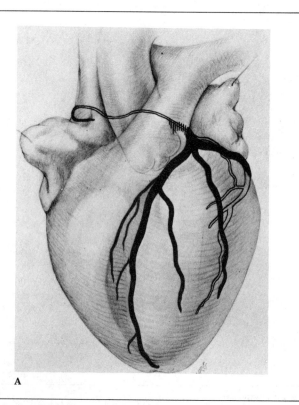

A

Fig. A-2. Left coronary artery (LCA) in left anterior oblique (A)
and right anterior oblique (B) views. A. The left main coronary artery
is dashed. Vessels on the near side are black (counterclockwise:
circumflex, followed by diagonals to the right, and septals toward
the left.) The obtuse marginal branches are outlined (far side).
B. Vessels on the far side are outlined (clockwise: left main, circumflex,
and left anterior descending [LAD] artery with three diagonal branches).
The septal branches of the LAD artery are in the interventricular
septum and are shaded. (From HL Abrams [ed.]. *Coronary
Arteriography: A Practical Approach.* Boston, 1983. Published by
Little, Brown and Company.)

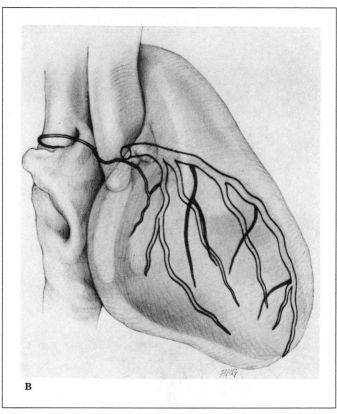

B

Fig. A-2 (continued)

Pulmonary Artery Segmental Branches

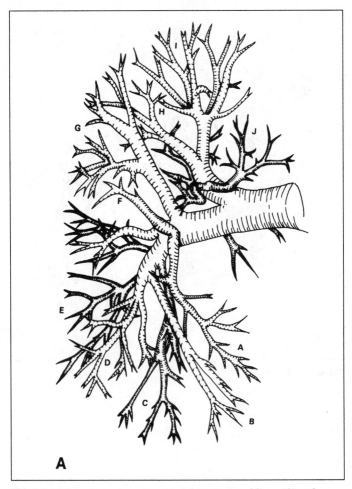

Fig. A-3. Right pulmonary artery in right anterior oblique (A) and left anterior oblique (B) projections. A = right middle lobe (RML) medial segment; B = right lower lobe (RLL) anterior basal segment; C = RLL lateral basal segment; D = RLL posterior basal segment; E = RLL medial basal segment; F = RML lateral segment; G = RLL superior segment; H = right upper lobe (RUL) posterior segment; I = RUL apical segment; J = RUL anterior segment. (Courtesy of SJ Singer, M.D.)

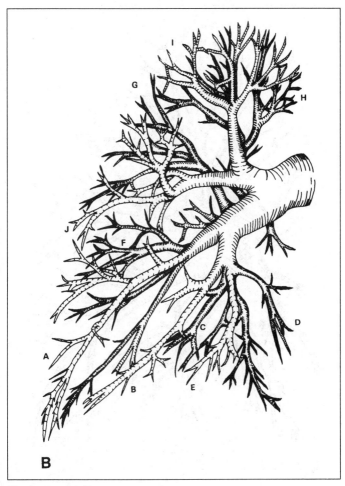

Fig. A-3 (continued)

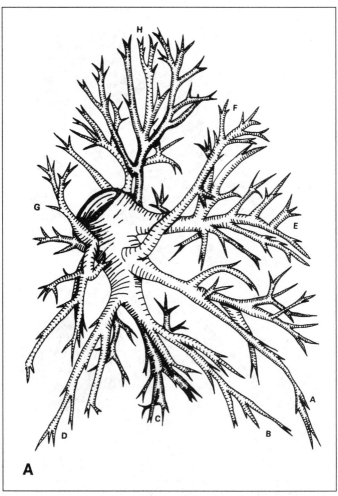

Fig. A-4. Left pulmonary artery in right anterior oblique (A) and left anterior oblique (B) projections. A = lingular inferior segment; B = left lower lobe (LLL) anteromedial basal segment; C = LLL lateral basal segment; D = LLL posterior basal segment; E = left upper lobe (LUL) anterior segment; F = lingular superior segment; G = LLL superior segment; H = LUL apical-posterior segment. (Courtesy of SJ Singer, M.D.)

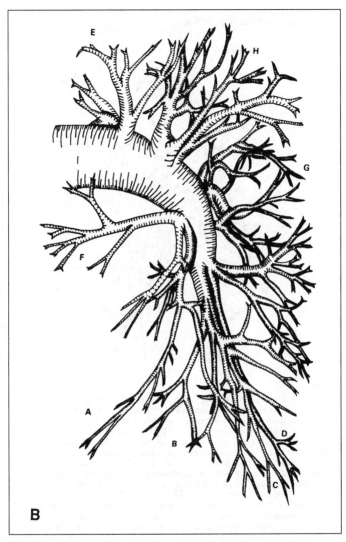

B

Fig. A-4 (continued)

Abdominal Aorta

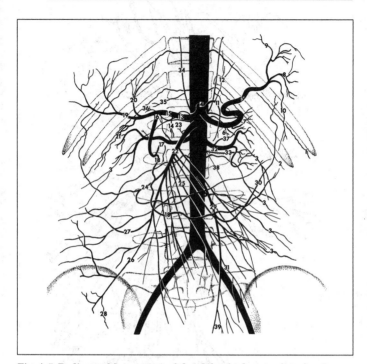

Fig. A-5. Radiographic anatomy of the abdominal aorta. Arteries: *1,*
intercostals; *2,* subcostals; *3,* lumbar; *4,* celiac; *5,* splenic; *6,* dorsal
pancreatic; *7,* pancreatica magna; *8,* terminal branches to spleen; *9,*
short gastric; *10,* left gastroepiploic; *11,* left gastric; *12,* esophageal;
13, common hepatic; *14,* right gastric; *15,* common hepatic; *16,*
gastroduodenal; *17,* anterosuperior pancreatic-duodenal; *18,* right
gastroepiploic; *19,* right hepatic; *20,* left hepatic; *21,* cystic; *22,* superior
mesenteric; *23,* inferior pancreatic-duodenal; *24,* middle colic; *25,*
intestinal; *26,* ileocolic; *27,* right colic; *28,* appendiceal; *29,* inferior
mesenteric; *30,* left colic; *31,* sigmoid; *32,* renal; *33,* accessory renal;
34, inferior phrenic; *35,* superior suprarenal; *36,* middle suprarenal;
37, inferior suprarenal; *38,* internal spermatic or ovarian; *39,*
superior hemorrhoidal. (From RF Muller, MM Figley. The arteries
of the abdomen, pelvis, and thigh. *AJR* 77:296, 1957. © by the American
Roentgenology Society.)

Common Locations of Abdominal Aortic Branches

Celiac artery	T_{12}–L_1 interspace (anterior aortic wall)
Superior mesenteric artery	Mid-L_1 (anterior aortic wall)
Renals	Upper border of L_2 (lateral aortic walls)
Inferior mesenteric artery	L_2–L_3 interspace (anterolateral wall)
Artery of Adamkiewicz	From intercostal or lumbar artery. T_8–L_4 (usually on left). Injection of NS or contrast may cause transverse myelitis

Selected Readings

Abrams HL. *Abrams' Angiography: Vascular and Interventional Radiology* (3rd ed.). Boston: Little, Brown, 1983.

Johnsrude IS, Jackson DC, Dunnick NR. *A Practical Approach to Angiography* (2nd ed.). Boston: Little, Brown, 1987.

Kadir S. *Diagnostic Angiography*. Philadelphia: Saunders, 1986.

Reuter SR, Redman HC, Cho KJ. *Gastrointestinal Angiography* (4th ed.). Philadelphia: Saunders, 1986.

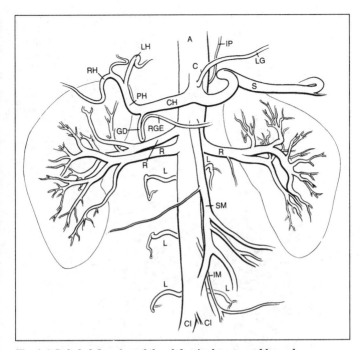

Fig. A-6. Labeled drawing of the abdominal aorta and branches.
Arteries: *A* = abdominal aorta; *C* = celiac; *LG* = left gastric;
IP = inferior phrenic; *S* = splenic; *CH* = common hepatic; *GD* =
gastroduodenal; *RGE* = right gastroepiploic; *PH* = proper hepatic;
RH = right hepatic; *LH* = left hepatic; *R* = renal; *SM* = superior
mesenteric; *IM* = inferior mesenteric; *L* = lumbar; *CI* = common
iliac. (Reprinted from R Dyer. *Handbook of Basic Vascular and
Interventional Radiology.* New York: Churchill Livingstone, 1993.
P. 65.)

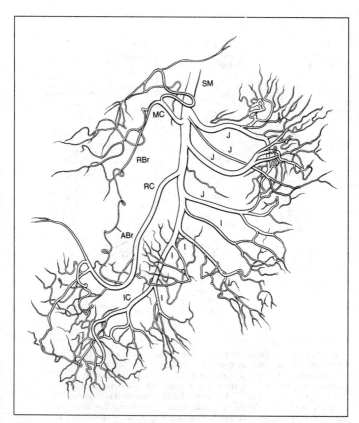

Fig. A-7. Labeled drawing of the superior mesenteric artery and branches. Arteries: *SM* = superior mesenteric; *MC* = middle colic; *RBr* = right branch of middle colic; *RC* = right colic; *J* = jejunal; *I* = ileal; *IC* = ileocolic; *ABr* = ascending branch of right colic. (Reprinted from R Dyer. *Handbook of Basic Vascular and Interventional Radiology.* New York: Churchill Livingstone, 1993. P. 100.)

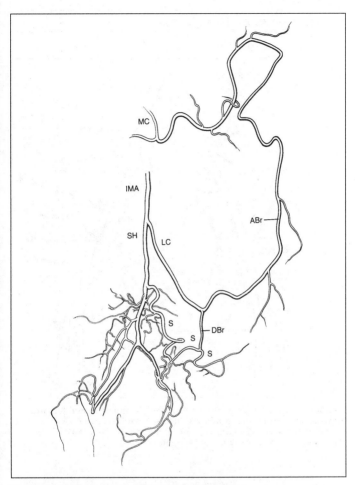

Fig. A-8. Labeled drawing of the inferior mesenteric artery.
Arteries: *IMA* = inferior mesenteric; *LC* = left colic; *SH* = superior
hemorrhoidal; *MC* = middle colic (filled retrogradely); *ABr* =
ascending branch left colic; *DBr* = descending branch left colic;
S = sigmoid. (Reprinted from R Dyer. *Handbook of Basic Vascular
and Interventional Radiology.* New York: Churchill Livingstone, 1993.
P. 108.)

Arteries of the Pelvis

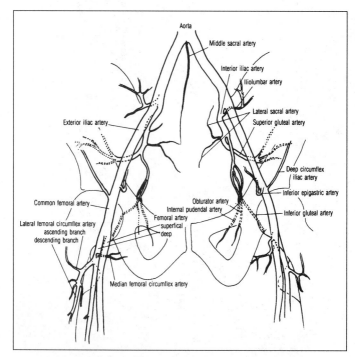

Fig. A-9. Arteriographic anatomy of the pelvic and proximal femoral branches. (From IS Johnsrude, DC Jackson, and NR Dunnick. *A Practical Approach to Angiography* [2nd ed.]. Boston, 1987. Published by Little, Brown and Company.)

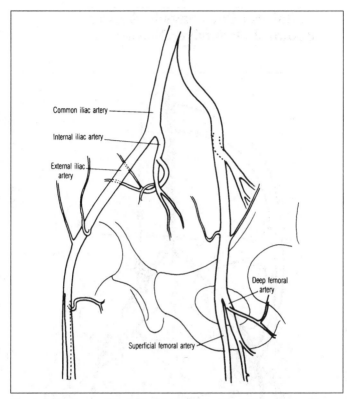

Fig. A-10. Right posterior oblique projection. The right common iliac and left common femoral bifurcations are better outlined in this projection. The origin of the left deep femoral artery branch (profunda femoris) may be hidden on the anteroposterior projection. With the patient in the supine position, elevate the symptomatic side to uncover hidden pathology in the profunda femoris. (From IS Johnsrude, DC Jackson, and NR Dunnick. *A Practical Approach to Angiography* [2nd ed.]. Boston, 1987. Published by Little, Brown and Company.)

Collateral Pathways in Aorto-Ilio-Femoral Occlusive Disease

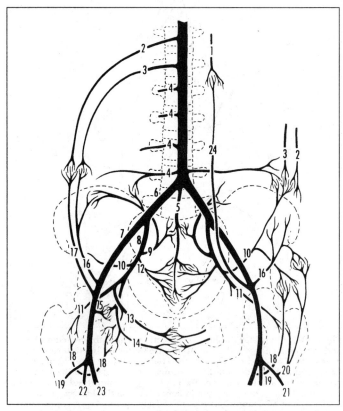

Fig. A-11. Schematic diagram of the major potential parietal pathways of collateral circulation demonstrated in aorto-ilio-femoral occlusive disease. Arteries: *1,* superior epigastric; *2,* intercostal; *3,* subcostal; *4,* lumbar; *5,* middle sacral; *6,* common iliac; *7,* external iliac; *8,* internal iliac; *9,* iliolumbar; *10,* superior gluteal; *11,* inferior gluteal; *12,* lateral sacral; *13,* obturator; *14,* internal pudendal; *15,* external pudendal; *16,* deep iliac circumflex; *17,* superficial iliac circumflex; *18,* medial femoral circumflex; *19,* lateral femoral circumflex; *20,* lateral ascending branch; *21,* lateral descending branch; *22,* profunda femoris; *23,* superficial femoral; *24,* inferior epigastric. (From RF Muller, MM Figley. The arteries of the abdomen, pelvis, and thighs. *AJR* 77:296, 1957. © by the American Roentgenology Society.)

Common Collateral Pathways

Circuit	Collaterals
SFA occlusion	PFA to popliteal
Common iliac: IMA	IMA to hemorrhoidals to internal iliac to external iliac
SMA: IMA	Mid-colic to left colic artery and vice versa (via marginal artery of Drummond; Arc of Riolan)
Celiac: SMA	Pancreatic-duodenal
Subclavian artery occlusion	Intercostals to distal subclavian artery
Lower abdominal aorta or aortic bifurcation occlusion	Lumbar arteries to internal iliac (via iliolumbar and superior gluteal branches) or external iliac art (via deep iliac circumflex or inferior epigastric arteries)
	Superior or inferior mesenteric artery to internal iliac artery (via hemorrhoidal and vesicular or rectal arteries)
	Internal mammary to external iliac artery (via superior and inferior epigastric arteries)

Selected Readings

Abrams HL. *Abrams' Angiography: Vascular and Interventional Radiology* (3rd ed.). Boston: Little, Brown, 1983.

Johnsrude IS, Jackson DC, Dunnick NR. *A Practical Approach to Angiography* (2nd ed.). Boston: Little, Brown, 1987.

Kadir S. *Diagnostic Angiography.* Philadelphia: Saunders, 1986.

Reuter SR, Redman HC, Cho KJ. *Gastrointestinal Angiography* (4th ed.). Philadelphia: Saunders, 1986.

Arteries of the Extremities

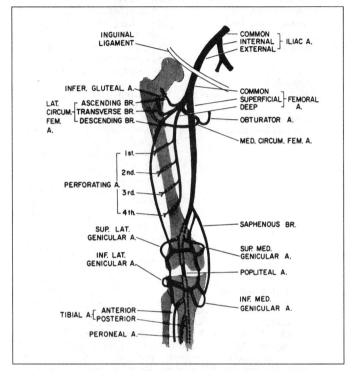

Fig. A-12. A composite drawing of the normal anatomy of the femoral artery, its branches, the distal runoff arteries, and the potential collateral vessels. (From HL Abrams. *Abrams Angiography* [3rd ed.]. Boston, 1983. Published by Little, Brown and Company.)

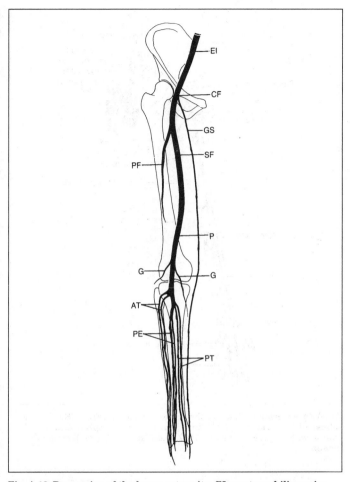

Fig. A-13. Deep veins of the lower extremity. *EI* = external iliac vein; *CF* = common femoral vein; *GS* = greater saphenous vein; *PF* = profunda femoris (deep femoral) vein; *SF* = superficial femoral vein; *P* = popliteal vein; *G* = gastrocnemius veins; *AT* = anterior tibial veins; *PE* = peroneal veins; *PT* = posterior tibial veins. (Reprinted from R Dyer. *Handbook of Basic Vascular and Interventional Radiology.* New York: Churchill Livingstone, 1993. P. 188.)

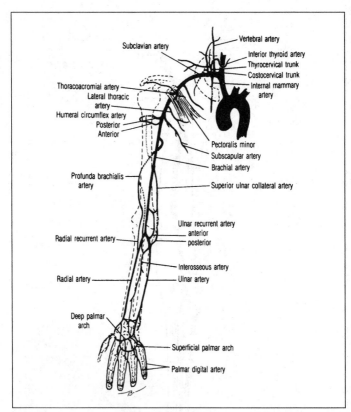

Fig. A-14. Arterial anatomy of the upper extremity. (From IS Johnsrude, DC Jackson, NR Dunnick. *A Practical Approach to Angiography* [2nd ed.]. Boston, 1987. Published by Little, Brown and Company.)

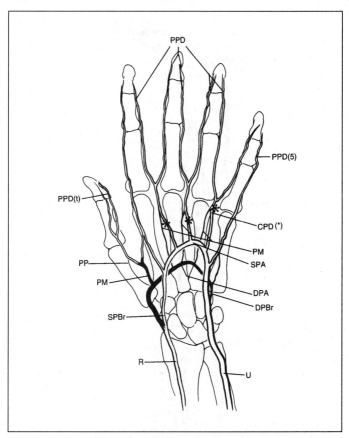

Fig. A-15. The classic arterial anatomy of the hand. Anatomic variation in the hand vasculature is commonplace. *R* = radial artery; *DPA* = deep palmar arch; *PP* = princeps policis artery; *PPD(t)* = proper palmar digital artery (thumb) from deep palmar arch; *U* = ulnar artery; *SPA* = superficial palmar arch; *CPD* = common palmar digital arteries (from superficial arch); *PM* = palmar metacarpal arteries (from deep arch); *PPD* = proper palmar digital arteries; *PPD(5)* = proper palmar digital artery (fifth finger) from superficial arch; *SPBr* = superficial palmar branch (from ulnar artery); *DPBr* = deep palmar branch (from radial artery). (Reprinted from R Dyer. *Handbook of Basic Vascular and Interventional Radiology.* New York: Churchill Livingstone, 1993. P. 132.)

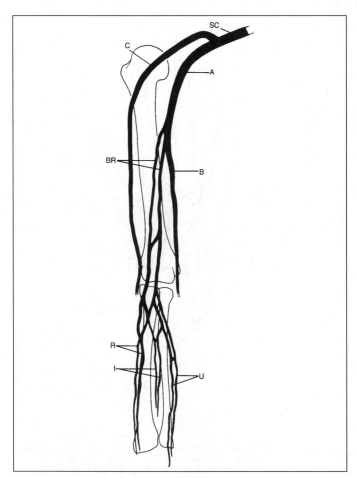

Fig. A-16. Veins of the upper extremity. *SC* = subclavian vein; *A* = axillary vein; *C* = cephalic vein; *B* = basilic vein; *BR* = brachial veins; *R* = radial veins; *I* = interosseous veins; *U* = ulnar veins. (Reprinted from R Dyer. *Handbook of Basic Vascular and Interventional Radiology.* New York: Churchill Livingstone, 1993. P. 160.)

Hemodynamic Monitoring and Cardiovascular Pressures

Michael G. Flater

Hemodynamic monitoring is an essential component of cardiopulmonary and peripheral angiographic procedures, and provides assessment of hemodynamic status by direct intracardiac, intravascular, and pulmonary arterial pressure monitoring. Right heart pressure analysis is often performed during cardiac catheterization and pulmonary angiography. Systemic arterial pressure is analyzed during cardiac catheterization and in angiographic evaluation of the peripheral vasculature, particularly when a stenosis is present. Identification of characteristic pressure waveforms and analysis of the component deflections can provide the angiographer with valuable information about cardiac output, ventricular function, valvular function, pulmonary function, and fluid volume status.

Overview

1. **Considerations**
   a. **Advantages**
      (1) Continuous real-time display of intracardiac and intravascular waveforms.
      (2) Allows early recognition of hemodynamic changes in response to fluid volume, pharmacological effect, and operator maneuvers.
      (3) Promotes early intervention and evaluation of treatments.
   b. **Disadvantages**
      (1) Increased risk to patients including embolization, vascular trauma, perforation, infection, and dysrhythmias.
      (2) Errors in measurement are possible, especially if the operator is not thoroughly proficient in the calibration, operation, and troubleshooting of the system.
2. **Instrumentation and applications**
   a. **Components**
      (1) Catheter/cannula
      (2) Noncompliant tubing
      (3) Fluid medium
      (4) Manifold and stopcock assembly
      (5) Transducer/strain gauge
      (6) Pressure amplifier
      (7) Oscilloscope/monitor
      (8) Printer
   b. **Characteristics**
      (1) Sensitivity: Relationship between the transducer signal input and amplifier output.
      (2) Frequency response: Variation in amplifier sensitivity over the range of input frequencies.

(3) Natural frequency: Frequency of oscillation in a system with no damping.

(4) Damping: Electrical or mechanical dissipation of the natural frequency.

(5) Resonance

    (a) Oscillations within the fluid column that occur as multiples of the natural frequency.

    (b) The sum of the pressure-wave frequency and the system-resonant frequency can result in distortion of the waveform.

c. Factors influencing frequency response/optimal damping

(1) Lumen radius: Optimal catheter ID $\geq$ 1.17 mm (18-gauge or 7 Fr.).

(2) Length of tubing: Optimal catheter and tubing length $\leq$ 100 cm.

(3) Compliance

    (a) Use noncompliant catheters and tubing.

    (b) Tighten all connections and ensure against leaks.

    (c) Establish good contact between the transducer diaphragm and the dome membrane (disposable type).

    (d) Carefully flush the entire system to ensure that all air bubbles are removed.

    (e) Practice frequent or continuous (3–6 ml/hr) flushing to prevent thrombus formation.

    (f) Secure the transducer in a vibration-free mount.

3. Errors in pressure measurement
a. Resonance and damping

(1) **Underdamping:** Transmission of all frequency components of the signal. Underdamping may result from

    (a) Stiff tubing

    (b) Air bubbles

    (c) Air trapped between the transducer diaphragm and the dome membrane (disposable type)

(2) **Overdamping:** Reduction in amplitude of the major components of the signal. Overdamping may result from

    (a) Small ID tubing

        (i) Restricts movement of the fluid column.

        (ii) Wave energy is lost in overcoming frictional resistance to motion.

    (b) Compliant tubing. Wave energy is absorbed in the luminal compression process.

    (c) Air bubbles. Greater compressibility of air absorbs pressure-wave energy; the result is reduced amplitude and waveform distortion.

    (d) Contrast media, blood, and high viscosity fluids result in viscous dampening of the pressure waveform.

(e) Coagulation effectively narrows the luminal diameter, and results in increased frictional resistance.

(f) Loose connections result in loss of wave energy as volume escapes the closed system.

b. Zero reference level

(1) Catheter tip and zero reference point must be at the same level.

(2) Intracardiac reference point at midchest in the supine patient: One half the AP chest measurement at the angle of Louis.

(3) Zero reference point must be modified with changes in patient position.

c. Transducer calibration

(1) Calibrate the transducer prior to each procedure.

(2) Calibrate all transducers in the system simultaneously.

(3) Reference the transducer with a mercury or digital manometer.

(4) Verify linearity of response using 25 mm Hg, 50 mm Hg, and 100 mm Hg.

d. Artifact

(1) Catheter tip motion

(2) End-pressure artifact

(3) Peripheral augmentation

(4) Respiratory variation

4. Troubleshooting errors in pressure measurement

a. General principles

(1) Perform component troubleshooting in a logical and systematic manner to expedite resolution of the problem.

(2) Flush through the zero line.

(3) Verify the integrity of the external components

(a) Tighten all connections.

(b) Purge the system with fluid to remove all air bubbles.

(4) Assess the integrity of the transducer.

(5) Revise catheter position and preserve lumen patency.

b. Underdamping

(1) Air bubbles in the catheter.

(a) Aspirate air bubbles with a syringe.

(b) Forward-flush the catheter with isotonic solution.

(2) Air bubbles in the tubing or transducer dome: Flush the system with solution to purge the system of air.

(3) High system resonance: Use short, noncompliant, large-bore catheter tubing.

c. Overdamping

(1) Air bubbles in the catheter

(a) Aspirate air bubbles with a syringe.

(b) Forward-flush the catheter with isotonic solution.

(2) Air bubbles in the tubing or transducer dome:

Flush the system with solution to purge the system of air.

(3) Blood or coagulation products in the catheter.

(a) Gently aspirate the catheter with a syringe.

(b) Forward-flush the catheter only if able to freely aspirate blood.

(4) Loss of system integrity

(a) Tighten all connections and replace faulty elements.

(b) Flush the system with solution to purge the system of air.

(5) Catheter position (in contact with vessel wall, kinked, vasospastic): Pull back, reposition, or remove catheter if necessary.

d. Pressure lower than clinically suggested

(1) Zero reference level above the phlebostatic axis: Check axis and level if necessary; verify level after a change in patient position.

(2) Transducer drift has occurred: Calibrate the transducer.

e. Pressure higher than clinically suggested

(1) Zero reference level below the phlebostatic axis: Check axis and level if necessary; verify level after a change in patient position.

(2) Increased intrathoracic pressure, Valsalva, pain or anxiety.

(a) Assess patient; reassure and medicate as appropriate.

(b) Measure pressures with patient off ventilator, if possible, or during the expiratory phase of ventilation.

f. Pressure gradient greater than expected: Air bubble can give a false zero level; flush through the zero line.

g. Loss of waveform

(1) Kink in the catheter or tubing

(a) Inspect catheter and tubing system.

(b) Replace catheter or unkink tubing.

(2) Improper stopcock position: Return stopcock(s) to proper position.

(3) Defective transducer: Recalibrate transducer and replace if necessary.

(4) Defective amplifier: Replace the amplifier.

h. Artifact

(1) Catheter tip motion (whip): Acceleration of the fluid in the catheter is caused by motion of the catheter tip and may produce pressure changes of $\pm$ 10 mm Hg. This is difficult to avoid; maximize catheter stability.

(2) End-pressure artifact: Flow of blood artifactually elevates pressure measured from an end hole catheter; this usually occurs in large vessels near the heart and may augment the pressure 3–15 mm Hg. Use a multiple side hole catheter in the left heart; avoid pointing the end-hole catheter toward high-velocity flow.

(3) Peripheral augmentation: Reflected waves in small vessels augment peak systolic and pulse pressures. Reverse systolic gradient (peripheral arterial > aortic) may be 20–50 mm Hg. Use pullback techniques when reverse gradient is observed.

Right Heart Catheterization

Right heart pressures are most frequently obtained using flow-directed, balloon-tip catheters. Common insertion sites include the internal jugular vein, subclavian vein, brachial vein, and femoral vein, the latter being the preferred site for most percutaneous procedures. Meticulous aseptic technique is essential to minimize the potential for nosocomial infection.

TECHNIQUE

1. Flush the catheter lumen; purge all air from the system using isotonic saline solution.
2. Verify balloon integrity
   a. Submerge the catheter tip in solution and inflate the balloon.
   b. Inspect for leaks or defects such as eccentricity.
3. Obtain venous access; insert an introducer sheath.
4. Advance the catheter to the central venous system. Inflate balloon with 1.5 cc of carbon dioxide, although many operators prefer the accessibility of room air; the balloon should never be inflated with air when intracardiac or intrapulmonary shunting is suspected.
5. Advance the catheter to the right atrium
   a. Continue to advance the catheter with the balloon inflated; the right atrium is approximately 40 cm from the femoral insertion site.
   b. Deflate the balloon and record phasic and mean right atrial pressure.
6. Advance the catheter to the right ventricle
   a. Inflate the balloon and advance the catheter across the tricuspid valve; tricuspid regurgitation may impede this maneuver.
   b. Position the catheter at a nonarrhythmogenic site within the right ventricular apex; the right ventricle apex is approximately 50 cm from the femoral insertion site.
   c. Deflate the balloon and record phasic right ventricular pressure.
7. Advance the catheter to the pulmonary artery
   a. Inflate the balloon.
   b. Apply counterclockwise torque to the catheter until the balloon is directed superiorly toward the right ventricular outflow tract.
   c. Withdraw the catheter slowly.
   d. Advance the catheter while the right ventricular systolic ejection wave assists in directing the balloon across the pulmonic valve.
      (1) Deep inspiration may facilitate this maneuver.

        (2) Carefully monitor the ECG for right bundle branch block.

           (a) In the patient with underlying left bundle branch block, complete heart block may ensue.

           (b) Emergent placement of a temporary ventricular pacing lead may be necessary should complete heart block occur.

8. Advance the catheter to the pulmonary capillary wedge position.

    a. Continue to advance the catheter with the balloon inflated (approximately 65 cm from the femoral insertion site) until the catheter is no longer free in the pulmonary artery and a discernible change in the pressure waveform is observed. Avoid excessive dampening of the pressure waveform.

    b. Record phasic and mean wedge pressures with the balloon inflated.

    c. Deflate the balloon and withdraw the catheter 3–5 cm to the main pulmonary artery.

    d. Record phasic and mean pulmonary artery pressures.

The practice of recording right heart pressures when continuous pressure monitoring is not required can be expedited by introducing the catheter into the venous system, inflating the balloon, and advancing the catheter to the pulmonary capillary wedge position. The right heart pressures are continuously recorded as the balloon is deflated, and the catheter is slowly withdrawn to the right atrium, pausing in the main pulmonary artery and again in the right ventricle for the duration of the selected chamber recording. The transducer is opened to atmospheric pressure at the beginning and again at the end of the recording to verify the accuracy of the recording. This technique is not used when it is necessary to exchange the catheter over a wire for selective catheter placement in the pulmonary vasculature.

COMPLICATIONS

1. Segmental pulmonary infarction

    a. May result from distal migration of the catheter tip to the peripheral pulmonary vasculature and spontaneous catheter-tip wedging.

    b. May also result if the balloon ruptures in the right heart, and the air embolus migrates to the distal pulmonary vasculature.

2. Pulmonary arterial perforation

    a. May result from prolonged balloon inflation; balloon inflation times should be minimal. There is a higher risk for pulmonary arterial perforation in patients who are female, elderly, anticoagulated, hypothermic, or have pulmonary hypertension; limit the number of PCWP measurements, and limit the inflation time to two respiratory cycles or 10 to 15 seconds.

    b. May occur following overdistension of the vessel

        (1) The balloon should not be inflated above the recommended volume as overdistension of the vessel may result in vascular trauma.

   (2) Pulmonary artery pressure should be monitored prior to inflation to verify that the catheter is in the pulmonary artery and has not migrated distally.

      (a) Discontinue balloon inflation on recognition of the transition from a PA to a PCWP trace.

      (b) If the catheter inflates with less than 1.5 cc of gas, deflate the balloon and withdraw it 1–2 cm before inflating.

      (c) Fluoroscopic evaluation of catheter position is recommended.

   c. Monitor the patient for signs and symptoms of pulmonary artery perforation

      (1) Hemoptysis

      (2) Pain

      (3) Respiratory distress.

3. Embolization results from catheter thrombus formation and consequent embolization.

   a. Pulmonary arterial catheters should be flushed regularly with a heparinized solution to minimize thrombus formation.

   b. Thrombosis is predominant in long-term indwelling central catheters.

4. Cardiac dysrhythmias

   a. May occur during catheter insertion and removal.

   b. May result from retrograde migration of the catheter tip into the right ventricle following balloon deflation.

   c. Electrocardiographic monitoring is essential during insertion, manipulation, and removal of the catheter.

      (1) Transient premature ventricular depolarizations are predominant.

      (2) Some lethal dysrhythmias may result.

      (3) Right bundle branch block may result.

      (4) Complete heart block may result, especially in the patient with underlying left bundle branch block. Prophylactic placement of a temporary pacing lead in patients with left bundle branch block may be prudent.

5. Infection, sepsis, and endocarditis: A risk of nosocomial infection exists with any invasive procedure. The risk may be substantially decreased by using proper aseptic technique during preparation, vascular access, and insertion and manipulation of the catheter:

   a. Shaving and preparation of the puncture site with an iodinated antimicrobial agent

   b. Proper handwashing

   c. Use of sterile garments and gloves is essential.

6. Right ventricular perforation is a rare complication and may be avoided by ensuring that the balloon is inflated prior to its advancement through the heart.

7. Pneumothorax is a rare complication, which has been reported following catheter placement via the internal jugular and subclavian vein approaches.

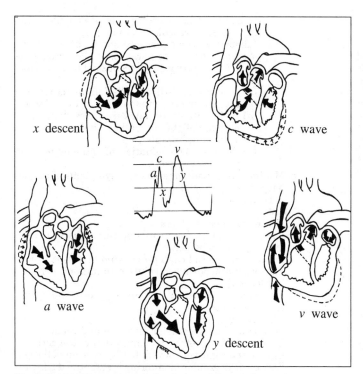

Fig. B-1. Atrial component deflections and the cardiac cycle.

Intracardiac and Pulmonary Pressure Waveform Analysis
(Fig. B-1)

1. Right atrium

    a. Pressure: mean RA = 0–8 mm Hg. See Fig. B-2.

    b. Waveform analysis

        (1) a wave. Right atrial contraction (follows the ECG p wave by approximately 80 ms).

        (2) x descent. Right atrial relaxation and downward movement of the AV junction.

        (3) c wave. Upward movement of the tricuspid valve toward the right atrium at the onset of right ventricular systole; follows the a wave by a period equal to the ECG PR interval. (This deflection is not always present; best visualized in the presence of ECG PR prolongation.)

        (4) v wave. Passive venous filling of the right atrium during right ventricular systole while the tricuspid valve is closed (occurs at the end of the ECG T-wave). The peak of the v wave occurs at the end of right ventricular systole when the tricuspid valve is closed.

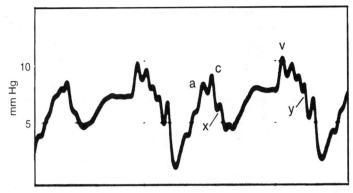

Fig. B-2

> **(5) y descent.** Rapid atrial emptying following the opening of the tricuspid valve.

2. Right ventricle

    a. Pressure: RV = 15–30/0–8 mm Hg. See Fig. B-3. Right ventricular end-diastolic pressure (RVEDP) equals right atrial (RA) pressure since they essentially form a common chamber during diastole when the tricuspid valve is open. RVEDP does not equal RA pressure in the presence of tricuspid valve disease.

    b. Waveform analysis

        (1) Isovolumetric contraction

            (a) The onset of right ventricular systole occurs at the peak of the ECG R wave.

            (b) The rapid upstroke of the systolic component is a result of right ventricular contraction against closed tricuspid and pulmonic valves.

        (2) Ejection

            (a) Right ventricular pressure exceeds pulmonary arterial pressure, the pulmonic valve opens, and blood is ejected into the pulmonary artery.

            (b) Rapid ejection phase occurs from the opening of the pulmonic valve to the peak of right ventricular systolic pressure.

            (c) Reduced ejection phase follows from the peak of right ventricular systolic pressure to the closure of the pulmonic valve.

        (3) Isovolumetric relaxation

            (a) When the pressure in the pulmonary artery exceeds that of the right ventricle, the pulmonic valve closes.

            (b) Isovolumetric relaxation follows, and the negative waveform deflection continues.

            (c) The opening of the tricuspid valve marks the end of isovolumetric relaxation and the onset of right ventricular diastole.

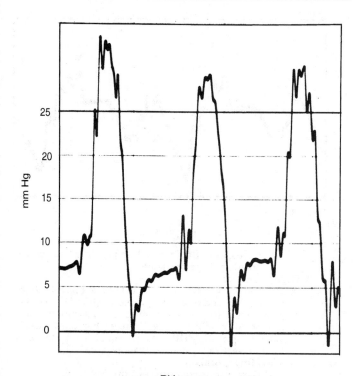

RV pressure

Fig. B-3

    (4) Rapid ventricular filling occurs from the opening of the tricuspid valve until diastasis is achieved. Rapid negative deflection results from right ventricular relaxation.

    (5) Reduced ventricular filling/diastasis

        (a) Slow filling of the right ventricle occurs until systole and is distinguished by a gradual rise in right atrial and right ventricular pressures and right ventricular volume.

        (b) The static baseline is inscribed as RV and RA pressures are equal throughout the phase.

        (c) Right ventricular end-diastolic pressure is measured at the peak of the T wave.

3. Pulmonary artery

    a. Pressure: PA = 15–30/4–12 mm Hg; mean PA = 9–18 mm Hg. See Fig. B-4. Pulmonary artery (PA) systolic pressure equals right ventricular (RV) systolic pressure, since they essentially form a common chamber during systole when the pulmonic valve in open. PA systolic pressure does not equal RV systolic pressure in the presence of pulmonary stenotic valve disease.

    b. Waveform analysis

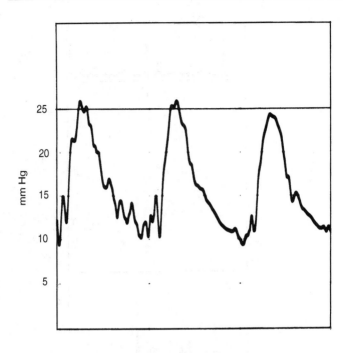

PA pressure

Fig. B-4

        (1) Systole
           (a) The rise in pulmonary artery pressure occurs
               as blood as ejected from the right ventricle
               into the pulmonary artery.
           (b) The peak of the systolic wave occurs during
               the ECG T wave.
           (c) The right ventricular and pulmonary artery
               pressures continue to increase until the right
               ventricle begins to relax.
        (2) Diastole
           (a) The right ventricular and pulmonary artery
               pressures decrease until the pressure in the
               pulmonary artery exceeds that of the right
               ventricle and the pulmonic valve closes. This
               produces the dicrotic notch, which marks the
               onset of right ventricular isovolumetric re-
               laxation.
           (b) Pressure continues to fall until right ventricu-
               lar contraction occurs and the cycle repeats.
    4. Pulmonary capillary wedge
      a. Pressure: mean PCWP = 2–10 mm Hg. See Fig. B-5.
        (1) Inflating the balloon occludes a small branch of
            the pulmonary artery and permits the retrograde

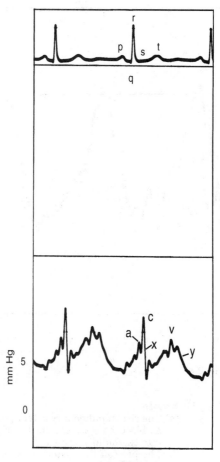

PCW pressure

Fig. B-5

transmission of the left atrial pressure wave through the pulmonary vasculature.
(2) PCWP equals left atrial (LA) pressure when there is no obstruction between the pulmonary artery and the left atrium throughout the cardiac cycle.
(3) Pulmonary capillary wedge pressure (PCWP) equals pulmonary artery diastolic (PAD) pressure because they are at equilibrium during diastole.
(4) PCWP does not equal PAD pressure during certain conditions including increased pulmonary vascular resistance, positive end-expiratory pressure (PEEP) ventilation, and diffuse pulmonary disease states.

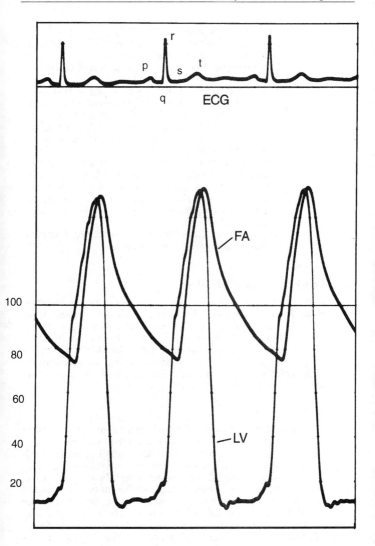

LV pressure with
systemic arterial (FA)
pressure superimposed

Fig. B-6

b. Waveform analysis (see Fig. B-1)

(1) a wave. Left atrial contraction (follows the ECG P wave by approximately 240 ms).

(2) x descent. Left atrial relaxation and downward movement of the AV junction.

(3) c wave. Upward movement of the mitral valve toward the left atrium at the onset of left ventricular systole; follows the a wave by a period equal to the ECG PR interval. (This deflection is not always present; best visualized in the presence of ECG PR prolongation.)

(4) v wave. Passive venous filling of the left atrium during left ventricular systole while the mitral valve is closed (occurs after the inscription of the ECG T wave). Peak of the v wave occurs at the end of ventricular systole, when the left atrium is maximally filled.

(5) y descent. Rapid left atrial emptying following the opening of the mitral valve.

Left Heart Catheterization

Aortic and left ventricular pressures are commonly recorded using a pigtail catheter. The pigtail catheter, by design, reduces the potential for vascular and cardiac trauma, i.e., perforation of the heart or great vessels. Its multiple sidehole design allows diffuse opacification of a large chamber with angiographic contrast material, while decreasing the potential for endocardial or intimal staining. The details of left heart catheterization are given in Chap. 4.

TECHNIQUE

1. The pigtail catheter is flushed with heparinized solution before being introduced into the arterial system.

2. Because of its circular design, the pigtail catheter is advanced over a guidewire to the central aorta.

3. The wire is removed, and the catheter is flushed with care.

4. Central aortic pressure is measured prior to advancing to the left ventricular apex. A moderate to severely stenotic aortic valve may obstruct progression to the left ventricle, thus requiring use of a guidewire to traverse the annulus.

5. The pigtail catheter is advanced over the wire to a nonarrhythmogenic position in the left ventricle.

COMPLICATIONS (see Chap. 4)

1. Embolization

a. May result from catheter microthrombi formation and subsequent embolization to the brain, viscera, or extremities. Arterial catheters should be flushed regularly with a heparinized solution to minimize thrombus formation.

b. May result from fragmentation of intraventricular thrombi. Exercise careful technique to minimize this risk. Risk is increased in patients with known arteriosclerotic disease, valvular stenotic disease, heart failure, atrial fibrillation, or hypercoagulability; anticoagulation is recommended to minimize this risk.

2. Cardiac dysrhythmias may occur during catheter insertion and removal. Electrocardiographic monitoring is essential during catheter and wire manipulations within the left ventricle. Transient premature ventricular depolarizations are predominant. Some lethal dysrhythmias or left bundle branch or fascicular block may result. Complete heart block may result in the patient with underlying right bundle branch block.

3. Infection, sepsis, and endocarditis. A risk of nosocomial infection exists with any invasive procedure. The risk may be substantially decreased by using **proper aseptic technique** during preparation, vascular access, and insertion and manipulation of the catheter:

   a. Shaving and preparation of the puncture site with an iodinated antimicrobial agent
   b. Proper handwashing
   c. Use of sterile garments and gloves is essential.

4. Perforation of the aorta or left ventricle is a rare complication; pigtail catheter design minimizes this risk.

Intracardiac Pressure Waveform Analysis

1. **Left ventricle**
   a. **Pressure:** (LV = 100–140/3–12 mm Hg). See Figs. B-6 and B-7.
      (1) Left ventricular end-diastolic pressure is an indicator of left ventricular function. LVEDP affects myocardial fiber length and reflects the compliance of the left ventricular myocardium during diastole and therefore the left atrial pressure necessary to fill the ventricle just prior to systole.
      (2) Left ventricular end-diastolic pressure (LVEDP) equals left atrial (LA) pressure, which equals pulmonary capillary wedge pressure (PCWP) when there is no obstruction between the pulmonary artery and the left ventricle while the mitral valve is open during diastole (see Fig. B-7).
      (3) Pulmonary capillary wedge pressure will not reflect LVEDP under certain conditions including mitral valve disease, increased alveolar pressure as is generated with positive end-expiratory pressure (PEEP) ventilation, pulmonary venous obstruction, pulmonary hypertension, left atrial myxoma, and cor triatriatum.
      (4) Left ventricular (LV) systolic pressure equals aortic systolic pressure when there is no obstruction between the left ventricle and the aorta while the aortic valve is open during left ventricular systole.
      (5) Left ventricular systolic pressure will not equal aortic systolic pressure in the presence of aortic stenosis or asymmetrical septal hypertrophy (ASH), also known as idiopathic hypertrophic subaortic stenosis (IHSS).

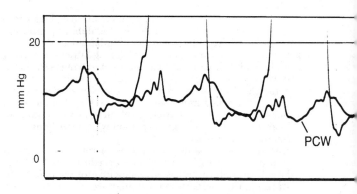

LVEDP and PCW superimposed

Fig. B-7

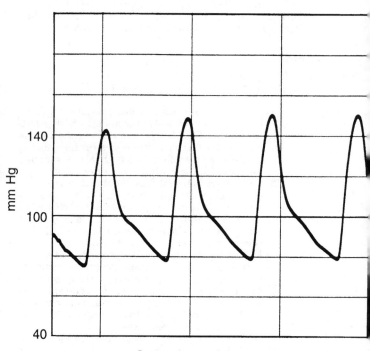

Systemic arterial pressure

Fig. B-8

2. Waveform analysis
a. Isovolumetric contraction
   (1) The onset of left ventricular systole occurs at the peak of the ECG R wave.
   (2) The rapid upstroke of the systolic component is a result of left ventricular contraction against closed mitral and aortic valves.

b. Ejection
   (1) Left ventricular pressure exceeds aortic pressure, the aortic valve opens, and blood is ejected into the aorta.
   (2) Rapid ejection phase occurs from the opening of the aortic valve to the peak of left ventricular systolic pressure.
   (3) Reduced ejection phase follows from the peak of left ventricular systolic pressure to the closure of the aortic valve.

c. Isovolumetric relaxation
   (1) When the pressure in the aorta exceeds that of the left ventricle, the aortic valve closes.
   (2) Isovolumetric relaxation follows, and the negative waveform deflection continues.
   (3) The opening of the mitral valve marks the end of isovolumetric relaxation and the onset of left ventricular diastole.

d. Rapid ventricular filling occurs from the opening of the mitral valve until diastasis is achieved. Rapid negative deflection results from left ventricular relaxation.

e. Reduced ventricular filling/diastasis
   (1) Slow filling of the left ventricle occurs until systole and is distinguished by a gradual rise in left atrial and left ventricular pressures and left ventricular volume.
   (2) The static baseline is inscribed as LV and LA pressures are equal throughout the phase.
   (3) Left ventricular end-diastolic pressure is measured at the peak of the T-wave.

3. Central aorta
a. Pressure: Ao = 100–140/60–90 mm Hg; mean Ao = 70–105 mm Hg. See Figs. B-6 and B-8. Systemic arterial systolic pressure equals aortic systolic pressure, which equals left ventricular systolic pressure while the aortic valve is open during left ventricular systole. These pressures may not be equal in the presence of aortic valve disease, aortic disease, or peripheral arterial disease.

b. Waveform analysis
   (1) Systole
      (a) The rise in aortic pressure occurs as blood is ejected from the left ventricle into the aorta and distally to the systemic vasculature.
      (b) This occurs during the ECG T wave.
      (c) The left ventricular and aortic pressures continue to increase until the left ventricle begins to relax.

(2) **Diastole**

  (a) The left ventricular and aortic pressures decrease until the pressure in the aorta exceeds that of the left ventricle and the aortic valve closes. This produces the dicrotic notch, which marks the onset of left ventricular isovolumetric relaxation.

  (b) Pressure continues to fall until left ventricular contraction occurs and the cycle repeats.

Clinical Significance of Waveforms

1. Right atrial pressure
   a. Mean = 0–8 mm Hg
   (1) Elevated
     (a) RV failure
     (b) Pericardial effusion/tamponade
     (c) Acute ventricular septal defect (VSD)
     (d) Tricuspid stenosis
     (e) Pulmonary embolus
     (f) Pulmonary hypertension
     (g) Hypervolemia
   (2) Elevated on inspiration (Kussmaul's sign)
     (a) RV infarct
     (b) Tricuspid insufficiency
     (c) Constrictive pericarditis
   (3) Decreased
     (a) Hypovolemia/dehydration
   (4) Decreased on inspiration
     (a) Pericardial effusion
   (5) Equalization of RA and LA (PCW)
     (a) Severe atrial septal defect (ASD)
     (b) Constrictive/restrictive cardiomyopathy
   (6) Equal to or exceeding PCW
     (a) Acute RV infarct
   (7) Dissociation of atrial and ventricular waveform components
     (a) Ebstein's anomaly (atrialization of the right ventricle)
   b. a wave = 2–8 mm Hg
   (1) Absent
     (a) Atrial fibrillation
     (b) Atrial flutter
     (c) Atrial standstill
   (2) Elevated
     (a) Increased resistance to RV filling
     (b) Pulmonary hypertension
     (c) Tricuspid stenosis
     (d) Decreased RV compliance
     (e) Constrictive pericarditis
     (f) Tricuspid insufficiency
     (g) Pulmonic stenosis
     (h) Right ventricular hypertrophy
   (3) Cannon waves (regular)
     (a) Atrial contraction against a closed tricuspid valve

          (i) Nodal rhythms
          (ii) AV node reentrant tachycardia
    (4) Cannon waves (irregular)
       (a) AV dissociation and wave summation (shortened diastole)
          (i) Wide-complex tachycardia (highly suggestive of VT)
       (b) Complete heart block
       (c) Ventricular pacing
    (5) Cannon waves (single)
       (a) Ventricular ectopy
    (6) Mechanical flutter waves
       (a) Atrial flutter (approximately 300/min)
  c. x descent
    (1) Prominent
       (a) Pericardial effusion
       (b) RV infarct
       (c) Volume expansion therapy
  d. v wave
    (1) Large
       (a) Tricuspid insufficiency
       (b) Constrictive pericarditis
       (c) Atrial septal defect
       (d) Atrial fibrillation
       (e) Hypervolemia
  e. y descent
    (1) prominent/rapid
       (a) Tricuspid insufficiency
       (b) Constrictive pericarditis
       (c) RV infarct
       (d) Volume expansion therapy
    (2) Attenuated/absent
       (a) Pericardial effusion
2. Right ventricular pressure
  a. Systolic = 15–30 mm Hg
    (1) Elevated
       (a) Pulmonary hypertension
       (b) Pulmonic stenosis
       (c) Ventricular septal defect
    (2) Decreased
       (a) CHF
       (b) Pericardial tamponade
       (c) Hypovolemia
  b. End-diastolic = 0–8 mm Hg
    (1) Elevated
       (a) RV failure
       (b) Chronic CHF
       (c) Pulmonary insufficiency
       (d) Constrictive pericarditis
       (e) Pericardial tamponade
       (f) Hypervolemia
    (2) Decreased
       (a) Tricuspid stenosis
       (b) Hypovolemia
    (3) Square root sign (early rapid diastolic dip with a mid-diastolic plateau)

        (a) Constrictive pericarditis
        (b) Restrictive cardiomyopathy
        (c) Moderate to severe RV failure
        (d) Bradycardia (artifactual)
    (4) Equalization (RVEDP and PAD within 4 mm Hg)
        (a) Restrictive constrictive cardiomyopathy
        (b) Shock
    (5) a-wave attenuation/absence
        (a) Tricuspid stenosis
        (b) Tricuspid insufficiency (in decreased RV compliance)
        (c) Atrial fibrillation
        (d) Atrial flutter
        (e) Atrial standstill
3. Pulmonary arterial pressure
  a. Mean PA = 9–17 mm Hg
  b. Peak systolic = 15–30 mm Hg
    (1) Elevated
        (a) Increased pulmonary flow
            (i) L-R shunt
        (b) Increased pulmonary vascular resistance
            (i) Parenchymal pulmonary disease
            (ii) Pulmonary stenosis
            (iii) Pulmonary embolus
            (iv) Primary or secondary pulmonary hypertension
        (c) Increases with PCW, PV, LA, or LVEDP
            (i) Mitral stenosis
            (ii) Mitral insufficiency
            (iii) LV failure
    (2) Decreased
        (a) Hypovolemia
        (b) Pulmonic stenosis
        (c) Ebstein's anomaly
        (d) Hypoplastic right heart syndrome
        (e) Tricuspid stenosis
        (f) Tricuspid atresia
  c. PA diastolic = 4–14 mm Hg
    (1) PAD > mean PCW
        (a) Primary pulmonary disorder (PAD − PCW > 6 mm Hg)
    (2) PAD < mean PCW
        (a) Acute mitral insufficiency
4. Pulmonary capillary wedge pressure (PCW)/left atrial (LA) pressure
  a. Mean PCW = 2–12 mm Hg
    (1) Elevated
        (a) Mitral stenosis
        (b) Mitral insufficiency
        (c) LV failure
        (d) Left ventricular hypertrophy
        (e) Decreased LV compliance
        (f) Increased pulmonary vascular resistance
        (g) "Overwedged" catheter

    (h) During negative pressure phase of PEEP/
     CPAP ventilation
    (i) Hypervolemia
   (2) Decreased
    (a) Hypovolemia
  b. a wave = 3–10 mm Hg
   (1) Absent
    (a) Atrial fibrillation
    (b) Atrial flutter
    (c) Atrial standstill
   (2) Elevated
    (a) Increased resistance to LV filling
     (i) Systemic hypertension
     (ii) Mitral stenosis
     (iii) Mitral insufficiency
     (iv) Aortic stenosis
     (v) Left ventricular hypertrophy
   (3) Cannon waves (regular)
    (a) Atrial contraction against a closed mitral
     valve
     (i) Nodal rhythms
     (ii) AV node reentrant tachycardia
   (4) Cannon waves (irregular)
    (a) AV dissociation and wave summation (short-
     ened diastole)
     (i) Wide-complex tachycardia (highly sug-
      gestive of VT)
    (b) Complete heart block
    (c) Ventricular pacing
   (5) Cannon waves (single)
    (a) Ventricular ectopy
   (6) Mechanical flutter waves
    (a) Atrial flutter (approximately 300/min)
  c. v wave
   (1) Elevated
    (a) Mitral insufficiency
    (b) Atrial fibrillation
    (c) Constrictive pericarditis
    (d) Hypervolemia
  d. y descent
   (1) Prominent
    (a) Mitral insufficiency
    (b) Constrictive pericarditis
    (c) Attenuated/absent
    (d) Pericardial effusion
 5. Left ventricular (LV) pressure
  a. Systolic = 100–140 mm Hg
   (1) Elevated
    (a) Systemic hypertension
    (b) Aortic stenosis
    (c) Aortic insufficiency
   (2) Decreased
    (a) Hypovolemia
    (b) CHF
    (c) Pericardial tamponade

6. End-diastolic = 3–12 mm Hg
   a. Elevated
      (1) Left ventricular failure
      (2) Left ventricular hypertrophy
      (3) Decreased LV compliance
         (a) Aortic insufficiency
         (b) Constrictive pericarditis
         (c) Pericardial tamponade
         (d) Endocardial fibrosis
   b. Decreased
      (1) Hypovolemia
      (2) Mitral stenosis
   c. Square root sign (early rapid diastolic dip with middiastolic plateau)
      (1) Constrictive pericarditis
      (2) Restrictive cardiomyopathy
      (3) Moderate to severe LV failure
      (4) Bradycardia (artifact)
   d. A wave attenuation/absence
      (1) Severe aortic insufficiency
      (2) Mitral stenosis
      (3) Mitral insufficiency
      (4) Atrial fibrillation
      (5) Atrial flutter
      (6) Atrial standstill
7. Aortic (Ao) pressure/systemic arterial pressure
   a. Mean = 70–105 mm Hg
   b. Peak systolic = 100–140 mm Hg
      (1) Elevated
         (a) Systemic hypertension
         (b) Aortic sclerosis
         (c) Elevated catecholamine states
         (d) Anxiety
      (2) Decreased
         (a) Aortic stenosis
         (b) Decreased cardiac output
         (c) Shock
   c. Diastolic = 60–90 mm Hg
      (1) Elevated
         (a) Systemic hypertension
   d. Pulse pressure
      (1) Wide
         (a) Systemic hypertension
         (b) Aortic insufficiency
         (c) Large L-R shunt
            (i) Patent ductus arteriosus
            (ii) Aortopulmonary fistula
            (iii) Truncus arteriosus communis
            (iv) Perforated sinus of Valsalva aneurysm
      (2) Narrow
         (a) Aortic stenosis
         (b) CHF
         (c) Pericardial tamponade
         (d) Shock

(3) Arterial pulsus bisferiens (spiked)
  (a) Aortic insufficiency
  (b) Idiopathic hypertrophic subaortic stenosis
(4) Pulsus paradoxus (> 10 mm Hg decrease in systolic pressure on inspiration)
  (a) Pericardial tamponade
(5) Pulsus parvus et tardus (weak pulse that rises and falls slowly)
  (a) Aortic stenosis
(6) Pulsus alternans (alternating weak/strong arterial pressure)
  (a) Congestive heart failure
  (b) Cardiomyopathy

Respiratory Effects

Variation in intracardiac and pulmonary pressures may result with changes in intrathoracic pressure.

1. All pressures: There may be cyclical variation in the amplitude of both the phasic and mean tracings of the systemic, ventricular, and pulmonary arterial pressures. The amplitude of pressure may be accentuated in the presence of significant pulmonary disease, severe heart failure, or during mechanical ventilation.
2. Atrial pressures: Mean right atrial pressure and mean left atrial and pulmonary capillary wedge pressures decrease on inspiration. The a- and v-waves and x- and y-descent are prominent during inspiration.

Selected Readings

Barash PG, Cullen BF, Stoelting RK (eds). *Clinical Anesthesia.* Philadelphia: Lippincott, 1989.

Bustin D (ed). *Hemodynamic Monitoring.* Norwalk, CT: Appleton Century Crofts, 1986.

Grossman W (ed). *Cardiac Catheterization and Angiography* (3rd ed.). Philadelphia: Lea & Febiger, 1986.

Robin E. The cult of the Swan-Ganz catheter. *Ann Intern Med* 103:445–449, 1985.

Sharkey SW. Beyond the wedge: Clinical physiology and the Swan-Ganz catheter. *Am J Med* 83:111–121, 1987.

Swan HJC, Ganz W, Forrester JS et al. Catheterization of the heart in man with use of a flow-directed-balloon-tipped catheter. *N Engl J Med* 283:447–451, 1970.

Woods SL (ed). *Cardiovascular Critical Care Nursing.* Philadelphia: Churchill Livingstone, 1983.

Normal Laboratory Values*

Krishna Kandarpa

Blood chemistries	Normal range
Sodium	139–147 mEq/L
Potassium	3.6–5.0 mEq/L
Chloride	102–113 mEq/L
Carbon dioxide	22–30 mEq/L
Blood urea nitrogen	7–22 mg/dl
Creatinine	0.6–1.3 mg/dl (female)
	0.8–1.5 mg/dl (male)
Total bilirubin	1.0 mg/dl
Direct bilirubin	0.3 mg/dl
Alkaline phosphatase	16–95 IU/L
Lactic acid dehydrogenase	88–196 IU/L
Serum glutamic oxaloacetic transaminase	22–47 IU/L
Cholesterol	130–260 mg/dl
Triglycerides	150 mg/dl
	190 mg/dl (> 40 years)

Blood chemistries	Normal range
Total protein	6.4–8.1 gm/dl
Albumin	4.1–5.5 gm/dl
Calcium	2.21–2.52 mEq/L (@ pH = 7.4 and 37°C)
Inorganic phosphorus	2.3–4.3 mg/dl
Glucose	70–112 mg/dl
Uric acid	2.2–7.3 mg/dl (female)
	3.9–8.3 mg/dl (male)

Arterial blood gases	Normal range
Arterial:	
pH	7.35–7.45
CO_2 (mEq/L)	22–30
PCO_2 (mm Hg)	36–47
PO_2 (mm Hg)	65–95
O_2 (% saturation)	93–97.5
Venous:	
pH	7.32–7.42
CO_2 (mEq/L)	25–29
PCO_2 (mm Hg)	42–55

Coagulation profile	
Prothrombin time (PT)	10–13 seconds
Partial thromboplastin time (PTT)	22–35 seconds
Thrombin time	18–25 seconds
Bleeding time	2–9 minutes

*Table is adapted from *Brigham and Women's Hospital Laboratory Manual.* Boston, 1995.

| Activated clotting time | 150 seconds |
| Platelet count | 150,000–450,000/μl |

Lytic state profile

Fibrinogen	170–410 mg%
Fibrin split products	10 μg/ml
Euglobin lysis time	90–300 minutes (adults)
	400 minutes (children)

Endocrine-hypertension

| Vanillylmandelic acid (VMA) (urine) | 0–10 mg/24 hours |
| Renin activity (low salt, upright) | 2.5–14.0 mg/ml/hour |

Standard Angiography/ Interventional Procedure Tray Contents

Eileen M. Bozadjian

Content	Use
Needles	
25-gauge × ⅝ in. (1)	Lidocaine injection
22-gauge × 1 in. (1)	
18-gauge × 1 in. (1)	Aspiration of lidocaine from vial
18-gauge × 2¾ in. (1)	Percutaneous access
Syringes	
Luer-Lok 10 ml (2)	Flush
Luer-Lok 20 ml (3)	Flush
Fingertip control Luer-Lok 10 ml (1)	Local anesthesia
Stopcock, plastic one-way (1)	For proximal end of catheter
Scalpel, no. 11 blade (1)	Skin incision
Hemostat, 5-in. curved mosquito (1)	Division of superficial soft tissues

Closed intravascular flush administration set with three-way stopcock to gravity drainage waste reservoir system (1)
Large basin with sterile solution for wire/catheter placement (1)
Large bowl (1) for disposal of sharp objects
Small cup (1) for table contrast (Hypaque 60%: 50 ml)
Sponges (gauze) 4 in. × 4 in. (20)
Sterile cloth towels (6)
Sterile table covers, drapes, gowns
Towel clips (3)
Solutions (flush/irrigation)
  1000-ml NS with 3000 units heparin (2 bags)

The Whitaker Test

John E. Aruny

Indications

1. The patient with a dilated renal pelvis in whom a ureteropelvic junction obstruction is suspected. The patient should already have had an intravenous urogram, a radionuclide renogram, and a diuretic renogram with the diagnosis still in doubt.
2. Persistence of a dilated renal pelvis and ureter following surgical reimplantation of a ureter or pyloplasty for a ureteropelvic junction obstruction.
3. A child with hydroureter, urinary tract infection, and a voiding cystogram that does not demonstrate vesicoureteral reflux [1].

Contraindications

1. Coagulopathy that cannot be corrected.
2. Untreated or unresponsive urinary tract infection.

Preprocedure Preparation

1. Obtain informed consent from the patient or parents if the patient is a minor.
2. Arrange for general anesthesia or heavy conscious sedation from the anesthesia department if the patient is a child.

Procedure (see Fig. E-1)

1. Using sterile technique, place a catheter into the urinary bladder. An appropriately sized Foley balloon catheter can be used in an adult or older child and a pediatric feeding tube can be used in an infant. The end of the catheter is connected to a manometer or pressure transducer connected to a chart recorder or digital pressure monitor.
2. Establish IV access for the administration of sedation as needed.
3. Establish access to the renal collecting system with the standard aseptic technique. The needle(s) are positioned within a large calix or the renal pelvis. There are three methods that can be used to perfuse and monitor pressures in the renal pelvis.
   a. A 22-gauge needle is placed within the renal collecting system with care not to allow the tip to rest up against the wall. Sharp rise and fall of the pressure tracing is a good indicator that the needle tip is against the wall of the collecting system. A three-way stopcock is attached to the end of the needle with one channel attached to the perfusion pump and one end to the pressure-measuring device. Intermittent pressure readings are obtained during short periods when the

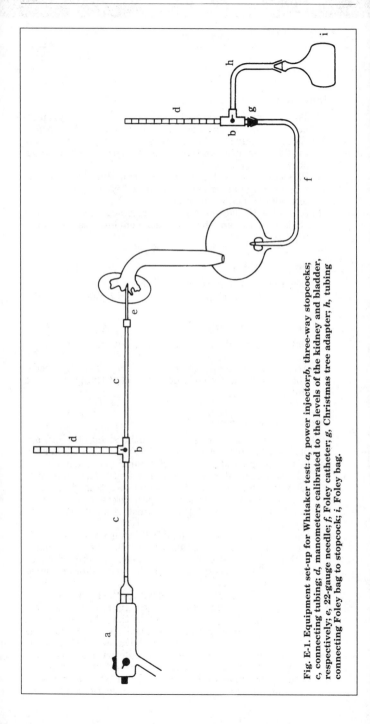

Fig. E-1. Equipment set-up for Whitaker test: *a*, power injector; *b*, three-way stopcocks; *c*, connecting tubing; *d*, manometers calibrated to the levels of the kidney and bladder, respectively; *e*, 22-gauge needle; *f*, Foley catheter; *g*, Christmas tree adapter; *h*, tubing connecting Foley bag to stopcock; *i*, Foley bag.

pump is not connected to the needle. At the end of the procedure the resistance of the needle is determined by running the infusion at 10 ml/min with the needle at the height of the pressure transducer or manometer, while measuring the pressure. This is the pressure drop across the needle secondary to the inherent resistance of its small caliber and must be taken into account when calculating the final gradient [2].

Alternatively, one may use a larger 18-gauge needle with a side-arm adapter attached to the needle. This allows simultaneous pressure monitoring during perfusion.

   b. Two 22-gauge needles are placed within the renal pelvis. One needle is used to measure pressures and the other is used for the infusion of saline and contrast. If the test is to be done on an outpatient basis, the single 22-gauge needle technique appears to offer the safest approach.
   c. A double-lumen needle has been described by Epstein [3] to allow for simultaneous continuous infusion and pressure monitoring.
4. Set the height of the transducer or manometer to the estimated height of the patient's kidney in the the prone position. The height of the second manometer or transducer used for bladder pressure measurements is set at the same level.
5. Record the resting bladder pressure, which is normally below 10 cm water.
6. Begin the infusion of dilute contrast (contrast : saline; 1 : 2 or 1 : 3) at 10 ml/minute in adults or older children and 5 ml/minute in infants. The infusion requires a continuous infusion pump.
7. During the infusion, the contrast allows fluoroscopy and spot films to be taken that show the progress of the infusion and to visualize any areas of anatomic narrowing. It is also important to know when to begin taking pressure measurements. This equilibrium point is when the renal pelvis and ureter are fully distended and the flow of fluid being pumped into the renal pelvis is equal to the amount of fluid leaving it. At the flow rate of 10 ml/minute, this may take considerable time in a dilated collecting system.
8. Once the system is in equilibrium, simultaneous pressures are measured in the renal pelvis and urinary bladder. In some cases, increasing the infusion rate to as high as 20 ml/minute may evoke an obstructive pressure gradient not seen at infusion rates of 10 ml/minute. Also in cases of a neurogenic bladder or following reimplantation of ureters it may be of value to measure pressures with the bladder empty and then distended.

Postprocedure Management

1. Following the completion of the test, the needle(s) may be removed. If the pressure gradient confirms that the kidney is obstructed, the access may be turned into a percutaneous nephrostomy drain if necessary.

2. If the needle(s) are removed, the patient is watched for 4 hours and then discharged if there are no complications.
3. If a nephrostomy tube is placed, the patient may be admitted for an overnight stay in the hospital for pain control and to observe for prolonged hematuria. However, if the urine is clear and tube placement was tolerated well, the patient may be discharged home on oral pain medication. The patient is instructed to return the next day for follow-up evaluation.

Results [4–7]

1. Pressure differences of less than 15 cm water are normal. Pressure differences greater than 22 cm water are abnormal and indicate obstructed upper tract.
2. Pressure gradients between 15 and 22 cm water measured at flow rates of 10 ml/minute are indeterminate. It has been shown that perfusion rates as high as 20 ml/minute will resolve many of the cases that fall into the indeterminate zone [8].
3. When positive, spot films are used to document the site of obstruction.
4. When a 22-gauge needle system is used, the resistance of the needle itself must be corrected for in measuring the pressure gradient between the kidney and bladder. The formula is:

Renal pelvic pressure − needle pressure − bladder pressure
= Gradient between renal pelvis and the bladder.

Complications

1. Infection.
2. Bleeding, usually transient hematuria.
3. Extravasation of contrast, self-limiting.

References

1. Whitaker RH, Johnston JH. A simple classification of wide ureters. *Br J Urol* 47:781, 1976.
2. Amis ES, Pfister RC, Newhouse JH. Resistances of various renal instruments used in ureteral perfusion. *Radiology* 143:267, 1982.
3. Epstein DH, et al. Double-lumen needle for percutaneous ureteral pressure-flow studies. *Radiology* 172:569, 1989.
4. Witherow RN, Whitaker RH. The predictive accuracy of antegrade pressure flow studies in equivocal upper tract obstruction. *Br J Urol* 53:496–499, 1981.
5. Whitaker RH. Methods of assessing obstruction in dilated ureters. *Br J Urol* 45:15–22, 1973.
6. Whitaker RH. An evaluation of 170 diagnostic pressure flow studies of the upper urinary tract. *J Urol* 121:602–604, 1979.
7. Whitaker RH, Chir M. The Whitaker test. *Urol Clin North Am* 6:529–539, 1979.
8. Pfister RC, Newhouse JH, Yoder IC. Effect of flow rates on ureteral perfusion results. *AJR* 135:209, 1980.

Calculating Creatinine Clearance from Serum Creatinine

John E. Aruny

Males

$$\frac{\text{Weight (kg)} \times (140 - \text{age})}{72 \times \text{serum creatinine (mg/100ml)}} = \text{Cr clearance cc/min}$$

Females

0.9 × value for males
Normal Cr clearance index = 80–110 cc/min/1.73 m^2

Index

Index

Note: Page numbers in *italic* type indicate figures; page numbers followed by t indicate tables.